ACP | MKSAP® 18

Medical Knowledge Self-Assessment Program®

Nephrology

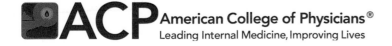

ACP American College of Physicians®
Leading Internal Medicine, Improving Lives

Welcome to the Nephrology Section of MKSAP 18!

In these pages, you will find updated information on the clinical evaluation of kidney function, fluids and electrolytes, acid-base disorders, hypertension, chronic tubulointerstitial nephritis, glomerular diseases, kidney manifestations of deposition diseases, genetic disorders and kidney disease, acute kidney injury, kidney stones, the kidney in pregnancy, and chronic kidney disease. All of these topics are uniquely focused on the needs of generalists and subspecialists *outside* of nephrology.

The core content of MKSAP 18 has been developed as in previous editions—all essential information that is newly researched and written in 11 topic areas of internal medicine—created by dozens of leading generalists and subspecialists and guided by certification and recertification requirements, emerging knowledge in the field, and user feedback. MKSAP 18 also contains 1200 all-new peer-reviewed, psychometrically validated, multiple-choice questions (MCQs) for self-assessment and study, including 108 in Nephrology. MKSAP 18 continues to include *High Value Care* (HVC) recommendations, based on the concept of balancing clinical benefit with costs and harms, with associated MCQs illustrating these principles and HVC Key Points called out in the text. Internists practicing in the hospital setting can easily find comprehensive *Hospitalist*-focused content and MCQs, specially designated in blue and with the ⊞ symbol.

If you purchased MKSAP 18 Complete, you also have access to MKSAP 18 Digital, with additional tools allowing you to customize your learning experience. MKSAP Digital includes regular text updates with new, practice-changing information, 200 new self-assessment questions, and enhanced custom-quiz options. MKSAP Complete also includes more than 1200 electronic, adaptive learning–enhanced flashcards for quick review of important concepts, as well as an updated and enhanced version of Virtual Dx, MKSAP's image-based self-assessment tool. As before, MKSAP 18 Digital is optimized for use on your mobile devices, with iOS- and Android-based apps allowing you to sync between your apps and online account and submit for CME credits and MOC points online.

Please visit us at the MKSAP Resource Site (mksap.acponline.org) to find out how we can help you study, earn CME credit and MOC points, and stay up to date.

On behalf of the many internists who have offered their time and expertise to create the content for MKSAP 18 and the editorial staff who work to bring this material to you in the best possible way, we are honored that you have chosen to use MKSAP 18 and appreciate any feedback about the program you may have. Please feel free to send any comments to mksap_editors@acponline.org.

Sincerely,

Patrick Alguire

Patrick C. Alguire, MD, FACP
Editor-in-Chief
Senior Vice President Emeritus
Medical Education Division
American College of Physicians

Nephrology

Committee

Michael J. Ross, MD, Section Editor[2]
Chief, Division of Nephrology
Professor of Medicine
Professor of Developmental and Molecular Biology
Albert Einstein College of Medicine
Montefiore Medical Center
Bronx, New York

Andrew S. Bomback, MD, MPH[2]
Assistant Professor of Medicine
Division of Nephrology
Columbia University Medical Center
New York, New York

Steven Coca, DO, MS[2]
Associate Professor of Medicine
Division of Nephrology
Icahn School of Medicine at Mount Sinai
New York, New York

Derek M. Fine, MD[2]
Associate Professor of Medicine
Division of Nephrology
Johns Hopkins University School of Medicine
Baltimore, Maryland

Susan Hedayati, MD, MSc[1]
Professor of Medicine, Division of Nephrology
Yin Quan-Yuen Distinguished Professorship in Nephrology
Associate Vice Chair for Research, Department of Internal
  Medicine
Director of Nephrology Translational and Population Health
  Research
University of Texas Southwestern Medical Center
Dallas, Texas

Harold M. Szerlip, MD, FACP[2]
Director, Nephrology Division
Baylor University Medical Center at Dallas
Dallas, Texas

Ashita Tolwani, MD, MSc[2]
Professor of Medicine
Division of Nephrology
University of Alabama at Birmingham
Birmingham, Alabama

Editor-in-Chief

Patrick C. Alguire, MD, FACP[2]
Senior Vice President Emeritus, Medical Education
American College of Physicians
Philadelphia, Pennsylvania

Deputy Editor

Davoren Chick, MD, FACP[2]
Senior Vice President, Medical Education
American College of Physicians
Philadelphia, Pennsylvania

Nephrology Reviewers

Faris A. Ahmed, MD, FACP[1]
Ayoola O. Akinbamowo, MBBS, FACP[1]
Fahad Aziz, MD[1]
Olurotimi J. Badero, MBchB, FACP[1]
Krishna M. Baradhi, MBBS, FACP[1]
Gautam Kantilal Bhanushali, MD, FACP[1]
Omar Hamze, MD, FACP[1]
Mira T. Keddis, MD, FACP[1]
Zeid J. Khitan, MD, FACP[1]
Wei Ling Lau, MD[2]

Hospital Medicine Nephrology Reviewers

Corinne A. Ahmar, MD, FACP[1]
Rahul S. Koushik, MBBS, FACP[1]

Nephrology ACP Editorial Staff

Megan Zborowski[1], Senior Staff Editor, Self-Assessment and
  Educational Programs
Margaret Wells[1], Director, Self-Assessment and Educational
  Programs
Becky Krumm[1], Managing Editor, Self-Assessment and
  Educational Programs

ACP Principal Staff

Davoren Chick, MD, FACP[2]
Senior Vice President, Medical Education

Acknowledgments

The American College of Physicians (ACP) gratefully acknowledges the special contributions to the development and production of the 18th edition of the Medical Knowledge Self-Assessment Program® (MKSAP® 18) made by the following people:

Graphic Design: Barry Moshinski (Director, Graphic Services), Michael Ripca (Graphics Technical Administrator), and Jennifer Gropper (Graphic Designer).

Production/Systems: Dan Hoffmann (Director, Information Technology), Scott Hurd (Manager, Content Systems), Neil Kohl (Senior Architect), and Chris Patterson (Senior Architect).

MKSAP 18 Digital: Under the direction of Steven Spadt (Senior Vice President, Technology), the digital version of MKSAP 18 was developed within the ACP's Digital Products and Services Department, led by Brian Sweigard (Director, Digital Products and Services). Other members of the team included Dan Barron (Senior Web Application Developer/Architect), Chris Forrest (Senior Software Developer/Design Lead), Kathleen Hoover (Senior Web Developer), Kara Regis (Manager, User Interface Design and Development), Brad Lord (Senior Web Application Developer), and John McKnight (Senior Web Developer).

The College also wishes to acknowledge that many other persons, too numerous to mention, have contributed to the production of this program. Without their dedicated efforts, this program would not have been possible.

MKSAP Resource Site (mksap.acponline.org)

The MKSAP Resource Site (mksap.acponline.org) is a continually updated site that provides links to MKSAP 18 online answer sheets for print subscribers; access to MKSAP 18 Digital; Board Basics® e-book access instructions; information on Continuing Medical Education (CME), Maintenance of Certification (MOC), and international Continuing Professional Development (CPD) and MOC; errata; and other new information.

International MOC/CPD

For information and instructions on submission of international MOC/CPD, please go to the MKSAP Resource Site (mksap.acponline.org).

Continuing Medical Education

The American College of Physicians is accredited by the Accreditation Council for Continuing Medical Education (ACCME) to provide continuing medical education for physicians.

The American College of Physicians designates this enduring material, MKSAP 18, for a maximum of 275 *AMA PRA Category 1 Credits*™. Physicians should claim only the credit commensurate with the extent of their participation in the activity.

Up to 25 *AMA PRA Category 1 Credits*™ are available from December 31, 2018, to December 31, 2021, for the MKSAP 18 Nephrology section.

Learning Objectives

The learning objectives of MKSAP 18 are to:

- Close gaps between actual care in your practice and preferred standards of care, based on best evidence
- Diagnose disease states that are less common and sometimes overlooked and confusing
- Improve management of comorbid conditions that can complicate patient care
- Determine when to refer patients for surgery or care by subspecialists
- Pass the ABIM Certification Examination
- Pass the ABIM Maintenance of Certification Examination

Target Audience

- General internists and primary care physicians
- Subspecialists who need to remain up to date in internal medicine
- Residents preparing for the certifying examination in internal medicine
- Physicians preparing for maintenance of certification in internal medicine (recertification)

ABIM Maintenance of Certification

Check the MKSAP Resource Site (mksap.acponline.org) for the latest information on how MKSAP tests can be used to apply to the American Board of Internal Medicine (ABIM) for Maintenance of Certification (MOC) points following completion of the CME activity.

Successful completion of the CME activity, which includes participation in the evaluation component, enables the participant to earn up to 275 medical knowledge MOC points in the ABIM's MOC program. It is the CME activity provider's responsibility to submit participant completion information to ACCME for the purpose of granting MOC credit.

Earn Instantaneous CME Credits or MOC Points Online

Print subscribers can enter their answers online to earn instantaneous CME credits or MOC points. You can submit your answers using online answer sheets that are provided at mksap.acponline.org, where a record of your MKSAP 18 credits will be available. To earn CME credits or to apply for MOC points, you need to answer all of the questions in a test and earn a score of at least 50% correct (number of correct answers divided by the total number of questions). Please note that if you are applying for MOC points, you must also enter your birth date and ABIM candidate number.

Take either of the following approaches:

1. Use the printed answer sheet at the back of this book to record your answers. Go to mksap.acponline.org, access the appropriate online answer sheet, transcribe your answers, and submit your test for instantaneous CME credits or MOC points. There is no additional fee for this service.

2. Go to mksap.acponline.org, access the appropriate online answer sheet, directly enter your answers, and submit your test for instantaneous CME credits or MOC points. There is no additional fee for this service.

Earn CME Credits or MOC Points by Mail or Fax

Pay a $20 processing fee per answer sheet and submit the printed answer sheet at the back of this book by mail or fax, as instructed on the answer sheet. Make sure you calculate your score and enter your birth date and ABIM candidate number, and fax the answer sheet to 215-351-2799 or mail the answer sheet to Member and Customer Service, American College of Physicians, 190 N. Independence Mall West, Philadelphia, PA 19106-1572, using the courtesy envelope provided in your MKSAP 18 slipcase. You will need your 10-digit order number and 8-digit ACP ID number, which are printed on your packing slip. Please allow 4 to 6 weeks for your score report to be emailed back to you. Be sure to include your email address for a response.

If you do not have a 10-digit order number and 8-digit ACP ID number, or if you need help creating a user-name and password to access the MKSAP 18 online answer sheets, go to mksap.acponline.org or email custserv@acponline.org.

Disclosure Policy

It is the policy of the American College of Physicians (ACP) to ensure balance, independence, objectivity, and scientific rigor in all of its educational activities. To this end, and consistent with the policies of the ACP and the Accreditation Council for Continuing Medical Education (ACCME), contributors to all ACP continuing medical education activities are required to disclose all relevant financial relationships with any entity producing, marketing, re-selling, or distributing health care goods or services consumed by, or used on, patients. Contributors are required to use generic names in the discussion of therapeutic options and are required to identify any unapproved, off-label, or investigative use of commercial products or devices. Where a trade name is used, all available trade names for the same product type are also included. If trade-name products manufactured by companies with whom contributors have relationships are discussed, contributors are asked to provide evidence-based citations in support of the discussion. The information is reviewed by the committee responsible for producing this text. If necessary, adjustments to topics or contributors' roles in content development are made to balance the discussion. Further, all readers of this text are asked to evaluate the content for evidence of commercial bias and send any relevant comments to mksap_editors@acponline.org so that future decisions about content and contributors can be made in light of this information.

Resolution of Conflicts

To resolve all conflicts of interest and influences of vested interests, ACP's content planners used best evidence and updated clinical care guidelines in developing content, when such evidence and guidelines were available. All content underwent review by peer reviewers not on the committee to ensure that the material was balanced and unbiased. Contributors' disclosure information can be found with the list of contributors' names and those of ACP principal staff listed in the beginning of this book.

Hospital-Based Medicine

For the convenience of subscribers who provide care in hospital settings, content that is specific to the hospital setting has been highlighted in blue. Hospital icons (H) highlight where the hospital-only content begins, continues over more than one page, and ends.

High Value Care Key Points

Key Points in the text that relate to High Value Care concepts (that is, concepts that discuss balancing clinical benefit with costs and harms) are designated by the HVC icon [HVC].

Educational Disclaimer

The editors and publisher of MKSAP 18 recognize that the development of new material offers many opportunities for error. Despite our best efforts, some errors may persist in print. Drug dosage schedules are, we believe, accurate and in accordance with current standards. Readers are advised, however, to ensure that the recommended dosages in MKSAP 18 concur with the information provided in the product information material. This is especially important in cases of new, infrequently used, or highly toxic drugs.

Application of the information in MKSAP 18 remains the professional responsibility of the practitioner.

The primary purpose of MKSAP 18 is educational. Information presented, as well as publications, technologies, products, and/or services discussed, is intended to inform subscribers about the knowledge, techniques, and experiences of the contributors. A diversity of professional opinion exists, and the views of the contributors are their own and not those of the ACP. Inclusion of any material in the program does not constitute endorsement or recommendation by the ACP. The ACP does not warrant the safety, reliability, accuracy, completeness, or usefulness of and disclaims any and all liability for damages and claims that may result from the use of information, publications, technologies, products, and/or services discussed in this program.

Publisher's Information

Disclaimer Regarding Direct Purchases from Online Retailers

CME and/or MOC for MKSAP 18 is available only if you purchase the program directly from ACP. CME credits and MOC points cannot be awarded to those purchasers who have purchased the program from non-authorized sellers such as Amazon, eBay, or any other such online retailer.

Unauthorized Use of This Book Is Against the Law

MKSAP 18 ISBN: 978-1-938245-47-3
Nephrology ISBN: 978-1-938245-57-2

Printed in the United States of America.

For order information in the U.S. or Canada call 800-ACP-1915. All other countries call 215-351-2600 (Monday to Friday, 9 AM – 5 PM ET). Fax inquiries to 215-351-2799 or email to custserv@acponline.org.

Errata

Errata for MKSAP 18 will be available through the MKSAP Resource Site at mksap.acponline.org as new information becomes known to the editors.

Table of Contents

Glomerular Diseases

Kidney Manifestations of Deposition Diseases

Genetic Disorders and Kidney Disease

Acute Kidney Injury

Kidney Stones

The Kidney in Pregnancy

Chronic Kidney Disease

Nephrology High Value Care Recommendations

The American College of Physicians, in collaboration with multiple other organizations, is engaged in a worldwide initiative to promote the practice of High Value Care (HVC). The goals of the HVC initiative are to improve health care outcomes by providing care of proven benefit and reducing costs by avoiding unnecessary and even harmful interventions. The initiative comprises several programs that integrate the important concept of health care value (balancing clinical benefit with costs and harms) for a given intervention into a broad range of educational materials to address the needs of trainees, practicing physicians, and patients.

HVC content has been integrated into MKSAP 18 in several important ways. MKSAP 18 includes HVC-identified key points in the text, HVC-focused multiple choice questions, and, for subscribers to MKSAP Digital, an HVC custom quiz. From the text and questions, we have generated the following list of HVC recommendations that meet the definition below of high value care and bring us closer to our goal of improving patient outcomes while conserving finite resources.

High Value Care Recommendation: A recommendation to choose diagnostic and management strategies for patients in specific clinical situations that balance clinical benefit with cost and harms with the goal of improving patient outcomes.

Below are the High Value Care Recommendations for the Nephrology section of MKSAP 18.

- The random (spot) urine protein-creatinine ratio and albumin-creatinine ratio are sufficiently accurate for screening and monitoring proteinuria.
- Urinalysis should not be used for detection of bladder cancer in asymptomatic patients.
- Ultrasonography is the most commonly used imaging modality in the evaluation of the kidneys and upper urinary tract because of its safety, cost effectiveness, and availability.
- Obtaining blood pressure measurements outside of the clinical setting for diagnostic confirmation is recommended before starting treatment.

- Non-dialytic palliative therapy is a reasonable option for elderly patients with end-stage kidney disease and multiple comorbidities, with treatment focusing on symptom management and quality of life.
- Use of the potassium exchange resin, sodium polystyrene sulfonate, is controversial; its effectiveness is limited, and it produces adverse gastrointestinal effects.
- Initial antihypertensive treatment for black patients with or without diabetes mellitus includes a thiazide diuretic or calcium channel blocker.
- Kidney biopsy is required to diagnose and classify lupus nephritis, which guides therapy.
- Kidney ultrasonography, rather than other imaging modalities, should be obtained for suspected urinary tract obstruction or when the underlying cause of acute kidney injury is unclear.
- Normal pregnancy is associated with decreased blood pressure, increased glomerular filtration rate with decreased serum creatinine, and increased proteinuria.
- In properly selected individuals, peritoneal dialysis allows patients to preserve their independence and offers outcomes similar to those seen with hemodialysis (see Item 19).
- Patients with newly diagnosed primary membranous glomerulopathy are observed for 6 to 12 months while on conservative therapy to allow time for possible spontaneous remission before initiating immunosuppression (see Item 38).
- Nonpharmacologic therapy alone is especially useful for prevention of hypertension, including in adults with elevated blood pressure, and for management of high blood pressure in adults with milder forms of hypertension (see Item 105).
- There is no benefit in starting renal replacement therapy (RRT) in asymptomatic patients or at an arbitrary estimated glomerular filtration rate cutoff compared with careful clinical management and initiating RRT for symptoms or metabolic abnormalities that are refractory to medical treatment (see Item 108).

Nephrology

Clinical Evaluation of Kidney Function

Assessment of Kidney Function

The kidney selectively removes waste while retaining needed substrate, maintains fluid and electrolyte homeostasis, and regulates blood pH. Glomerular filtration rate (GFR) measures total nephron filtration of blood and therefore correlates closely with toxin removal and overall kidney function. Early loss of kidney function is difficult to detect because nephron loss is not initially accompanied by GFR changes due to compensation through hypertrophy and hyperfiltration. Other markers of disordered glomerular filtration, such as proteinuria and hematuria, are also indicators of kidney disease that may precede any evidence of reduced filtration.

Biochemical Markers of Kidney Function

Although numerous methods for estimating kidney function are available (**Table 1**), serum creatinine and serum cystatin C are the primary biomarkers used to estimate GFR.

Serum Creatinine

Serum creatinine is the most extensively used measure of kidney function. Creatinine is freely filtered by the glomerulus, without metabolism or reabsorption. Therefore, changes in serum creatinine primarily reflect changes in GFR. However, the relationship of serum creatinine to GFR is nonlinear; significant losses in kidney function at higher GFR may be masked by only small changes in serum creatinine, and small filtration changes at lower GFR are associated with large changes in serum creatinine (**Figure 1**). Creatinine is also secreted into urine by the proximal tubule, and the contribution of secretion to total creatinine excretion increases as GFR declines. Therefore, when measured creatinine clearance is used to estimate GFR, secreted creatinine will contribute to overestimation of true GFR. With complete loss of kidney function (anuria), serum creatinine typically increases by about 1.0 mg/dL (88.4 μmol/L) per day in patients with average muscle mass.

Creatinine is a metabolite of creatine, which is mostly present in skeletal muscle. Persons with higher muscle mass (such as younger people, men, and black persons) have a higher serum creatinine compared with less muscular persons with the same GFR. Loss of muscle mass seen with aging, muscle wasting, malnutrition, or amputation will result in lower serum creatinine despite stable GFR. In persons with decreased muscle mass, serum creatinine therefore tends to overestimate the GFR.

Some medications reduce proximal tubule secretion of creatinine. Such drugs include cimetidine, trimethoprim, cobicistat, and dolutegravir. Resulting increases in serum creatinine occur despite stable GFR. Reassessment of the serum creatinine level 1 week after identification of the increase will confirm the drug's effect.

Serum Cystatin C

Cystatin C is produced by all nucleated cells, freely filtered by glomeruli, and catabolized by tubules. Compared with serum creatinine, serum cystatin C levels are less affected by age, sex, or muscle mass but may be increased by acute disease (such as malignancy, inflammation, or HIV infection). Changes in serum cystatin C may identify small decreases in kidney function better than serum creatinine. Formulas using cystatin C to estimate GFR are helpful for patients in whom creatinine-based GFR may be inaccurate.

Blood Urea Nitrogen

Blood urea nitrogen (BUN) is a product of protein metabolism. Levels increase with reduced GFR and with increased urea reabsorption caused by renal hypoperfusion. BUN is also affected by protein intake and by changes in catabolic rate as caused by glucocorticoids, starvation, or stress. Persons with liver disease have abnormally low levels. BUN may be useful in detecting renal hypoperfusion because elevation of BUN from increased reabsorption is disproportionate to the rise in serum creatinine level.

Estimation of Glomerular Filtration Rate

Creatinine-based formulas are used to estimate GFR by adjusting for factors that affect serum creatinine and creatinine clearance. These formulas take into account the effects of age, race, sex, and muscle mass (estimated by weight) on serum creatinine levels (see Table 1).

The Chronic Kidney Disease Epidemiology (CKD-EPI) Collaboration creatinine equation is the most widely used method for estimating GFR and is the most accurate equation for most persons, particularly when GFR >60 mL/min/1.73 m². A newer CKD-EPI creatinine-cystatin C equation is the most accurate when serum cystatin creatinine-cystatin C is known. CKD-EPI equations presume standard body surface area and therefore require adjustment for very large or small persons.

The Modification of Diet in Renal Disease (MDRD) study equation does not accurately estimate high GFRs. It performs similarly to the CKD-EPI equation at GFRs

TABLE 1. Methods for Estimating Kidney Function		
Method	**Applications**	**Considerations**
Serum Creatinine		
	Most frequently used assessment of kidney function	Nonlinear relationship with GFR Nonkidney effects on blood levels (muscle mass, drugs affecting secretion)
Serum Cystatin C		
	More accurate in elderly population and patients with cirrhosis due to their low muscle mass More accurate in those with an increase in muscle mass Sensitive to mild changes in GFR	Levels are affected by diabetes mellitus, thyroid disease, inflammation, glucocorticoid use, malignancy, HIV infection
Chronic Kidney Disease Epidemiology (CKD-EPI) Collaboration Equation[a]		
CKD-EPI Creatinine		
Variables include serum creatinine, age, race, and gender: $eGFR = 141 \times min(S_{Cr}/\kappa, 1)^{\alpha}$ $\times max(S_{Cr}/\kappa, 1)^{-1.209}$ $\times 0.993^{Age}$ $\times 1.018$ [if female] $\times 1.159$ [if black]	More accurate than MDRD and CGE equations in elderly population and in those with eGFR >60 mL/min/1.73 m^2	Preferred formula for calculating creatinine-based eGFR
CKD-EPI Cystatin C		
Variables include serum cystatin C, age, and gender: $eGFR = 133 \times min(S_{Cr}/\kappa, 1)^{-0.499}$ $\times max(S_{Cr}/\kappa, 1)^{-1.328}$ $\times 0.996^{Age}$ $\times 0.932$ [if female]	Can be used as confirmatory test for CKD. May be more accurate than creatinine-based equation in those with muscle wasting, chronic illness, or high muscle mass.	Helpful in estimating GFR in those taking drugs that affect creatinine secretion (such as cobicistat, dolutegravir, bictegravir, trimethoprim, and cimetidine)
CKD-EPI Creatinine-Cystatin C		
Equation uses same variables as CKD-EPI creatinine but different exponents and includes serum cystatin C: $eGFR = 135 \times min(S_{Cr}/\kappa, 1)^{\alpha}$ $\times max(S_{Cr}/\kappa, 1)^{-0.601}$ $\times min(S_{Cys}/0.8, 1)^{-0.375}$ $\times max(S_{Cys}/0.8, 1)^{-0.711}$ $\times 0.995^{Age}$ $\times 0.969$ [if female] $\times 1.08$ [if black]	Creatinine-cystatin C combination provides most accurate eGFR in most patient populations	—
Modification of Diet in Renal Disease (MDRD) Study Equation[a]		
Variables include serum creatinine, age, race, and gender: $eGFR = 175 \times (S_{Cr})^{-1.154}$ $\times (age)^{-0.203}$ $\times 0.742$ [if female] $\times 1.212$ [if black]	Similar accuracy as CKD-EPI when eGFR is 15-60 mL/min/1.73 m^2	Most accurate (but similar to CKD-EPI) when eGFR is 15-60 mL/min/1.73 m^2 Underestimates GFR when GFR >60 mL/min/1.73 m^2

(Continued on the next page)

TABLE 1.	Methods for Estimating Kidney Function *(Continued)*	
Method	**Applications**	**Considerations**
Creatinine Clearance (CrCl)		
$U_{Cr}V/S_{Cr} = U_{Cr}$ (mg/dL) $\times$ 24-hour urine volume (mL/24 h)/S_{Cr} (mg/dL) $\times$ 1440 (min/24 h)	Useful in pregnancy, extremes of age and weight, amputees, malnourished and cirrhotic patients (situations where creatinine is low so CKD-EPI and MDRD will overestimate GFR)	Overestimates GFR 10%-20% Overestimation worsens with lower GFR (due to increased ratio of creatinine secretion to filtration) Over- or undercollection limits accuracy
Cockcroft-Gault Equation (CGE)		
Variables include serum creatinine, body weight, age, and gender: CrCl = (140 − age) × (weight in kg) × (0.85 if female)/(72 × S_{Cr})	Improved accuracy when age is <65 years	Most accurate when eGFR is 15-60 mL/min/1.73 m² Underestimates GFR in obesity Overestimates GFR when BMI <25
Radionuclide Kidney Clearance Scanning		
Iothalamate GFR scan or diethylenetriamine pentaacetic acid (DTPA) GFR scan	Useful in kidney donor evaluation if eGFR is borderline for donation or other times when accurate prediction is essential	Most precise method; expensive

CKD = chronic kidney disease; eGFR = estimated glomerular filtration rate; GFR = glomerular filtration rate; S_{Cr} = serum creatinine (mg/dL); S_{Cys} = serum cystatin C (mg/L); U_{Cr} = urine creatinine (mg/dL).

α = −0.329 for females, -0.411 for males; κ = 0.7 for females, 0.9 for males; min = minimum of S_{Cr}/κ or 1; max = maximum of S_{Cr}/κ or 1.

[a]Mathematical equations recommended by the National Kidney Foundation Kidney Disease Outcomes Quality Initiative for estimation of GFR.

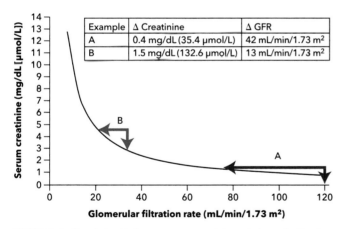

Example	Δ Creatinine	Δ GFR
A	0.4 mg/dL (35.4 μmol/L)	42 mL/min/1.73 m²
B	1.5 mg/dL (132.6 μmol/L)	13 mL/min/1.73 m²

FIGURE 1. The relationship between serum creatinine and glomerular filtration rate (GFR). Example A illustrates that a small increase in the serum creatinine level in the reference range (in this case, 0.8 to 1.2 mg/dL [70.7-106.1 μmol/L]) reflects a relatively large change in GFR (120 to 78 mL/min/1.73 m²). Example B illustrates that a relatively greater increase in the serum creatinine level (in the high range of 3.0 to 4.5 mg/dL [265.2-398 μmol/L]) reflects a proportionately smaller change in GFR (35 to 22 mL/min/1.73 m²).

GFR. The MDRD study equation also requires adjustment for large or small body surface area.

The Cockcroft-Gault equation (CGE) is the least accurate method. It remains in use for drug dosing because it was used in pharmacokinetic studies for most medications.

Creatinine clearance obtained by using 24-hour urine collection is a better measure of GFR than serum creatinine, but it is not recommended for routine estimation of GFR because it is affected by the accuracy of collection and by creatinine secretion.

Radionuclide imaging provides the most accurate measurement of GFR and is the gold standard in research. It is useful for accurate determination of GFR during evaluation of kidney donors, evaluation of recipients for other organs, or assessment of the differential GFR of each kidney before nephrectomy.

KEY POINTS

- Serum creatinine changes nonlinearly with glomerular filtration rate (GFR), and significant losses in kidney function at higher GFR may cause only small changes in serum creatinine.

- The Chronic Kidney Disease Epidemiology (CKD-EPI) Collaboration equation is the most widely used equation to estimate glomerular filtration rate (GFR); it is the most accurate equation for most persons, particularly in the elderly and those with a GFR >60 mL/min/1.73 m².

<60 mL/min/1.73 m². Clinical laboratories that use the MDRD do not report GFRs >60 mL/min/1.73 m²; therefore, physicians may not be aware of the presence of kidney disease. However, an increasing serum creatinine level, proteinuria, or other urine abnormalities should alert the clinician to the presence of kidney disease despite high

Interpretation of the Urinalysis

Urine dipstick and urine microscopy are indicated in the evaluation of both acute and chronic kidney disease (**Table 2**). Analysis is best performed on a fresh specimen within 30 to 60 minutes of voiding. Midstream collection is preferred with a clean catch in women and uncircumcised men.

Urine Dipstick

See Table 2 for details on urine dipstick.

Specific Gravity

Specific gravity measures hydration status and reflects the kidney's ability to concentrate urine.

pH

Low urine pH may occur in persons eating high-protein diets. High alkaline pH ≥7.0 can occur in strict vegetarians and in persons with infections caused by urea-splitting organisms. Urine pH may be inappropriately high in some forms of renal tubular acidosis (type 1 distal) but may be appropriately low in others (type 4 distal).

TABLE 2.	Findings on Urinalysis	
	Normal Range	**Comments**
Dipstick		
Specific gravity	1.005-1.030	Low: dilute urine from excess hydration; impaired urine concentration (diabetes insipidus; sickle cell nephropathy; acute tubular injury)
		High: volume depletion; renal hypoperfusion; excretion of hypertonic solute (glycosuria; contrast dye)
pH	5.0-6.5	Low/acidic: high protein diets; increases risk for uric acid and cystine calculi; type 4 distal RTA; some type 2 proximal RTA
		High/alkaline: urease-splitting organisms (most commonly *Proteus* species; other potential organisms include *Escherichia coli* and *Pseudomonas*, *Klebsiella*, and some staphylococcal species); low acid ingestion; type 1 distal RTA; some type 2 RTA; increases risk for struvite and calcium phosphate calculi
Blood/heme pigments	None	Positive: hemoglobin or myoglobin; absence of erythrocytes suggests myoglobinuria or intravascular hemolysis
		False positive: alkaline urine (pH >9)
Protein	None to trace	Dipsticks primarily detect albumin; concentration dependent (trace positive can be normal in a concentrated specimen); not sufficiently sensitive to detect moderately increased albuminuria
		Graded as trace (10-30 mg/dL), 1+ (30 mg/dL), 2+ (100 mg/dL), 3+ (300 mg/dL), 4+ (>1000 mg/dL)
Glucose	None	Positive: plasma glucose exceeds ~180 mg/dL (10.0 mmol/L); proximal tubule defect (Fanconi syndrome); pregnancy (lower excretion threshold)
Ketones	None	Detects acetone and acetoacetic acid, not β-hydroxybutyrate
		Positive: diabetic ketoacidosis; starvation; vomiting; pregnancy
Leukocyte esterase	None	Enzyme found in leukocytes; indicates pyuria (possibly from UTI); positive test requires ≥5 leukocytes/hpf
Nitrites	None	Produced by bacteria from nitrates
		Positive: suggests UTI
		Negative: does not rule out UTI (specific but not sensitive)
Microscopic		
Erythrocytes	0-2/hpf	Urine microscopy should be performed to evaluate erythrocyte morphology
Leukocytes	0-4/hpf	The presence of any leukocytes may be abnormal depending on clinical circumstances
Squamous epithelial cells	<15/hpf	Increased epithelial cells indicates contamination
Casts	None or hyaline	Hyaline casts: indicative of poor kidney perfusion
		Granular casts: acute tubular injury
		Erythrocyte casts: glomerular bleeding/glomerulonephritis
		Leukocyte casts: infection; acute interstitial nephritis
Crystals (see Table 3)	None	Most common are calcium oxalate, calcium phosphate, uric acid, and struvite

RTA = renal tubular acidosis; UTI = urinary tract infection.

Blood

Dipsticks detect peroxidase activity of blood and free heme pigments (hemoglobin and myoglobin). Three or more erythrocytes result in a positive test (1+ blood). A positive test in the absence of erythrocytes in the urine sediment may indicate myoglobinuria (due to rhabdomyolysis) or hemoglobinuria (due to intravascular hemolysis, transfusion, or shear stress related to mechanical heart valve and perivalvular leak). False-positive tests may occur with other substances with peroxidase activity, including peroxidase-expressing bacteria and drugs such as rifampin or chloroquine. Ascorbic acid can cause a false-negative result. Medications (rifampin, phenytoin) or food (beets) can cause red-colored urine that is heme negative.

Protein

Although various proteins may be present in urine, the dipstick preferentially detects albumin. Because dipsticks are dependent on urine concentration, false negatives may result from dilute urine and false positives from highly concentrated urine. Because moderately increased albuminuria (microalbuminuria) may go undetected by dipstick, direct quantification of albuminuria and/or proteinuria using a random (spot) protein-creatinine ratio or albumin-creatinine ratio or a 24-hour urine collection is required in high-risk patients. False-positive tests can occur with highly alkaline urine specimens.

Glucose

Glucosuria typically occurs when plasma glucose exceeds 180 mg/dL (10.0 mmol/L). Glucosuria in the absence of hyperglycemia suggests proximal tubular dysfunction, as seen with myeloma or exposure to drugs (including tenofovir disoproxil fumarate and sodium-glucose cotransporter-2 inhibitors such as empagliflozin and canagliflozin). Glucosuria may be present in normal pregnancy due to changes in tubular threshold for glucose reabsorption.

Ketones

Ketonuria is most commonly seen in starvation, diabetic ketoacidosis, and alcoholic ketoacidosis. Urine ketones are also seen in salicylate toxicity and isopropyl alcohol poisoning. Urine dipstick detects acetone and acetoacetate but not β-hydroxybutyrate; therefore, in diabetic ketoacidosis and alcoholic ketoacidosis where β-hydroxybutyrate is the primary ketone, the dipstick underestimates ketone excretion. False-positive tests may occur with drugs containing sulfhydryl groups, such as captopril.

Leukocyte Esterase and Nitrites

Leukocyte esterase is an enzyme present in leukocytes. A positive test suggests pyuria (≥5 leukocytes/hpf).

A positive nitrite test signifies the presence of gram-negative bacteria (*Escherichia coli*; *Klebsiella*, *Enterobacter*, *Citrobacter*, and *Proteus* species) capable of converting urine nitrates into nitrites. The test is falsely negative if there is inadequate contact time for urine nitrates with the bacteria. The nitrite test is negative in urinary tract infection (UTI) caused by nonconverting organisms (*Enterococcus*, *Staphylococcus*, *Streptococcus*, or *Haemophilus* species).

The presence of both leukocyte esterase and nitrites on urine dipstick is highly predictive of a UTI; conversely, the absence of both has a high negative predictive value for a UTI.

Bilirubin

Bilirubin should be absent from the urine when serum levels are normal. Conjugated, water-soluble bilirubin is excreted in the urine in severe liver disease or obstructive hepatobiliary disease.

Urobilinogen

Gut bacteria produce urobilinogen through metabolism of bilirubin. Urobilinogen is then absorbed via portal circulation and excreted in urine. Increased urobilinogen is associated with hemolytic anemia or parenchymal liver disease. Decreased levels are seen with severe cholestasis and obstructive disease.

KEY POINTS

- Because moderately increased albuminuria (microalbuminuria) may go undetected by dipstick, direct quantification using a random (spot) protein-creatinine ratio or albumin-creatinine ratio or a 24-hour urine collection is required in high-risk patients.

- The urine nitrite test is negative in urinary tract infections caused by nonconverting organisms (*Enterococcus*, *Staphylococcus*, *Streptococcus*, or *Haemophilus* species).

- The presence of both leukocyte esterase and nitrites on urine dipstick is highly predictive of a urinary tract infection (UTI); conversely, the absence of both has a high negative predictive value for a UTI.

HVC

Urine Microscopy

Microscopic assessment of urine sediment (**Figure 2**) is indicated for patients with abnormalities on dipstick and in those with acute kidney injury, newly diagnosed chronic kidney disease, or suspected glomerulonephritis. See Table 2 for details on urine microscopy.

Erythrocytes

Erythrocyte morphology may indicate their origin (see Figure 2). Isomorphic erythrocytes (round and of consistent size) suggest a nonglomerular origin as a result of infection, mass, cyst, or stone. Glomerular bleeding may be associated with erythrocyte fragmentation, leading to dysmorphic appearances with significant variability. Acanthocytes, a form of dysmorphic erythrocytes characterized by vesicle-shaped protrusions, are most suggestive of a glomerular source of bleeding and should result in prompt

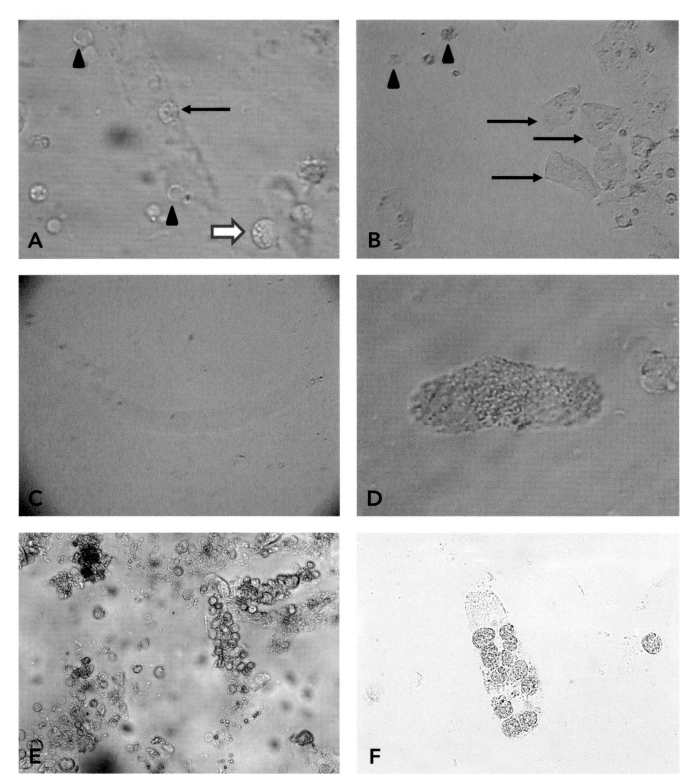

FIGURE 2. Findings on urine microscopy. **A**, Erythrocytes (*black arrowheads*). Also shown is a leukocyte (*black arrow*) embedded in a cast, as well as a tubular cell (*white arrow*). **B**, Leukocytes (*black arrowheads*): Note the large relative size of squamous epithelial cells (*black arrows*). **C**, Hyaline cast. **D**, Granular cast. **E**, Erythrocyte cast. **F**, Leukocyte cast.

evaluation for glomerulonephritis (**Figure 3**). See Clinical Evaluation of Hematuria for more information.

Leukocytes

The presence of ≥5 leukocytes in the urine sediment indicates pyuria, which is most commonly caused by a UTI. Sterile pyuria is the presence of urine leukocytes in the setting of negative urine culture; common causes include vaginitis and cervicitis in women, prostatitis in men, acute interstitial nephritis (AIN), kidney stones, kidney transplant rejection, and, less commonly, UTIs due to organisms that do not grow by standard culture techniques (*Chlamydia* species, *Mycobacterium tuberculosis*, *Ureaplasma urealyticum*). The absence of leukocytes does not rule out AIN.

Eosinophils

Urine eosinophils suggest interstitial nephritis, atheroembolic disease, glomerulonephritis, small-vessel vasculitis, UTI, prostatic disease, or parasitic infections. Poor sensitivity and specificity limit the utility of urine eosinophils in the diagnosis of interstitial nephritis.

Epithelial Cells

Renal tubular, transitional, and squamous epithelial cells may be seen on urinalysis (see Figure 2). Renal tubular epithelial cells are round with central nuclei and are 1.5 to 3 times larger than leukocytes. Their presence in the context of granular casts suggests acute tubular necrosis. Transitional epithelial cells are slightly larger than renal tubular epithelial cells and may be binucleate; they originate anywhere from the renal pelvis to the proximal urethra. Squamous epithelial cells are the largest epithelial cells, and are flat and irregular with small central nuclei; they are derived from the distal urethra or external genitalia, and their presence in large numbers (>15/hpf) denotes contamination by genital secretions.

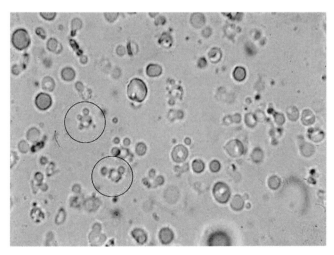

FIGURE 3. Urine microscopy demonstrating acanthocytes, indicated in the red circles. Acanthocytes, a form of dysmorphic erythrocytes characterized by vesicle-shaped protrusions, are most suggestive of glomerular bleeding.

Courtesy of J. Charles Jennette, MD.

Casts

The backbone of all urine casts is a matrix composed of Tamm-Horsfall protein (uromodulin). These cylindrical casts form in the distal tubular lumen. Any cells or debris in casts were present in the tubule at the time of cast formation, therefore originating from a more proximal part of the nephron. Erythrocyte casts are highly suggestive of glomerulonephritis. Leukocyte casts may be present in AIN and infections (pyelonephritis). Pigmented or granular (muddy brown) casts contain tubular cell debris (**Figure 4**) and are present in acute tubular necrosis. The severity of acute kidney injury correlates with the number of casts and presence of renal tubular epithelial cells.

Crystals

Crystalluria results from the supersaturation of solutes in concentrated urine. These solutes are derived from metabolic disorders, inherited diseases, or drugs. **Table 3** describes features of common crystals. Certain drugs can crystallize in concentrated urine and when used in high doses, including sulfadiazine, sulfamethoxazole, intravenous acyclovir, methotrexate, and atazanavir.

KEY POINTS

- Isomorphic erythrocytes suggest a nonglomerular origin of blood; dysmorphic erythrocytes, particularly acanthocytes, suggest a glomerular origin.
- Erythrocyte casts are highly suggestive of glomerulonephritis, leukocyte casts may be present in acute interstitial nephritis and infections, and granular (muddy brown) casts are present in acute tubular necrosis.

Measurement of Albumin and Protein Excretion

Assessment for urine protein is indicated in patients with any suspected kidney disease. Concurrent increased serum creatinine or abnormal findings on urine sediment raise concern for active kidney disease in any patient with proteinuria.

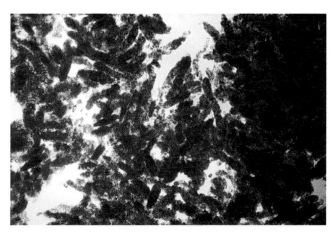

FIGURE 4. Tubular injury (for example, acute tubular necrosis) may lead to deposition of pigmented epithelial tubular debris in the proteinaceous matrix of the cast, with the formation of pigmented or granular (muddy brown) casts.

TABLE 3. Urine Crystals

Type	Morphology	Associated Conditions	Image
Calcium oxalate	Envelope; dumbbell; needle	Hypercalciuria; hyperoxaluria; ethylene glycol poisoning	
Calcium phosphate	Prism; needle; star-like clumps	Distal renal tubular acidosis; urine pH >6.5; tumor lysis syndrome; acute phosphate nephropathy	
Uric acid	Rhomboid; needle; rosette; barrels; hexagonal plates	Hyperuricemia; gout; diabetes mellitus; obesity; tumor lysis syndrome; urine pH <6.0	
Struvite (magnesium ammonium phosphate)	Coffin-lid	Alkaline urine due to chronic urinary tract infection with urease-producing organisms	
Cystine	Hexagonal	Cystinuria	

Assays to detect protein in the urine include urine dipstick, random (spot) urine protein-creatinine ratio or albumin-creatinine ratio, and 24-hour urine collections. Due to the challenges of 24-hour urine collections, the random urine albumin-creatinine ratio and protein-creatinine ratio have been widely adopted. Both random tests adequately determine the presence of albuminuria, but the urine protein-creatinine ratio also detects nonalbumin proteins. Random collections correlate well with timed collections and are sufficiently accurate for screening and monitoring proteinuria despite inaccuracies due to diurnal fluctuations of urine protein and interindividual differences in urine creatinine excretion. **Table 4** outlines the definitions of proteinuria and albuminuria as well as normal values.

Urine albumin, when present at high levels, indicates glomerular injury; conversely, the absence of albuminuria essentially excludes most glomerular diseases. Smaller proteins are filtered at the level of the glomerulus but are reabsorbed by the proximal tubule; their presence in urine generally indicates tubulointerstitial disease. Light chains present at high levels, such as in monoclonal gammopathy, are detected on urine protein electrophoresis or free light chain assay.

Transient, nonpathologic, usually small elevations in urine protein can occur with acute illness or fever, rigorous exercise, and pregnancy. Orthostatic proteinuria is a benign proteinuria that increases when the patient is upright but decreases when the patient is recumbent. This condition is more common in adolescents but should be considered in those up to age 30 years. Split urine collection (daytime versus nighttime collection that includes first morning void) can evaluate this diagnosis.

ACP recommends against screening for chronic kidney disease, including screening for proteinuria in asymptomatic adults without risk factors for chronic kidney disease, because there is no evidence of benefit from early treatment to outweigh the harms of screening, including false-positive results and unnecessary testing and treatment. However, screening

TABLE 4. Definitions of Proteinuria and Albuminuria

Total Urine Protein

Urine Collection Method	Normal	Clinical Proteinuria
24-Hour Excretion	<150 mg/24 h	≥150 mg/24 h
Spot Urine Protein-Creatinine Ratio[a]	≤150 mg/g ≈ ≤150 mg/24 h	>150 mg/g ≈ >150 mg/24 h

Urine Albumin

Urine Collection Method	Normal[b]	Moderately Increased Albuminuria (Microalbuminuria)[b,c]	Severely Increased Albuminuria (Macroalbuminuria)[b,c]
24-Hour Excretion	<30 mg/24 h	30-300 mg/24 h	>300 mg/24 h
Conventional Spot Urine Dipstick[d]	Negative	Negative	Positive
Albumin-Specific Spot Urine Dipstick[e]	<3.0 mg/dL Negative	≥3.0 mg/dL Positive	Positive
Spot Urine Albumin-Creatinine Ratio[a]	<30 mg/g ≈ <30 mg/24 h	30-300 mg/g ≈ 30-300 mg/24 h	>300 mg/g ≈ >300 mg/24 h

[a]Because of the difficulty of obtaining a 24-hour urine collection, urine protein-creatinine ratio or urine albumin-creatinine ratio on random (spot) urine samples is used to estimate 24-hour excretion. Measurement of either urine protein or albumin concentration in a sample is divided by the creatinine concentration of the same sample to derive a unitless value. These ratios correlate well with the 24-hour excretion of protein or albumin. Although these calculations are technically dimensionless, they may be expressed by different laboratories with their units of calculation, such as mg/g (mg protein or albumin/g creatinine) or with units to reflect the proportional 24-hour excretion amount (mg or g protein or albumin/g creatinine).

[b]Chronic kidney disease classification categories A1, A2, and A3 correspond to normal (or mildly increased), moderately increased, and severely increased albuminuria, respectively.

[c]The newer terminology of "moderately increased albuminuria" and "severely increased albuminuria" has been adopted due to the finding that even relatively low levels of urine protein have been associated with significant cardiovascular risk and risk of progression of underlying kidney disease.

[d]Conventional urine dipsticks are more sensitive for detection of albumin than non-albumin proteins; the detection limit is approximately 30 mg/dL, although they are not highly accurate for determining the degree of albuminuria if present.

[e]Urine dipsticks designed specifically to detect small amounts of albuminuria. Similar to conventional urine dipsticks, these dipsticks detect albumin above a concentration threshold but are sensitive to the presence of albumin at lower levels and can be used to indicate the presence of moderately increased albuminuria.

for proteinuria may be considered in high-risk patients, such as hypertensive, diabetic, and older patients.

In patients with diabetes mellitus, urine albumin screening is recommended due to its ability to detect early disease. The American Diabetes Association recommends yearly assessment in patients with type 2 diabetes, and assessment after 5 years of disease in patients with type 1 diabetes. Because there is no evidence that monitoring proteinuria levels in patients taking ACE inhibitors or angiotensin receptor blockers is beneficial or that reduced proteinuria levels translate into improved outcomes, ACP recommends against testing for proteinuria in adults with or without diabetes who are currently taking an ACE inhibitor or an angiotensin receptor blocker.

Urine protein electrophoresis can characterize proteins, allowing for classification of the proteinuria as glomerular or tubular. It also detects monoclonal gammopathy, although it is less sensitive than light chain assay.

KEY POINTS

HVC
- The random (spot) urine protein-creatinine ratio and albumin-creatinine ratio correlate with 24-hour urine collections and are sufficiently accurate for screening and monitoring proteinuria.
- High urine albumin levels indicate glomerular injury; the absence of albuminuria excludes most glomerular diseases.

Clinical Evaluation of Hematuria

Hematuria is defined as the presence of ≥3 erythrocytes/hpf in the urine sediment and may be microscopic (detectable only on urine testing) or macroscopic (grossly visible). Hematuria is most often of nonglomerular origin. A glomerular origin is suggested by concurrent proteinuria, presence of dysmorphic erythrocytes, increased serum creatinine or decrease in estimated GFR (eGFR), or systemic signs and symptoms. Evaluation of hematuria is outlined in **Figure 5**.

Urinalysis should not be used for cancer screening in asymptomatic adults. However, a single incidental finding of hematuria is sufficient to warrant further investigation. Evaluation should be pursued even in patients with bleeding diatheses or those taking antiplatelet or anticoagulation therapy. If menstruation, viral illness, vigorous exercise, or some other benign cause is suspected, urinalysis should be repeated after the cause is resolved. If infection is confirmed, urinalysis should be repeated after treatment to document resolution of hematuria.

In a patient with asymptomatic microscopic hematuria, it is important to assess kidney function, erythrocyte morphology, and urine protein to evaluate for a nephrologic cause, particularly glomerulonephritis. The absence of proteinuria generally rules out a glomerular process; exceptions include very mild glomerular disease (most often IgA nephropathy) or thin glomerular basement membrane disease related to a type

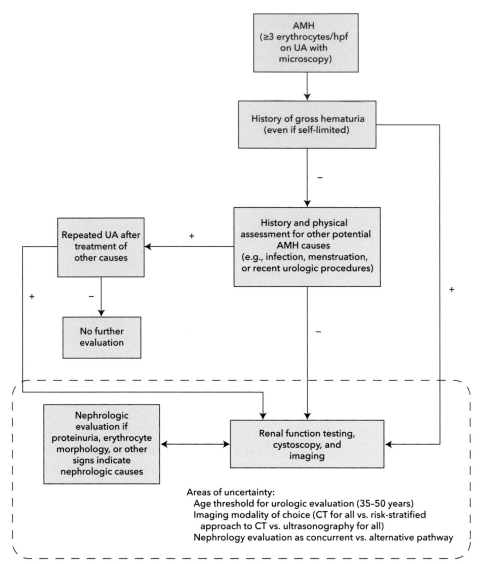

FIGURE 5. Summary of the American College of Physicians recommendations for the evaluation of patients with hematuria. AMH = asymptomatic microscopic hematuria; UA = urinalysis.

Reprinted with permission from Nielsen M, Qaseem A; High Value Care Task Force of the American College of Physicians. Hematuria as a marker of occult urinary tract cancer: advice for high-value care from the American College of Physicians. Ann Intern Med. 2016;164:488-97. [PMID: 26810935] Copyright 2016, American College of Physicians.

IV collagen defect that may present as isolated hematuria. Systemic signs and symptoms raise suspicion for nephrologic disease, particularly those associated with rheumatologic disorders and rapidly progressive glomerulonephritis.

Macroscopic hematuria should prompt urology referral even if self-limited, with further evaluation of nephrologic disease and malignancy as indicated.

If a nephrologic cause of hematuria is not suggested, hematuria may indicate a malignancy. The American Urological Association (AUA) guidelines recommend that patients older than 35 years or those with risk factors for malignancy undergo evaluation for malignancy. Although CT urography (contrast CT with kidney-specific imaging) has the highest sensitivity and specificity for renal malignancy, noncontrast helical CT is more appropriate if a kidney stone is suspected. Ultrasonography is a reasonable first imaging step because of availability, lower cost, and no ionizing radiation. MRI with contrast is useful when CT contrast studies cannot be performed. Cystoscopy is indicated when imaging is negative. ACP and the AUA recommend against obtaining urine cytology in the initial evaluation of hematuria. **H**

KEY POINTS

- Urinalysis should not be used for detection of bladder cancer in asymptomatic patients. **HVC**

- Hematuria requires thorough evaluation because of potentially life-threatening causes, such as rapidly progressive glomerulonephritis and urinary tract malignancy.

- Evaluation of nonglomerular hematuria in patients older than 35 years or those with risk factors for urologic malignancy includes CT urography unless contraindicated; if imaging is negative, cystoscopy should be performed.

Imaging Studies

Ultrasonography is the most commonly used kidney imaging modality. It is easily available, safe, and relatively inexpensive. Ultrasonography can demonstrate hydronephrosis, kidney size and cortical thickness, echogenicity, and presence of cysts and tumors. Absence of hydronephrosis quickly rules out obstruction in most cases. Echogenicity is the ability of a tissue to "bounce back" or return the ultrasound signal and is recognized as brighter shades on the sonogram image. Echogenicity is nonspecific but implies acute or chronic parenchymal disease. Additionally, ultrasonography can measure pre- and postvoid bladder residual, for evaluation of bladder dysfunction or outlet obstruction. Ultrasonography is also useful for uncomplicated nephrolithiasis; a positive ultrasound may be adequate for initial diagnosis. Ultrasonography is less useful in evaluating diseases (including stones) of the mid or distal ureter. Doppler ultrasonography may detect renal artery stenosis or renal vein thrombosis, but is highly user dependent.

CT is appropriate for patients with a nondiagnostic ultrasound or a more complicated presentation. Noncontrast helical CT is the gold standard for diagnosis of nephrolithiasis, and is appropriate for evaluating renal colic. Most stones can be detected, including small stones and those in the distal ureter not detected on ultrasound. It may provide information regarding stone composition and, because the entire urinary tract and abdomen is visualized, alternative diagnoses may be suggested.

CT urography (contrast-enhanced kidney-specific CT) is the test of choice for patients with unexplained hematuria and allows characterization of renal tumors and cysts. CT with contrast is valuable for imaging the renal vasculature. The use of contrast confers risk for contrast-induced nephropathy, particularly in patients with an eGFR <50 mL/min/1.73 m².

MRI with contrast is an alternative for evaluation of renal masses and cysts when CT cannot be performed. MR angiography for detection of renal artery stenosis, and venography for detection of renal vein thrombosis, can be performed with or without gadolinium-based contrast, although contrast provides optimal imaging. MR angiography and CT angiography have mostly replaced standard angiography of renal arteries. Due to concerns for nephrogenic systemic fibrosis (NSF), gadolinium contrast must be avoided in patients with an eGFR <30 mL/min/1.73 m². In life-threatening situations in which benefit outweighs the risk for NSF, MRI is performed with low doses of stable gadolinium agents. See MKSAP 18 Dermatology for more information on NSF.

Radionuclide imaging provides the most accurate measurement of GFR and is the gold standard in research (see Estimation of Glomerular Filtration Rate).

KEY POINTS

HVC
- Ultrasonography is the most commonly used imaging modality in the evaluation of the kidneys and upper urinary tract because of its safety, cost effectiveness, and availability.
- CT urography is the test of choice for patients with unexplained hematuria and allows characterization of renal tumors and cysts; noncontrast helical CT is the gold standard for diagnosis of nephrolithiasis, and CT with contrast is valuable in imaging the renal vasculature.

Kidney Biopsy

Clinical and laboratory features are often insufficient for definitive diagnosis of kidney disease. Kidney biopsy may therefore be essential for diagnosis and management. Indications include glomerular hematuria, severely increased albuminuria, acute or chronic kidney disease of unclear cause (in the absence of atrophic kidneys), and kidney transplant dysfunction or monitoring. AIN and atheroembolic disease may require biopsy for diagnosis because they frequently present only with increased serum creatinine. Classes of lupus nephritis are also distinguished through biopsy.

Percutaneous kidney biopsy with ultrasonography or CT guidance is most common. Open or laparoscopic surgical biopsy is performed when percutaneous biopsy is not possible. Contraindications to percutaneous biopsy include the uncooperative patient, bleeding diatheses (including antiplatelet use or anticoagulation), uncontrolled hypertension, poor kidney visualization, atrophic kidneys, and active UTI. Solitary kidney and pregnancy require weighing of risks and benefits.

The most common risks of biopsy are bleeding and injury to surrounding organs. The most common major complications (occurring in <3% of cases) are need for transfusion or angiography with or without embolization, as well as hemodynamic instability. Minor complications include pain and hematuria. Kidney loss and death are very rare complications.

KEY POINT

- Indications for kidney biopsy include glomerular hematuria, severely increased albuminuria, kidney disease of unclear cause, and kidney transplant dysfunction or monitoring.

Fluids and Electrolytes
Osmolality and Tonicity

The osmolality of a solution is determined by the number of solutes per kilogram. In serum or plasma, osmolality can be measured by freezing point depression or calculated using the following formula:

$$2 \times [Na^+] + \text{Glucose (mg/dL)}/18 + \text{Blood Urea Nitrogen (mg/dL)}/2.8 + \text{Ethanol if present (mg/dL)}/4.6$$

If using international units: $2 \times [Na^+] + \text{Urea (mmol/L)} + \text{Glucose (mmol/L)} + \text{Ethanol (mmol/L)}$

Normal serum osmolality is between 275 and 295 mOsm/kg H₂O. The difference between measured osmolality and calculated osmolality (the osmolal gap) should be <10 mOsm/kg H₂O. A greater value suggests the presence of a low-molecular-weight alcohol. Because water moves freely between the intracellular and extracellular spaces based on the osmotic gradient, the osmolality of both compartments is virtually identical.

Tonicity is effective osmolality due to solutes that are not freely permeable across the cell membrane. Differences in tonicity determine the distribution of water between body compartments. The major solute determining plasma tonicity is sodium. Because urea and ethanol are freely permeable across the cell membrane, they do not contribute to tonicity or the movement of water.

Osmolality is tightly controlled within a narrow range by thirst and antidiuretic hormone (ADH; also known as vasopressin). ADH stimulates reabsorption of water in the collecting duct of the kidney. Increases in tonicity stimulate both thirst and ADH. As long as there is access to water, appropriate thirst, normal control of ADH, and a functioning nephron, serum osmolality should be maintained in the normal range. Disorders of osmolality reflect impaired water homeostasis. Because the body will defend volume status over tonicity, volume depletion (a decrease in total body sodium content) will stimulate ADH such that at any given osmolality, volume depletion will result in an exaggerated ADH response.

Disorders of Serum Sodium

Hyponatremia

Hyponatremia is defined as a serum sodium concentration <135 mEq/L (135 mmol/L). Evaluation begins with measurement of serum osmolality. Hyponatremia is then identified as hypertonic (osmolality >295 mOsm/kg H_2O), isotonic (osmolality 275-295 mOsm/kg H_2O), or hypotonic (osmolality <275 mOsm/kg H_2O) (**Figure 6**).

Evaluation

Symptoms caused by hyponatremia depend on both the rapidity and degree of decline in serum sodium. Acute hyponatremia in <48 hours provides inadequate time for the brain to adapt. A sudden drop in serum sodium causes water to move into the brain, producing cerebral edema and possible headaches, seizures, or death. More chronic declines that allow cells to regulate their volume by decreasing intracellular electrolytes may be asymptomatic.

Hypertonic Hyponatremia

Hypertonic hyponatremia (osmolality >295 mOsm/kg H_2O) results from an increased concentration of effective osmotic solute (typically glucose). The increase in osmolality pulls water out of cells, diluting the sodium. For every 100 mg/dL (5.6 mmol/L) increase in glucose, serum sodium decreases by 1.6 to 2.2 mEq/L (1.6-2.2 mmol/L).

Isotonic (Pseudo) Hyponatremia

Isotonic (pseudo) hyponatremia (osmolality 275-295 mOsm/kg H_2O) is a laboratory artifact. Normally, plasma is 93% water (in which solutes are dissolved) and 7% solids (proteins and lipids). The normal sodium concentration in the water phase is 154 mEq/L (154 mmol/L) (hence, normal saline has a sodium concentration of 154 mEq/L [154 mmol/L]). The lower normal value (around 140 mEq/L [140 mmol/L]) is approximately 7% less because electrolytes are reported as a concentration per liter of plasma/serum. Conditions such as severe hypertriglyceridemia or multiple myeloma that increase the solid phase decrease the sodium concentration in plasma.

Hypotonic Hyponatremia

Hypotonic hyponatremia (osmolality <275 mOsm/kg H_2O) reflects excess water for the sodium present and is further categorized by volume status into hypovolemic, hypervolemic, or isovolemic.

In hypovolemic hypotonic hyponatremia, renal sodium and water reabsorption are stimulated by sympathetic outflow, angiotensin, aldosterone, and ADH, leading to urine sodium concentration <20 mEq/L (20 mmol/L) and urine osmolality

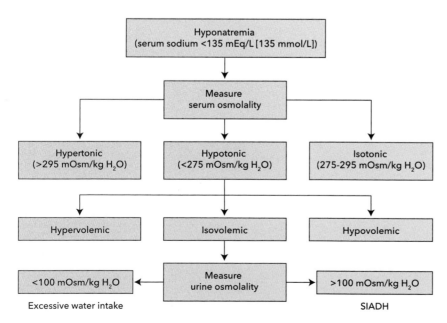

FIGURE 6. Evaluation of hyponatremia. SIADH = syndrome of inappropriate antidiuretic hormone secretion.

>300 mOsm/kg H_2O (except if taking diuretics). Common causes of volume depletion include gastrointestinal losses, excessive sweating, or renal salt wasting from diuretics.

In hypervolemic hypotonic hyponatremia resulting from heart failure or cirrhosis, effective circulating blood volume is inadequate despite total volume overload, resulting in similar urine chemistries.

Isovolemic hypotonic hyponatremia is secondary either to impaired dilution of urine or to water intake that exceeds the kidney's ability to excrete dilute urine. Urine osmolality distinguishes between these two entities. Urine osmolality <100 mOsm/kg H_2O indicates excessive water intake, as seen with psychogenic polydipsia or poor solute intake. Because the kidney cannot excrete pure water, a minimal solute concentration of 50 mOsm/kg H_2O is required. If solute intake is low while liquid intake remains high (as seen in beer potomania or chronic low food intake), water excretion is limited by available urinary solute.

Isovolemic hypotonic hyponatremia with urine osmolality >100 mOsm/kg H_2O can occur in patients with late-stage chronic kidney disease because of impairment of urine dilution, causing hyponatremia after excessive dietary fluid intake. Urine osmolality >100 mOsm/kg H_2O also occurs in isovolemic hypotonic hyponatremia due to the syndrome of inappropriate antidiuretic hormone secretion (SIADH) (**Table 5**). Medications are the most common cause of SIADH, with antidepressants and thiazide diuretics being the most common. 3,4-Methylenedioxymethamphetamine (ecstasy) is increasingly recognized as a cause of hyponatremia. This drug stimulates ADH and, because of the frequently associated fever and dry mouth, induces thirst. Hyponatremia has also been reported in inexperienced marathon runners who overhydrate. Of note, hyponatremia associated with thiazide diuretics, ecstasy, or extreme exertion occurs more frequently in women. A frequent finding in SIADH is a low serum urate level (<4.0 mg/dL [0.24 mmol/L]). Cortisol and thyroid hormone are required to suppress ADH; therefore, deficiencies of these hormones should be evaluated.

Management

Treatment of hypotonic hyponatremia is determined by the underlying pathogenesis. In patients with volume overload, treatment is targeted to the underlying disease process along with water restriction. In hypovolemia, volume expansion with isotonic saline will suppress ADH, thereby increasing water excretion with correction of the hyponatremia.

Treatment of isovolemic hypotonic hyponatremia is determined by the severity of symptoms and the rapidity of the decline.

Symptomatic patients with isovolemic hypotonic hyponatremia and an acute decrease in serum sodium should be treated with a 100-mL bolus of 3% saline to increase the serum sodium by 2.0 to 3.0 mEq/L (2.0-3.0 mmol/L). This is usually adequate to decrease cerebral edema and relieve symptoms. If symptoms persist, the bolus can be repeated once or twice at

TABLE 5.	Causes of the Syndrome of Inappropriate Antidiuretic Hormone Secretion
Cause	**Examples**
Drugs[a]	Thiazide diuretics
	Selective serotonin reuptake inhibitors
	Phenothiazines
	Haloperidol
	Clofibrate
	Carbamazepine
	Cyclophosphamide
	Tricyclic antidepressants
	Valproic acid
	Bromocriptine
	3,4-Methylenedioxymethamphetamine (ecstasy)
Malignancy	Small cell carcinoma
	Squamous cell carcinoma of the head and neck
Central nervous system disease	—
Pulmonary disease	—
Endocrine disorders	Glucocorticoid deficiency
	Myxedema
Idiopathic	—
Endurance exercise (marathon running)	—

[a]Drugs are the most common cause.

10-minute intervals as long as the serum sodium can be measured. If the acute decline in sodium is secondary to excess water intake, fluid restriction will rapidly correct the hyponatremia. Because it is often not possible to determine the acuity of the hyponatremia, some authorities recommend limiting the sodium increase in this population by using either hypotonic solutions or desmopressin.

In isovolemic hypotonic hyponatremia with a more chronic (>48 hours) decline in serum sodium, overly aggressive treatment can result in neuronal damage and osmotic demyelination. The serum sodium should not be increased >8.0 to 10 mEq/L (8.0-10 mmol/L) in 24 hours. If there is significant neurologic impairment (for example, seizures or coma), sodium can be acutely increased 2.0 to 4.0 mEq/L (2.0-4.0 mmol/L) using a bolus of 3% saline as long as the total increase remains ≤10 mEq/L (10 mmol/L) in 24 hours. Administration of potassium will also increase plasma sodium because it enters cells, increasing intracellular osmolality and causing water to move from the extracellular space into the intracellular space, thus raising the plasma sodium concentration.

In patients with asymptomatic isovolemic hypotonic hyponatremia or with only mild to moderate symptoms (headache, lethargy), water restriction is safe and effective.

CONT.

However, limiting fluid intake to <800 mL/24 h is often intolerable. If water restriction is not adequate, therapy is targeted at blocking ADH activity or increasing water excretion. Demeclocycline inhibits ADH action and can be used chronically but is frequently associated with photosensitivity and gastrointestinal symptoms. Tolvaptan, an ADH antagonist, is effective and usually well tolerated, but it is cost-prohibitive and its use is limited to 1 month because of potential liver toxicity. Loop diuretics can be used adjunctively to limit urine concentration, along with increased oral sodium intake. Oral urea, 15 to 30 g/d, is also effective in increasing water excretion, although its use is often limited by unpalatable taste. **H**

KEY POINTS

- Hyponatremia is divided into three categories: hypertonic (osmolality >295 mOsm/kg H_2O), isotonic (osmolality 275-295 mOsm/kg H_2O), or hypotonic (osmolality <275 mOsm/kg H_2O); hypotonic hyponatremia is further categorized by volume status (hypovolemic, hypervolemic, or isovolemic).

- Treatment of acute symptomatic isovolemic hypotonic hyponatremia consists of a 100-mL bolus of 3% saline; if the acute decline in serum sodium is secondary to excess water intake, fluid restriction will rapidly correct the hyponatremia.

- Overly aggressive treatment of chronic isovolemic hypotonic hyponatremia can result in neuronal damage and osmotic demyelination; therefore, serum sodium should not be increased >8.0 to 10 mEq/L (8.0-10 mmol/L) in 24 hours.

Hypernatremia

Hypernatremia is defined as a serum sodium concentration >145 mEq/L (145 mmol/L). Although less common than hyponatremia, hypernatremia is often seen in hospitalized patients and is associated with increased mortality in the critically ill.

Hypernatremia can be divided into three broad categories: inappropriate intake/administration of hypertonic solutions; loss of hypotonic fluids; and excessive water loss due to defects in ADH release or action. A detailed history and physical examination combined with measurement of urine electrolytes and osmolality help distinguish the pathogenesis of hypernatremia.

Evaluation

The most common cause of hypernatremia is loss of hypotonic body fluids with inadequate water replacement because of lack of access or absence of thirst (adipsia). Hypotonic losses may result from diarrhea, the respiratory tract, excessive sweating, or renal losses from osmotic diuresis (such as with glucosuria). If the losses are nonrenal, urine osmolality will be elevated to >600 mOsm/kg H_2O. In osmotic diuresis, urine osmolality is usually between 300 and 600 mOsm/kg H_2O. Hypotonic losses

with inadequate replacement result in intravascular volume depletion with orthostasis or frank hypotension.

Hypertonic hypernatremia can also occur with administration of excessive quantities of hypertonic saline or sodium bicarbonate, or with salt ingestion. The acute increase in sodium causes water to move out of cells, causing shrinkage and neurologic findings. Symptoms can range from lethargy to seizures and coma. Physical examination frequently reveals intravascular volume overload with elevated jugular venous pressure and pulmonary crackles.

Less commonly, hypernatremia may be secondary to either an inadequate release (central diabetes insipidus) or action of ADH (nephrogenic diabetes insipidus). Common symptoms are polydipsia and polyuria. Urine osmolality <300 mOsm/kg H_2O in a hypernatremic patient confirms the diagnosis. An increase in urine osmolality after a dose of desmopressin (ADH analogue) distinguishes between central and nephrogenic diabetes insipidus. Because solute loss is not excessive, hypernatremia from water loss is usually associated with minimal symptoms unless the sodium increases acutely.

Management

Management of hypernatremia is determined by the underlying pathogenesis. When secondary to acute hypertonic gains, treatment of hypernatremia needs to rapidly restore normal sodium concentration. Water can be administered as 5% dextrose, along with intravenous loop diuretics, to abrogate the volume overload. If available, hemodialysis can be considered.

If hypernatremia has occurred over >24 hours, the brain adapts by uptake of electrolytes and other osmotically active solutes. Therefore, to prevent cerebral edema during water infusion, the correction should be <10 mEq/L/24 h (10 mmol/L/d). The change in the serum sodium for each liter of infusate can be calculated using the formula:

(Infusate Sodium) − (Serum Sodium) ÷ (Total Body Water + 1)

If possible, water should be administered orally or by means of a nasogastric tube. Because dextrose-containing solutions may cause glycosuria and increased free water losses, it is important to monitor serum glucose and maintain it below 180 mg/dL (10 mmol/L). In the presence of hemodynamic compromise due to intravascular volume depletion, replacement fluid should be isotonic saline; otherwise, a hypotonic solution (half [0.45%] or quarter [0.22%] normal saline) can be used.

In patients with diabetes insipidus, the first step is determining whether the defect is secondary to a defect in ADH secretion or an ADH action. Central diabetes insipidus can be treated with intranasal or oral desmopressin, a synthetic analogue of vasopressin. Nephrogenic diabetes insipidus is more difficult to treat. Therapy is aimed at limited solute intake to decrease the amount of free water that the kidney can excrete and induction of mild volume depletion using a thiazide diuretic to increase salt and water reabsorption proximal to the collecting duct. **H**

- The most common cause of hypernatremia is loss of hypotonic body fluids with inadequate water replacement because of lack of access or adipsia.
- Treatment of hypernatremia secondary to acute hypertonic gains is aggressive, with rapid restoration of normal sodium concentration
- If hypernatremia has occurred over >24 hours, correction should be <10 mEq/L/24 h (10 mmol/L/d) to prevent cerebral edema.

H Disorders of Serum Potassium

Hypokalemia

Hypokalemia is defined as a serum potassium level <3.5 mEq/L (3.5 mmol/L). It can be divided into disorders of internal balance (movement of potassium between the intracellular and extracellular compartments) and disorders of external balance (potassium intake and output) (**Figure 7**). Serum potassium >3.0 mEq/L (3.0 mmol/L) is usually asymptomatic. Because the ratio of intracellular to extracellular potassium is the major determinant of the membrane potential of electrically active tissue, symptoms of hypokalemia include weakness or paralysis, decreased gastrointestinal motility or ileus with nausea, and cardiac arrhythmias. Electrocardiographic (ECG) manifestations include ST-segment depression, decreased T-wave amplitude, and increased U-wave amplitude. Severe hypokalemia can cause rhabdomyolysis.

Evaluation

The cause of hypokalemia can usually be determined from the history and simple laboratory evaluation. Rarely, hypokalemia is spurious, as can occur in leukemia when delayed sample processing allows large numbers of metabolically active leukocytes to take up potassium. In addition to leukocytosis, a clue to pseudohypokalemia is the lack of signs and symptoms associated with hypokalemia.

Hypokalemia can occur secondary to disordered internal balance. Insulin or β_2-agonists shift potassium into cells, causing an acute, transient, and modest hypokalemia that is usually asymptomatic. Ingestion of soluble barium or cesium salts, which block potassium exit from cells, can produce severely symptomatic hypokalemia with levels below 2.0 mEq/L (2.0 mmol/L). Increased cell production after repletion of vitamin B_{12} or folate in deficient individuals can also cause hypokalemia. Hypokalemic periodic paralysis, either an inherited autosomal dominant disorder or an acquired disorder seen in hyperthyroid patients usually of Japanese descent, may present with severe muscle weakness and paralysis.

Most cases of hypokalemia are due to disordered external balance with total body potassium depletion, secondary either to lack of potassium intake or to increased potassium excretion. Because the kidney can almost cease potassium excretion, only a severely compromised diet can cause hypokalemia. The major determinants of renal potassium secretion are distal tubular flow rate and aldosterone, both of which increase sodium reabsorption, increasing the electronegativity of the tubule lumen and promoting potassium secretion.

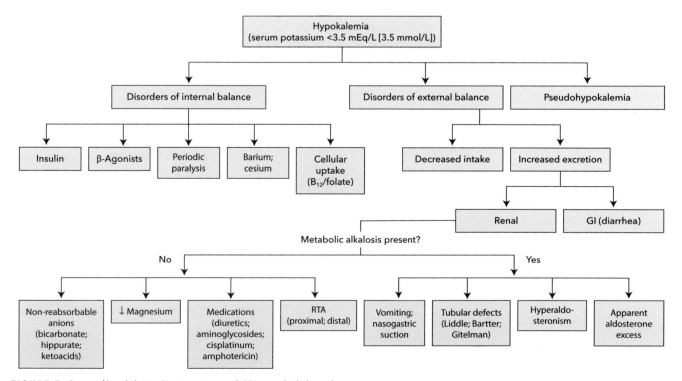

FIGURE 7. Causes of hypokalemia. GI = gastrointestinal; RTA = renal tubular acidosis.

Under normal conditions, distal flow and aldosterone levels are inversely related, thus preventing disruptions in potassium homeostasis by changes in intravascular volume.

The gold standard to distinguish between renal and extra-renal causes of total body potassium depletion is a 24-hour urine potassium <30 mEq/24 h (30 mmol/d); however, this test is often impractical. The preferred alternative is a spot urine potassium-creatinine ratio. A value <13 mEq/g identifies hypokalemia secondary to lack of intake, transcellular shifts, or gastrointestinal losses.

Gastrointestinal losses are usually caused by diarrhea or laxative abuse. Frequently, a concomitant metabolic acidosis is present. Renal potassium wasting may be caused by numerous disorders, including medications (most commonly diuretics), delivery of non-reabsorbable anions to the distal tubule (such as bicarbonate), aldosterone excess, hypomagnesemia, and tubular defects (see Figure 7).

Hyperaldosteronism is associated with hypertension and a metabolic alkalosis. Hypomagnesemia can cause potassium wasting, and renal potassium wasting also occurs in inherited tubular defects, including Liddle, Bartter, and Gitelman syndromes. In Liddle syndrome, increased sodium reabsorption in the distal nephron causes hypertension, metabolic alkalosis, and potassium wasting. Bartter and Gitelman syndromes are caused by mutations in transporters that mimic the effects of diuretics on the tubule. Finally, proximal and distal renal tubular acidosis is associated with potassium wasting.

Management

The total body potassium deficit is difficult to predict and can be up to 200 mEq (200 mmol) for each mEq/L decrease in plasma potassium. In patients with neuromuscular or cardiac symptoms, it is important to increase the potassium promptly. Intravenous potassium can be safely infused at 20 mEq/h (20 mmol/h). Infusion through a central vein can be increased to 40 mEq/h (40 mmol/h) with close monitoring. For mild hypokalemia (2.5-3.5 mEq/L [2.5-3.5 mmol/L]), oral supplementation using potassium chloride or potassium bicarbonate is usually adequate. Concurrent hypomagnesemia must be corrected to prevent ongoing potassium losses. In patients with potassium wasting, potassium-sparing diuretics can be helpful. When significant hypokalemia is secondary to acute transcellular shifts, total body potassium is normal and excessive potassium replacement may cause rebound hyperkalemia. [H]

Hyperkalemia

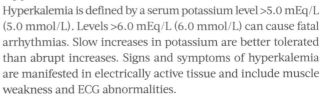

Hyperkalemia is defined by a serum potassium level >5.0 mEq/L (5.0 mmol/L). Levels >6.0 mEq/L (6.0 mmol/L) can cause fatal arrhythmias. Slow increases in potassium are better tolerated than abrupt increases. Signs and symptoms of hyperkalemia are manifested in electrically active tissue and include muscle weakness and ECG abnormalities.

Evaluation

Initial evaluation of hyperkalemia requires a history and physical examination, review of all medications, assessment of kidney function, and an ECG. Initial ECG manifestations include peaked precordial T waves and a shortened QT interval. With progression of hyperkalemia, lengthening of the PR interval, loss of the P wave, widening of the QRS complex, a sine wave pattern, and asystole may occur (**Figure 8**). However, ECG findings do not always correlate with the serum potassium level and do not necessarily progress in an orderly fashion.

During the clotting process, cells are disrupted with the release of intracellular potassium, and pseudohyperkalemia may occur in serum specimens when there are extreme elevations of leukocytes or platelets. In these cases, repeating a plasma specimen will be normal. A tight tourniquet or excessively clenched fist during blood draw can also cause local potassium release.

Hyperkalemia may be caused by transcellular shifts, as occur in states of insulin deficiency or hypertonicity or with the use of β_2-adrenergic blockers. Rapid breakdown of cells such as that seen in rhabdomyolysis or in tumor lysis from treatment of leukemias and lymphomas can acutely raise serum potassium levels.

Hyperkalemia usually results from increased intake with decreased renal excretion. Hyperkalemia frequently occurs with

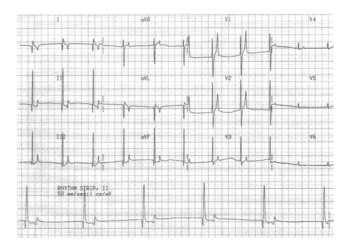

FIGURE 8. This electrocardiogram demonstrates tall, peaked T waves and decreased P waves, which are characteristic of hyperkalemia. T-wave peaking begins with mild to moderate elevations of serum potassium (5.5-7.0 mEq/L [5.5-7.0 mmol/L]) and tends to persist with more severe hyperkalemia. As serum potassium levels increase to above 7.0 to 8.0 mEq/L (7.0-8.0 mmol/L), decreases in P-wave amplitude and widening of the QRS complex are seen. With serum potassium levels above 9.0 to 10.0 mEq/L (9.0-10.0 mmol/L), the waveform will become sinusoidal, and cardiac arrest may follow.

CONT.

oliguric acute or chronic kidney disease with a glomerular filtration rate (GFR) <20 mL/min/1.73 m². Potassium-sparing diuretics (amiloride, triamterene, spironolactone) also commonly cause hyperkalemia through decreased excretion. Other medications that decrease potassium excretion include trimethoprim and pentamidine (by blocking the epithelial sodium channel) and NSAIDs (by decreasing renin). Hypoaldosteronism caused by inhibitors of the renin-angiotensin system, heparin, type 4 renal tubular acidosis (often seen in early diabetic nephropathy), or primary adrenal insufficiency also cause hyperkalemia, especially in the presence of excess potassium intake.

Management

Elevation in the serum potassium level >6.5 mEq/L (6.5 mmol/L), or >6.0 mEq/L (6.0 mmol/L) with ECG changes, should be promptly treated. Treatment is directed at stabilizing the cardiac membrane, shifting potassium into cells, and removing potassium from the body. Intravenous administration of calcium gluconate (100 mg) quickly antagonizes the effects of hyperkalemia on the cardiac membrane. Its duration of action is relatively short and therefore is never definitive therapy. Intravenous administration of insulin alone if serum glucose is >250 mg/dL (13.9 mmol/L) or with 10% dextrose will drive potassium into cells, and is effective for up to 6 hours. Potassium can also be shifted into cells using high-dose nebulized albuterol. Sodium bicarbonate therapy has fallen out of favor because it does not promote redistribution of potassium.

Definitive treatment of severe hyperkalemia must include removal of potassium from the body. In patients without severe kidney disease, loop diuretics can be effective. Use of the potassium exchange resin sodium polystyrene sulfonate is controversial; its effectiveness is limited, and it produces adverse gastrointestinal effects. Hemodialysis is the treatment of choice in patients with severe hyperkalemia and oliguric kidney disease.

In chronic hyperkalemia, limiting potassium intake may be beneficial. Increased sodium intake along with a thiazide or loop diuretic will increase potassium excretion. In hypoaldosteronism, fludrocortisone will normalize the potassium; however, it may cause elevated blood pressure and edema, and long-term effects of fludrocortisone are unknown. All potentially causative medications should be discontinued if possible. If necessary, newer potassium binders (such as patiromer) may allow continuation of essential medications. **H**

KEY POINTS

- Intravenous administration of calcium gluconate quickly antagonizes the effects of hyperkalemia on the cardiac membrane, but its duration of action is relatively short.
- Definitive treatment of severe hyperkalemia must include removal of potassium from the body; loop diuretics can be effective in patients without severe kidney disease, and hemodialysis is the treatment of choice in patients with severe hyperkalemia and oliguric kidney disease.

Disorders of Serum Phosphate

Hypophosphatemia

Hypophosphatemia is defined as a serum phosphate level <2.7 mg/dL (0.87 mmol/L). Phosphate (PO_4) is found primarily within bone and the intracellular space. Phosphate is required for metabolic pathways involved in energy production, cellular repair, and enzymatic activity. Mild hypophosphatemia is rarely symptomatic. Levels <2.0 mg/dL (0.65 mmol/L) are associated with muscle weakness. Severe hypophosphatemia (<1.0 mg/dL [0.32 mmol/L]) is associated with life-threatening symptoms, including delirium, seizures, coma, heart failure, respiratory failure, rhabdomyolysis, and hemolysis.

Evaluation

Hypophosphatemia results from transcellular shifts, decreased intake, or increased excretion. Movement of phosphorous into cells occurs with respiratory alkalosis, insulin treatment, or refeeding of starved individuals. Medications that bind phosphate in the gut (calcium, antacids) can decrease effective intake. Because the kidney can decrease phosphate excretion to very low levels, low dietary phosphate rarely causes hypophosphatemia without coexisting malnutrition. Increased excretion may be caused by diarrhea or renal wasting. Excretion of >100 mg of phosphate in a 24-hour urine collection or a fractional excretion of phosphate (FE_{PO_4}) >5% suggests renal wasting. FE_{PO_4} is calculated as follows:

$$FE_{PO_4} = (U_{PO_4} \times P_{Cr})/(P_{PO_4} \times U_{Cr}) \times 100$$

(where Cr = creatinine, P = plasma, PO_4 = phosphate, U = urine)

Renal losses of phosphate are seen in hyperparathyroidism and in proximal tubular dysfunction.

Management

Mild decreases in serum phosphate can be treated with oral sodium or potassium phosphate. Levels <2.0 mg/dL (0.65 mmol/L) should be treated with intravenous sodium phosphate. Calcitriol is sometimes required to increase intestinal absorption of phosphate.

KEY POINTS

- Severe hypophosphatemia (<1.0 mg/dL [0.32 mmol/L]) is associated with life-threatening symptoms, including delirium, seizures, coma, heart failure, respiratory failure, rhabdomyolysis, and hemolysis.
- Mild hypophosphatemia can be treated with oral sodium or potassium phosphate; levels <2.0 mg/dL (0.65 mmol/L) should be treated with intravenous sodium phosphate.

Hyperphosphatemia

Hyperphosphatemia is defined by a serum phosphate level >4.5 mg/dL (1.45 mmol/L). Causes include cellular lysis with release of phosphate, excessive intake, and/or decreased renal

CONT.

excretion. Symptoms are usually related to co-occurring hypocalcemia. Acute elevations in phosphate can cause precipitation of calcium phosphate in the kidney, resulting in phosphate nephropathy.

Evaluation

Hyperphosphatemia from reduced renal excretion does not occur due to reduced GFR unless patients have severe chronic kidney disease. Hypoparathyroidism decreases excretion through increased phosphate tubular reabsorption; hypocalcemia is often present. Rare defects in the action of fibroblast growth factor-23 (such as in tumoral calcinosis) also increase tubular reabsorption of phosphate.

Because phosphate is primarily an intracellular anion, widespread cellular damage as occurs in rhabdomyolysis and tumor lysis syndrome increases serum phosphate, especially if the GFR is decreased. Excessive phosphate intake rarely causes hyperphosphatemia because the kidney rapidly excretes phosphate. However, phosphate-containing cathartics can cause acute elevations in serum phosphate, especially in patients with reduced GFR.

Management

If kidney function is adequate, serum phosphate levels should normalize in 12 to 24 hours. If necessary, phosphate excretion can be increased with intravenous saline. In patients with acute kidney injury, dialysis may be necessary. Because many foods contain phosphate, dietary phosphate restriction is difficult. Therefore, patients with chronic hyperphosphatemia must often use agents that bind phosphate in the gut. **H**

> **KEY POINTS**
>
> - Causes of hyperphosphatemia include cellular lysis with release of phosphate, excessive intake, and/or decreased renal excretion from decreased glomerular filtration rate or increased tubular reabsorption (hypoparathyroidism).
> - If kidney function is adequate in patients with hyperphosphatemia, serum phosphate levels should normalize in 12 to 24 hours; if necessary, phosphate excretion can be increased with intravenous saline, and dialysis can be initiated for those with acute kidney injury.

H Disorders of Serum Magnesium

There are approximately 24 grams of magnesium in the body, with 99% residing intracellularly and within bone. Magnesium is essential for protein and nucleic acid synthesis, cell adhesion, enzyme reactions, and modulating channel activity.

Hypomagnesemia

Hypomagnesemia is defined by a serum magnesium level <1.7 mg/dL (0.7 mmol/L). Symptoms usually do not develop until serum magnesium is <1.2 mg/dL (0.5 mmol/L). Symptoms include tremors, fasciculations, muscle weakness,

carpopedal spasm, Chvostek (contraction of the ipsilateral facial muscles by tapping the facial nerve) and Trousseau (carpopedal spasm after inflation of blood pressure cuff above systolic blood pressure) signs, and seizures. Hypomagnesemia also appears to potentiate cardiac arrhythmogenicity due to hypokalemia, myocardial ischemia, and various drugs. In addition, hypomagnesemia causes hypokalemia due to renal potassium wasting, and it causes hypocalcemia by impeding parathyroid hormone release and action.

Evaluation

Hypomagnesemia results from decreased gastrointestinal absorption or increased renal secretion. History and physical examination often delineate the cause. More than 10 mg of magnesium in a 24-hour urine collection or a fractional excretion of magnesium (FE_{Mg}) >2% suggests renal wasting in the setting of hypomagnesemia. FE_{Mg} is calculated by using the following formula:

$$FE_{Mg} = ([U_{Mg} \times P_{Cr}]/[\{0.7 \times P_{Mg}\} \times U_{Cr}]) \times 100$$

(where Cr = creatinine, Mg = magnesium, P = plasma, U = urine. Magnesium is multiplied by 0.7 because only 70% of the magnesium is filtered.)

Causes of decreased magnesium absorption include severe malnutrition, diarrhea, and malabsorption. The use of proton pump inhibitors has become an important cause of hypomagnesemia, with most reported cases occurring after prolonged use; hypomagnesemia rapidly reverses upon discontinuation of the drug.

Hypomagnesemia from renal losses occurs with diuretics, cisplatin, aminoglycosides, or calcineurin inhibitors. Vascular endothelial growth factor inhibitors used in cancer treatment can cause significant magnesium wasting. Other causes of urine losses include volume expansion, alcohol ingestion, and diabetic ketoacidosis.

Management

If significant symptoms are present, 4 grams of magnesium sulfate should be infused over 12 hours and repeated if necessary. Less severe symptoms can be treated with 1 to 2 grams of intravenous magnesium sulfate. Importantly, half of acutely infused intravenous magnesium is excreted by the kidney; therefore, slow-release oral magnesium or nasogastric tube delivery may be better to replete mild to moderate degrees of hypomagnesemia. **H**

> **KEY POINTS**
>
> - Significant symptoms of hypomagnesemia usually develop when the serum magnesium level is <1.2 mg/dL (0.50 mmol/L); these include tremors, fasciculations, muscle weakness, carpopedal spasm, Chvostek and Trousseau signs, seizures, and cardiac arrhythmogenicity.
> - Treatment of significant symptoms of hypomagnesemia includes magnesium sulfate infusions; less severe symptoms can be treated with infusion or with slow-release oral magnesium.

Hypermagnesemia

Hypermagnesemia is defined by a serum magnesium level of >2.4 mg/dL (0.99 mmol/L).

Evaluation

Hypermagnesemia occurs infrequently and most commonly results from excessive intake in the setting of decreased kidney function. Numerous medications such as antacids and laxatives contain magnesium, and magnesium sulfate can be used in the treatment of refractory asthma and remains the treatment of choice for prevention of preeclampsia.

Symptoms of hypermagnesemia do not occur until levels are >5.0 mg/dL (2.1 mmol/L). Early symptoms include loss of deep tendon reflexes, progressing to flaccid paralysis at higher levels. Hypermagnesemia also results in hypotension from vascular relaxation. Laboratory analysis often shows hypocalcemia.

Management

Prevention is the key to management of hypermagnesemia. Hypermagnesemia is usually self-limited; magnesium-containing agents should be limited or avoided in individuals with kidney disease. Magnesium-containing medications should be discontinued, and magnesium excretion can be enhanced with saline diuresis. For more severe symptoms, intravenous calcium will antagonize the effects of magnesium. **H**

KEY POINTS

- Early symptoms of hypermagnesemia include loss of deep tendon reflexes, progressing to flaccid paralysis at higher levels.

- For patients with hypermagnesemia, all magnesium-containing medications should be discontinued, and magnesium excretion can be enhanced with saline diuresis; for more severe symptoms, intravenous calcium will antagonize the effects of magnesium.

Acid-Base Disorders

Overview

Acid-base balance is essential to appropriate function of the human body. Hydrogen ions are maintained within narrow limits and determine pH (**Table 6**). Alterations of acid-base

TABLE 6. Physiologic Levels of Tests Used in the Assessment of Acid-Base Status

	pH	PCO_2	Bicarbonate
Arterial blood	7.37-7.44	36-44 mm Hg (4.8-5.9 kPa)	22-26 mEq/L (22-26 mmol/L)
Venous blood	7.32-7.38	42-50 mm Hg (5.6-6.7 kPa)	23-27 mEq/L (23-27 mmol/L)

balance can have dire consequences; therefore, any change in pH results in a predictable response to limit that change.

Causes of acid-base disorders can be determined by using blood gas results (pH, PCO_2), serum bicarbonate measurements, and the serum anion gap. Arterial blood provides the most accurate measurement, although venous blood gases may be useful in following response to therapy. Venous gases are least useful in patients with shock, due to lower pH and higher PCO_2 values than in arterial gases.

Primary acid-base disorders are classified according to the underlying mechanism (metabolic or respiratory) and their effect on acid-base balance (acidosis or alkalosis) (**Figure 9**). Expected compensatory response to the primary disorder is then assessed (**Table 7**). A mixed acid-base disorder is present when measured values fall outside the range of the predicted compensatory response. The primary disorder is usually reflected by the blood pH, although a normal pH may occur in the context of a mixed disorder. Appropriate compensation may result in near-normal pH.

KEY POINTS

- Primary metabolic acidosis is defined by low serum bicarbonate and primary metabolic alkalosis by elevated serum bicarbonate.

- In primary respiratory acidosis, arterial PCO_2 is above the normal range; in primary respiratory alkalosis, PCO_2 is below normal.

Metabolic Acidosis

General Approach

Metabolic acidosis is detected by low pH and low serum bicarbonate. A stepwise approach to assessment supports appropriate diagnosis of the underlying acid-base disorder. First, both pH and PCO_2 are needed to confirm the primary disorder

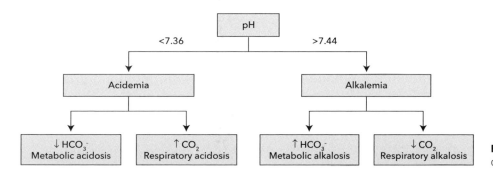

FIGURE 9. Classification of primary acid-base disorders.

TABLE 7. Compensation in Acid-Base Disorders	
Condition	**Expected Compensation**
Metabolic acidosis	Maximally compensated: expected $P_{CO_2} = (1.5)[HCO_3] + 8 \pm 2$ (Winter's formula)
	Measured P_{CO_2} > expected: complicating primary respiratory acidosis
	Measured P_{CO_2} < expected: complicating primary respiratory alkalosis
Metabolic alkalosis	For each ↑ 1.0 mEq/L (1.0 mmol/L) in [HCO$_3$], P_{CO_2} ↑ 0.7 mm Hg (0.09 kPa)
Respiratory acidosis	Acute: 1.0 mEq/L (1.0 mmol/L) ↑ [HCO$_3$] for each 10 mm Hg (1.3 kPa) ↑ in P_{CO_2}
	Chronic: 3.5 mEq/L (3.5 mmol/L) ↑ [HCO$_3$] for each 10 mm Hg (1.3 kPa) ↑ in P_{CO_2}
	[HCO$_3$] < expected value: complicating metabolic acidosis
	[HCO$_3$] > expected value: complicating metabolic alkalosis
Respiratory alkalosis	Acute: 2.0 mEq/L (2.0 mmol/L) ↓ [HCO$_3$] for each 10 mm Hg (1.3 kPa) ↓ in P_{CO_2}
	Chronic: 4.0-5.0 mEq/L (4.0-5.0 mmol/L) ↓ [HCO$_3$] for each 10 mm Hg (1.3 kPa) ↓ in P_{CO_2}
	[HCO$_3$] < expected value: complicating metabolic acidosis
	[HCO$_3$] > expected value: complicating metabolic alkalosis

because low serum bicarbonate may be a compensatory response to respiratory alkalosis.

Next, the serum anion gap is calculated to assess whether the low serum bicarbonate is due to loss of serum bicarbonate (no anion gap) or is a result of unmeasured anion (anion gap acidosis). The anion gap is calculated as follows:

Anion Gap = Serum Sodium (mEq/L) – (Serum Chloride [mEq/L] + Serum Bicarbonate [mEq/L])

The normal reference range for the anion gap is 8.0 to 10 mEq/L ± 2 mEq/L (8.0-10 mmol/L ± 2 mmol/L). In normal subjects, negatively charged albumin is a major contributor to the anion gap. Therefore, changes in albumin need to be taken into account. This is most important in the context of a low albumin wherein failure to correct the anion gap will result in underestimation of the true anion gap. The albumin-corrected anion gap (with normal albumin being 4.0 g/dL [40 g/L]) is calculated as follows:

Albumin-Corrected Anion Gap = Anion Gap + 2.5 × (Normal Albumin – Measured Albumin [g/dL])

If the corrected anion gap is increased, patients should next be assessed for coexistent normal anion gap acidosis or metabolic alkalosis. One method for detection of a coexistent additional acid-base disorder is to assess the ratio of the amount of anion gap abnormality (Δ anion gap) to the amount of bicarbonate abnormality (Δ bicarbonate), or the "delta-delta (Δ-Δ) ratio."

Δ-Δ Ratio = Δ Anion Gap/Δ Bicarbonate = (Anion Gap – 12)/ (25 – Bicarbonate)

A ratio of <0.5 to 1 may reflect the presence of concurrent normal anion gap metabolic acidosis, whereas a ratio of >2 may indicate the presence of metabolic alkalosis.

Patients with metabolic acidosis due to acute or chronic kidney disease may have either a normal anion gap or an increased anion gap, depending on severity of loss of nephron mass. When the glomerular filtration rate (GFR) decreases to

<45 mL/min/1.73 m², decreased urine ammonium excretion leads to a normal anion gap metabolic acidosis, often associated with hyperkalemia. When the GFR decreases to <15 mL/min/1.73 m², retention of sulfates, phosphates, and organic acids results in an increased anion gap metabolic acidosis. **H**

KEY POINTS

- Metabolic acidosis is detected by low pH and low serum bicarbonate levels.
- When metabolic acidosis is present, the anion gap is useful in assessing whether the decreased serum bicarbonate is due to an unmeasured organic anion (increased anion gap metabolic acidosis) or to a loss of bicarbonate (normal anion gap metabolic acidosis).
- Metabolic acidosis due to acute or chronic kidney disease may have either a normal anion gap or an increased anion gap, depending on severity of nephron loss.

Increased Anion Gap Metabolic Acidosis

Increased anion gap metabolic acidosis occurs when unmeasured anions accumulate. Lactic acidosis is the most common cause (**Table 8**). Less common causes include ketoacidosis (diabetic, alcoholic, or starvation), acute or chronic kidney injury, or poisoning (methanol, ethylene glycol, salicylate, or propylene glycol). The plasma osmolal gap may assist in identifying a cause. The plasma osmolal gap is the difference between the measured and calculated plasma osmolality. The calculated plasma osmolality is determined as follows:

Plasma Osmolality (mOsm/kg H$_2$O) = (2 × Serum Sodium [mEq/L]) + Plasma Glucose (mg/dL)/18 + Blood Urea Nitrogen (mg/dL)/2.8

A high osmolal gap (>10 mOsm/kg H$_2$O) indicates the presence of unmeasured osmoles such as methanol or ethylene glycol, which are metabolized to organic acids, thereby increasing the anion gap. A high osmolal gap is also seen in

TABLE 8. Causes of Lactic Acidosis

Condition	Cause	Clinical and Laboratory Manifestations	Treatment	Comments
Lactic Acidosis	See below.	Serum lactate level >4.0 mEq/L (4.0 mmol/L)	Treat underlying cause; sodium bicarbonate when arterial pH is <7.1 to raise pH to 7.2	Most common cause of increased anion gap metabolic acidosis
Type A lactic acidosis	Tissue hypoperfusion	Multisystem organ dysfunction typically present	Correct cause of hypoperfusion	—
Type B lactic acidosis				
Propofol	Propofol >4 mg/kg/h for >24 h	Rhabdomyolysis; hyperlipidemia; cardiogenic shock	Discontinue propofol; hemodialysis	Seen with continuous infusion, not bolus dosing
Metformin	Metformin use in patients with impaired kidney function	More likely to occur in those with acute kidney injury	Hemodialysis	Avoid in those with eGFR <30 mL/min/1.73 m²
HIV nucleoside reverse transcriptase inhibitor	Mitochondrial toxicity	Type B lactic acidosis	Discontinue medication; supportive care	Risk factors: female sex, pregnancy, obesity, poor liver function, lower CD4 count; mostly: ddl, d4T > AZT; rare: TFV, ABC, FTC, 3TC
Hematologic malignancy	Thought to be due to anaerobic metabolism in cancer cells	Type B lactic acidosis; hypoglycemia	Treat underlying malignancy	Portends very poor prognosis; seen in high-grade B-cell lymphomas
D-Lactic acidosis	Short-bowel syndromeᵃ; undigested carbohydrates in the colon are metabolized to D-lactate by bacteria	Intermittent confusion; slurred speech; ataxia; increased anion gap metabolic acidosis with normal serum lactate level	Antibiotics (e.g., metronidazole or neomycin) directed toward bowel flora; restriction of dietary carbohydrates	Diagnosis requires measurement of D-lactate because D-isomer is not measured by conventional assays for serum lactate

3TC = lamivudine; ABC = abacavir; AZT = zidovudine; d4T = stavudine; ddl = didanosine; eGFR = estimated glomerular filtration rate; FTC = emtricitabine; TFV = tenofovir.

ᵃAfter jejunoileal bypass or small-bowel resection.

pseudohyponatremia, in which plasma osmolality is normal while calculated osmolality is low. The patient's history should guide further testing for unmeasured anions.

Diabetic ketoacidosis usually presents with an increased anion gap metabolic acidosis due to accumulation of β-hydroxybutyrate and acetoacetate, although it may present with a normal anion gap due to excretion of ketoacids. Compensatory hyperventilation is characterized by increased tidal volume rather than increase in respiratory rate. Urine dipstick assays for ketones detect acetoacetate using the nitroprusside assay; however, β-hydroxybutyrate is the dominant ketoacid in diabetic ketoacidosis, so urine dipstick results can be falsely negative or underestimate the total ketone load (see MKSAP 18 Endocrinology and Metabolism).

Alcoholic ketoacidosis occurs in patients with chronic ethanol abuse who typically have a history of recent binge drinking, little food intake, and persistent vomiting. Liver chemistry test abnormalities may be present due to concomitant alcoholic hepatitis. Treatment with intravenous saline and intravenous glucose typically results in rapid resolution of ketones due to induction of insulin secretion and suppression of glucagon release. For patients with chronic malnutrition related to alcohol use, thiamine should be administered before glucose to decrease the risk of precipitating Wernicke encephalopathy.

Medication and toxin exposures that cause increased anion gap acidosis are described in **Table 9.**

KEY POINTS

- Lactic acidosis is defined as a serum lactate level >4.0 mEq/L (4.0 mmol/L); management includes treatment of the underlying cause and sodium bicarbonate when arterial pH is <7.1.

- Ethylene glycol or methanol ingestion should be suspected in patients with an increased anion gap acidosis associated with a serum bicarbonate level <10 mEq/L (10 mmol/L) and a plasma osmolal gap >10 mOsm/kg H₂O.

Normal Anion Gap Metabolic Acidosis

Normal anion gap metabolic acidoses most often result from gastrointestinal bicarbonate losses (diarrhea), kidney bicarbonate losses (type 2 renal tubular acidosis), or inability of the kidney to adequately excrete acid (types 1 and 4 renal tubular acidosis; chronic kidney disease). Although a patient history

TABLE 9. Medication and Toxin Exposures that Cause Increased Anion Gap Acidosis

Condition	Cause	Clinical and Laboratory Manifestations	Treatment	Comments
Ethylene glycol ingestion	Glycolic acid accumulation; calcium oxalate precipitation in renal tubules and crystals in the urine	Neurotoxicity/inebriation; AKI and flank pain due to precipitation of calcium oxalate in kidneys; hypocalcemic symptoms; cardiovascular collapse; pulmonary edema Serum bicarbonate level <10 mEq/L (10 mmol/L); plasma osmolal gap >10 mOsm/kg H_2O	Fomepizole IV hydration Hemodialysis: in severe acidemia, very large ingestions, severe CNS depression, AKI, systemic collapse Pyridoxine and thiamine: in suspected ethylene glycol toxicity Sodium bicarbonate	Found in antifreeze, solvents, cosmetics May be difficult to differentiate from methanol ingestion
Methanol ingestion	Formic acid accumulation	CNS damage; optic nerve/eye damage with blindness; inebriation less prominent than with ethylene glycol; papilledema; mydriasis; afferent pupillary defect; abdominal pain; pancreatitis Serum bicarbonate level <10 mEq/L (10 mmol/L); plasma osmolal gap >10 mOsm/kg H_2O	Fomepizole Hemodialysis: in severe acidemia, very large ingestions, severe CNS depression, any visual impairment Folic acid: in suspected methanol toxicity Sodium bicarbonate	Found in windshield-washing fluid, commercial solvents, paints, some antifreezes May be difficult to differentiate from ethylene glycol ingestion 80%-90% mortality rate with methanol ingestion; permanent blindness may occur
Salicylate toxicity	Salicylate anion accumulation; ingestion of as little as 10 grams of aspirin in adults	Respiratory alkalosis; tinnitus; nausea/vomiting; impaired mental status; cerebral edema and fatal brainstem herniation; tachypnea; low-grade fever; noncardiogenic pulmonary edema; hepatic injury; with severe intoxication, lactic acidosis or ketoacidosis	Bicarbonate infusion: alkalinization mitigates CNS toxicity; aim for urine pH >7.5 Hemodialysis: in AKI, impaired mental status, cerebral edema, serum salicylate levels >100 mg/dL with acute ingestion and levels >60 mg/dL with chronic ingestion, refractory acidemia, pulmonary edema	Toxicity can develop from ingestion or mucocutaneous exposure to salicylate preparations such as methyl salicylate (oil of wintergreen)
Propylene glycol toxicity	Large doses of propylene glycol (a solvent used for IV medications), most commonly lorazepam diluted in propylene glycol (80%)	AKI; anion gap metabolic acidosis with increased plasma osmolal gap; toxicity when propylene glycol levels >25 mg/dL or plasma osmolal gap >10 mOsm/kg H_2O	Discontinue the IV infusion Hemodialysis	Monitor acid-base status and serum osmolality when lorazepam doses >1 mg/kg/d; unlikely to develop if 24-h lorazepam dose is limited to <166 mg/d
Pyroglutamic (5-oxoproline) acidosis	Resulting from chronic acetaminophen ingestion; most common in critically ill patients, those with poor nutrition, liver disease, or CKD, and in vegetarians	Impaired mental status; on urine testing for organic anions, high concentrations of urine pyroglutamate (5-oxoproline)	Discontinue acetaminophen Consider N-acetylcysteine to regenerate depleted glutathione stores	Female preponderance (80%); genetic factors may play a role

AKI = acute kidney injury; CKD = chronic kidney disease; CNS = central nervous system; IV = intravenous.

may elucidate the cause, the urine anion gap may help to narrow down the cause.

The kidneys should increase acid excretion in response to acidemia. This is achieved primarily by increased tubular production of ammonia (NH_3) and secretion of protons, resulting in increased urine ammonium (NH_4^+). The amount of urine ammonium reflects the ability of the kidneys to respond appropriately to acidemia and indicates if the kidney is a cause of the acidosis. Because urine ammonium is difficult to obtain,

the urine anion gap is used as a surrogate to assess kidney acid excretion:

Urine Anion Gap = (Urine Sodium + Urine Potassium) – Urine Chloride

In patients with gastrointestinal losses of bicarbonate (diarrhea; laxative abuse) or those exposed to an acid load, urine NH_4^+ should increase. Ammonium cation excretion results in proportionately less excretion of sodium and

CONT.

potassium (the predominant urine cations). Chloride anion excretion continues with ammonium cation excretion to maintain electrical neutrality. In the context of increased urine NH_4^+ production, therefore, the urine anion gap will be negative (less than zero). A positive urine anion gap in a patient with acidemia suggests the presence of a distal renal tubular acidosis. Proton secretion in the distal nephron generates NH_4^+, and in distal renal tubular acidosis there is a defect in this proton secretion. Therefore, urine NH_4^+ will be low, with proportionately greater sodium and potassium excretion resulting in a positive urine anion gap.

The urine anion gap, together with serum potassium levels and urine pH, can help further distinguish the causes of normal anion gap metabolic acidosis (**Table 10**).

Type 2 (Proximal) Renal Tubular Acidosis

The primary defect in type 2 (proximal) renal tubular acidosis (RTA) is failure of the proximal tubule to adequately absorb filtered bicarbonate, resulting in bicarbonate loss and acidosis. Type 2 RTA is usually accompanied by other evidence of proximal tubular dysfunction, including Fanconi syndrome (glycosuria, phosphaturia, aminoaciduria, hypouricemia). As blood bicarbonate levels decrease, less bicarbonate is filtered and eventually the resorptive threshold is reached, such that serum bicarbonate levels stabilize (around 12-14 mEq/L [12-14 mmol/L]). Because the distal nephron functions appropriately in type 2 RTA, urine can still be acidified to a pH <5.5 and NH_4^+ production will be normal, usually making the urine anion gap negative. Hypokalemia is also often present due to increased distal tubular potassium secretion. This occurs because sodium accompanies bicarbonate to the distal tubule, where sodium is reabsorbed in exchange for potassium.

Alkali replacement is the mainstay of treatment for type 2 RTA. Thiazide diuretics may help by causing mild volume depletion with subsequent aldosterone-driven proximal reabsorption of sodium and bicarbonate.

Type 1 (Hypokalemic Distal) Renal Tubular Acidosis

In type 1 (hypokalemic distal) RTA, a distal tubular defect results in impaired excretion of hydrogen ions by the distal nephron (hence, low urine ammonium and positive urine

anion gap) with inability to acidify urine below a pH of 6.0. Serum bicarbonate may fall below 10 mEq/L (10 mmol/L) as levels fail to stabilize as is seen with type 2 (proximal) RTA; despite lower filtered bicarbonate, continued impairment in acid excretion will worsen the acidosis.

The most common causes include Sjögren syndrome and other tubulointerstitial diseases, including reflux uropathy and obstructive uropathy. Type 1 RTA can also be caused by medications such as amphotericin B and lithium and has been described in dysproteinemias, sickle cell disease, and Wilson disease.

Urinary potassium wasting in the setting of diminished proton secretion underlies the development of hypokalemia. Hypercalciuria and hyperphosphatemia are frequent in untreated type 1 RTA due to increased calcium and phosphate release from bone due to buffering of acid. Reduced tubular calcium resorption in the context of acidosis exacerbates hypercalciuria. Increased proximal reabsorption of citrate in the context of acidosis and hypokalemia causes hypocitraturia. Citrate usually inhibits calcium crystallization; therefore, hypocitraturia, in addition to hypercalciuria, increases the risk of calcium phosphate stones and nephrocalcinosis.

Treatment consists of potassium citrate, 1 mEq/kg/d (which is subsequently metabolized to bicarbonate), with the dose titrated to response.

Type 4 (Hyperkalemic Distal) Renal Tubular Acidosis

Type 4 (hyperkalemic distal) RTA is caused by aldosterone deficiency or resistance. Primary adrenal insufficiency (Addison disease) may cause aldosterone deficiency. Hyporeninemic hypoaldosteronism is a more common cause and may occur in the presence of various kidney diseases, most often diabetic nephropathy. Aldosterone resistance can occur in those with tubulointerstitial disease, including urinary obstruction, sickle cell disease, medullary cystic kidney disease, and kidney transplant rejection. Drug-induced type 4 RTA can be caused by numerous drugs that reduce aldosterone production, including ACE inhibitors, angiotensin receptor blockers, heparin, and cyclooxygenase-2 inhibitors.

Type 4 RTA is associated with a positive urine anion gap but a urine pH <5.5 (see Table 10). Hyperkalemia decreases NH_3 production (and therefore NH_4^+), resulting in a positive

TABLE 10. Diagnostic Approach to Normal Anion Gap Metabolic Acidosis			
Diagnosis	**Urine Anion Gap $(U_{Na} + U_K) - U_{Cl}$**	**Serum Potassium**	**Urine pH**
Ammonium chloride ingestion (acid load)	Negative	Normal	<5.5
Diarrhea and acidosis	Negative	Normal	<5.5
Type 2 (proximal) RTA[a]	Negative	Decreased	Variable[b]
Type 1 (hypokalemic distal) RTA	Positive	Decreased	>5.5
Type 4 (hyperkalemic distal) RTA	Positive	Increased	<5.5

RTA = renal tubular acidosis; U_{Cl} = urine chloride; U_K = urine potassium; U_{Na} = urine sodium.

[a]Type 2 (proximal) RTA is often associated with Fanconi syndrome (glycosuria, phosphaturia, aminoaciduria, hypouricemia).

[b]Patients with type 2 (proximal) RTA have normal distal renal tubular function and can acidify the urine once the serum bicarbonate drops to a point at which the filtered load of bicarbonate can be normally reabsorbed.

CONT.

urine anion gap. Even if the distal nephron is able to decrease urine pH appropriately, reduced NH_4^+ excretion will lead to insufficient acid excretion, generating a metabolic acidosis.

Treatment is focused on correcting the underlying cause if possible; offending medications should be discontinued when identified. Because many patients are also hypertensive and volume expanded, thiazide or loop diuretics may help increase bicarbonate and decrease serum potassium. Fludrocortisone can be used to replace mineralocorticoids in hyporeninemic hypoaldosteronism in those without hypertension or heart failure. Use of the potassium exchange resin sodium polystyrene sulfonate is controversial because its effectiveness is limited. The newer cation-exchanger patiromer is effective.

Mixed Forms of Renal Tubular Acidosis

Topiramate inhibits carbonic anhydrase in both proximal and distal tubules, causing the acquired form of RTA. Due to consequent high urine pH (>6.0) and hypocitraturia, topiramate is associated with increased risk for calcium phosphate stones. Rare hereditary carbonic anhydrase deficiencies also result in combined proximal and distal RTAs. **H**

> **KEY POINTS**
>
> - In type 2 (proximal) renal tubular acidosis, failure of the proximal tubule to adequately absorb filtered bicarbonate causes bicarbonate loss; treatment consists of alkali replacement and a thiazide diuretic.
>
> - In type 1 (hypokalemic distal) renal tubular acidosis, impaired distal hydrogen ion excretion causes citrate reabsorption and increases the risk for nephrocalcinosis; treatment consists of potassium citrate.
>
> - In type 4 (hyperkalemic distal) renal tubular acidosis, aldosterone deficiency or resistance causes hyperkalemia and decreased NH_4^+ excretion; treatment includes correction of the underlying cause and treatment of hyperkalemia.

H Metabolic Alkalosis

Metabolic alkalosis with high blood pH results either from a loss of acid or from administration or retention of bicarbonate (alkali). Metabolic alkalosis occurs in two phases: a generation phase in which the primary disorder (such as vomiting or the accumulation of alkali) occurs, and a maintenance phase in which typical renal compensatory excretion of excess bicarbonate is ineffective. The metabolic alkalosis generation phase usually involves the gastrointestinal (GI) tract (in vomiting-induced acid loss) or the kidney (typically a mineralocorticoid effect, either primary or in response to intravascular volume depletion, with resulting sodium and bicarbonate retention at the expense of acid and potassium secretion). Conditions that contribute to maintenance of metabolic alkalosis include volume contraction, ineffective arterial blood volume, hypokalemia, chloride depletion, and decreased glomerular filtration.

Symptoms of metabolic alkalosis are usually related to the underlying disorder. Coexisting hypokalemia markedly increases the risk for cardiac arrhythmias. Severe metabolic alkalosis (serum bicarbonate >50 mEq/L [50 mmol/L]) can cause hypocalcemia, hypoventilation, and hypoxemia, with potential neurologic consequences (seizures, delirium, stupor).

Thorough history and physical examination, including assessment of blood pressure and volume status, are essential to identifying the likely cause (**Figure 10**). Laboratory evaluation is based on urine chloride rather than urine sodium. Urine sodium can be high during appropriate compensatory urine bicarbonate excretion because sodium is the primary cation excreted with bicarbonate. Urine sodium measurement may also be misleading with diuretic use.

The most common causes of metabolic alkalosis are associated with chloride depletion: vomiting, nasogastric suction, and diuretic use. Although upper GI losses are far more common, lower GI chloride-secretory diarrheas (villous adenoma, congenital chloridorrhea) can rarely cause chloride depletion with bicarbonate retention. A "contraction alkalosis" results from loss of extracellular fluid containing low amounts of bicarbonate, leaving a contracted extracellular volume around a constant amount of existing circulating bicarbonate.

In patients with low urine chloride (<15 mEq/L [15 mmol/L]), normal/low intravascular volume, and normal/low extracellular volume, treatment consists of saline administration plus repletion of potassium (saline-responsive metabolic alkalosis) while addressing the primary cause of the alkalosis. In contrast, those with a low urine chloride (<15 mEq/L [15 mmol/L]) and normal/low intravascular volume but with an increased extravascular volume (heart failure, cirrhosis) have secondary hyperaldosteronism with sodium and bicarbonate retention manifested by edema; treatment is tailored to improving effective arterial blood volume and diuresis.

Mineralocorticoid excess presents with a high urine chloride (>15 mEq/L [15 mmol/L]) with elevated blood pressure and hypokalemia without volume overload (saline-resistant metabolic alkalosis). The lack of an overt increase in extravascular volume is often described as "aldosterone escape": after initial sodium retention, sodium balance is attained through spontaneous diuresis that returns vascular volume toward normal. Mineralocorticoid excess is treated with potassium repletion and treatment of the underlying condition.

Rarely, patients may have clinical features consistent with saline-responsive metabolic alkalosis but with a urine chloride of >15 mEq/L (15 mmol/L); ongoing diuretic use can present this way. Two autosomal recessive genetic conditions, Bartter and Gitelman syndromes, result in disordered renal sodium and chloride transporters and clinically mimic loop diuretic

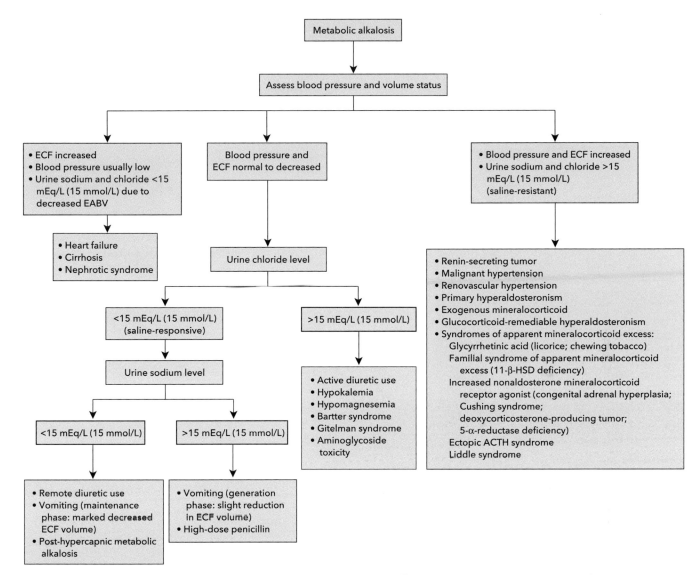

FIGURE 10. Assessment of metabolic alkalosis. ACTH = adrenocorticotropic hormone; EABV = effective arterial blood volume; ECF = extracellular fluid; HSD = hydroxysteroid dehydrogenase.

and thiazide diuretic use, respectively. These diagnoses should be considered only after urine diuretic screening.

KEY POINTS

- The most common causes of metabolic alkalosis are associated with chloride depletion: vomiting, nasogastric suction, and diuretic use.

- In metabolic alkalosis, blood pressure, volume status, and urine chloride are critical to identify the likely cause and to determine treatment.

Respiratory Acidosis

Respiratory acidosis is characterized by retention of arterial CO_2 (hypercapnia). The most common causes are inadequate ventilation (decreased central respiratory drive, thoracic neuromuscular dysfunction, musculoskeletal disorders), impaired arterial-alveolar gas exchange (pneumonia, pulmonary edema, interstitial lung diseases), and airway obstruction (COPD, status asthmaticus, upper airway obstruction).

With acute respiratory acidosis, excess CO_2 is initially buffered by water, leading to formation of hydrogen ions and bicarbonate. Thus, the acute arterial blood gas reveals increased P_{CO_2}, decreased pH, and a slight increase in bicarbonate. Over 3 to 5 days, compensatory increases in renal acid excretion (with bicarbonate reabsorption) reach a new steady state (see Table 7).

Clinical manifestations of respiratory acidosis are complicated by frequently associated hypoxemia. Symptoms are predominantly neurologic, including headache, anxiety, blurred vision, and tremor. Severe acidosis can cause confusion, somnolence, or seizures. Chronic respiratory acidosis may have milder neurologic effects such as memory loss, inattentiveness, or irritability. Cardiovascular manifestations include

CONT.

vasodilation and tachycardia that may evolve to cardiac arrhythmias and decreased cardiac output. Renal vasoconstriction with enhanced sodium retention occurs in severe respiratory acidosis, typically in those with severe lung disease and right-sided heart failure.

Treatment involves correcting the underlying mechanism if possible, and may necessitate mechanical ventilation to reduce CO_2 and oxygen supplementation. H

KEY POINTS

- In respiratory acidosis, arterial blood gases demonstrate elevated P_{CO_2} (hypercapnia), decreased pH, and increased bicarbonate.

- Symptoms of acute respiratory acidosis are predominantly neurologic and can include confusion, somnolence, or seizures; chronic respiratory acidosis may result in memory loss, inattentiveness, or irritability.

H Respiratory Alkalosis

Respiratory alkalosis is defined by a reduction in arterial P_{CO_2} (hypocapnia) due to increased ventilation. The most common causes of respiratory alkalosis are an enhanced respiratory drive (sepsis, hepatic failure, anxiety, iatrogenic hyperventilation, pregnancy, nicotine, salicylate intoxication, subarachnoid hemorrhage), hypoxemia, and pulmonary disease with stimulation of thoracic stretch receptors (pneumonia, acute respiratory distress syndrome, pulmonary embolism).

Acute hypocapnia leads to a rapid increase in arterial pH. However, immediate compensatory diffusion of hydrogen ions from intracellular stores, and subsequent reduction in serum bicarbonate through regeneration of CO_2, limits the magnitude of alkalosis. The typical arterial blood gas in this setting demonstrates a decrease in P_{CO_2}, an increase in pH, and a slight decrease in bicarbonate. Over 2 to 3 days, bicarbonate levels decrease further as compensatory kidney excretion of bicarbonate reaches a new steady state (see Table 7).

Respiratory alkalosis may cause increased cellular lactic acid production. Increases in negatively charged albumin may cause a mildly increased anion gap and decreased ionized calcium (from enhanced albumin binding). Finally, severe hypophosphatemia can occur due to a shift of phosphate from extracellular to intracellular fluid.

Clinical presentation includes underlying tachypnea and neurologic findings such as lightheadedness, numbness and paresthesias, cramps, confusion, and, rarely, seizures. An important consideration is the potential for salicylate intoxication, which in its early phases presents with mental status changes, respiratory alkalosis, and an increased anion gap metabolic acidosis.

Treatment of respiratory alkalosis is directed at correction of the primary disorder. Treatment of salicylate intoxication includes forced diuresis, urine alkalization, or hemodialysis. For anxiety-induced or psychogenic hyperventilation, increasing inspired P_{CO_2} by closed bag rebreathing may be effective.

In rare circumstances of severe alkalemia (pH >7.55) with hemodynamic instability, arrhythmias, or altered mental status, strategies to reduce bicarbonate include acetazolamide or controlled mechanical hypoventilation. H

KEY POINTS

- Respiratory alkalosis is associated with a decrease in P_{CO_2}, an increase in pH, and a slight decrease in bicarbonate.

- Salicylate intoxication presents in the early phase with mental status changes, respiratory alkalosis, and an increased anion gap metabolic acidosis; treatment includes forced diuresis, urine alkalization, or hemodialysis.

Hypertension
Epidemiology

In the United States, hypertension is second only to smoking as a risk factor for death and disability. In 2010, hypertension was the leading cause of death and disability-adjusted life-years worldwide. The prevalence of hypertension varies based on the cut-point used to define hypertension, with the prevalence increasing from 32% to 46% when the cutoff is changed from a blood pressure (BP) ≥140/90 mm Hg to ≥130/80 mm Hg. Prevalence increases as the population ages, such that in individuals without hypertension at age 45 years, the 40-year risk for developing hypertension is 93% for black adults, 92% for Hispanic adults, 86% for white adults, and 84% for Chinese adults. Overall, persons free of hypertension at 55 years have a 90% lifetime risk for developing hypertension. Although several clinical trials have revealed that treatment of hypertension with antihypertensive medications reduces cardiovascular events, hypertension control to a BP <140/90 mm Hg is achieved in only 50% of the U.S. population.

Consequences of Sustained Hypertension
End-Organ Injury

Exposure to chronic BP elevation and, in some cases, to hypertensive emergency (defined as severely elevated BP with symptoms or signs of acute target-organ damage) can significantly injure multiple organs.

Eye

Chronically elevated BP can lead to elevated arteriolar pressure, resulting in hypertensive retinopathy, which manifests as vasoconstriction and arteriolar narrowing (visualized as "arteriovenous nicking" or "copper wiring" on funduscopic examination), endothelial damage and retinal hemorrhage (or "flame hemorrhages"), and choroidopathy. Optic neuropathy may result from ischemia to the nerve fiber secondary to fibrinoid necrosis of vessels, manifesting as "cotton wool spots" or optic disc pallor.

Hypertensive emergency can lead to papilledema, resulting from leakage, ischemia, and fibrinoid necrosis of arterioles supplying the optic disc, causing optic nerve hemorrhage and swelling. Loss of visual acuity and blindness can occur.

Medium to Large Vessels

Long-standing hypertension can damage the vascular endothelium and, combined with elevated cholesterol and especially in the presence of diabetes mellitus, lead to peripheral vascular disease, including aortic aneurysms.

Hypertensive emergency may cause aortic aneurysmal rupture or aortic wall dissection.

Brain

Arteriosclerosis related to long-standing hypertension can cause distal ischemia, including transient ischemic attacks, lacunar infarctions, cerebrovascular accidents, and vascular neurocognitive disorder.

Hypertensive emergency has serious manifestations such as hemorrhagic stroke or subarachnoid hemorrhage from cerebral aneurysmal rupture, resulting in paralysis or fatality.

Heart

Left ventricular hypertrophy can occur as a compensatory mechanism, resulting in diastolic dysfunction, and can eventually lead to heart failure.

Hypertensive emergency can lead to acute myocardial infarction.

Kidney

Injury to the renal vasculature results in arteriosclerosis and atherosclerosis and, ultimately, hypertensive nephrosclerosis and chronic kidney disease (CKD). Hypertension is a major cause of CKD and end-stage kidney disease (ESKD), especially in black persons. Additionally, uncontrolled hypertension can increase the rate of CKD progression in patients with other underlying CKD causes, such as diabetic nephropathy.

Hypertensive emergency can cause acute kidney injury (AKI), with arteriolar proliferation (onion skinning), fibrinoid necrosis, and features of thrombotic microangiopathy.

Clinical Impact

Hypertension is one of the most significant but modifiable risk factors for cardiovascular disease, stroke, ESKD, and overall mortality. Systolic is more important than diastolic BP as an independent risk factor for coronary events, heart failure, stroke, and ESKD. Data suggest that BP-related cardiovascular disease, kidney disease, and vascular death risk is evident before development of hypertension per se; risk increases progressively throughout ranges of BP that were previously recognized as normal and are now referred to as "elevated blood pressure." Therefore, a large proportion of the U.S. population has BP below the traditional threshold for pharmacologic treatment but high enough to signify future risk. Worldwide, approximately 50% of strokes and of ischemic heart disease events are attributable to high BP, equivalent to 7.6 million premature deaths (13.5% of total) and 92 million disability-adjusted life-years (6% of total).

KEY POINTS

- Chronic elevation of blood pressure can lead to significant injury in multiple organs, including the eyes, blood vessels, brain, heart, and kidneys; hypertensive emergency is defined as severely elevated blood pressure and acute target-organ damage.

- Worldwide, approximately 50% of strokes and of ischemic heart disease events are attributable to high blood pressure.

Blood Pressure Measurement

Proper Technique

Repeat BP determinations with proper technique are necessary before making clinical decisions regarding management. Smoking, caffeinated beverages, or exercise within 30 minutes before BP measurements should be avoided. A properly calibrated and validated instrument using the oscillometric method (manual or calibrated automated device) should be employed. The patient should be quietly seated in a chair for ≥5 minutes, with the back supported, feet on the floor, legs uncrossed, and the arm bared and supported on a flat surface, with the upper arm at the heart level. The cuff size should be appropriately chosen to ensure that the bladder encircles at least 80% of the upper arm. Two common reasons for an elevated BP office reading include using a cuff that is too small or measuring the BP before the patient has rested in a seated position. At least two measurements should be taken and averaged, about 2 minutes apart; the process should be repeated if the initial measurements differ by more than 5 mm Hg. Office BP measurement(s) and the expected BP target should be communicated to the patient orally and in writing to increase awareness and adherence.

Auscultatory Blood Pressure Monitoring

The sphygmomanometer is placed on the arm with the lower cuff edge about 2 to 3 cm above the antecubital fossa. A stethoscope is placed over the brachial artery in the antecubital fossa. The cuff is inflated at least 30 mm Hg above the point at which the palpated brachial pulse disappears (estimated systolic BP). Systolic BP is recorded at the point at which the first sound is heard (or onset of the first Korotkoff sound), and diastolic BP is recorded at the point the sound disappears (or disappearance of all Korotkoff sounds).

Electronic Blood Pressure Monitoring

Electronic devices use the same oscillometric method as manual cuffs and may reduce the inter-individual variability of manual measurements. However, proper calibration is essential for accurate measurements, especially if used by the patient at home. In general, electronic devices underestimate systolic BP and overestimate diastolic BP compared with intra-arterial measurements, which is more of a problem than with nonautomated devices.

Ambulatory Blood Pressure Monitoring

Ambulatory blood pressure monitoring (ABPM) is an electronic BP measuring device that can be worn continuously for periods of 24 hours or longer and programmed to measure and record BP every 15 to 60 minutes during daytime wakefulness and nighttime sleep. Average 24-hour, daytime, and nighttime systolic and diastolic BP are also generally reported. Normal BP by ABPM includes a 24-hour average BP <115/75 mm Hg; daytime average BP <120/80 mm Hg; and nighttime average BP <100/65 mm Hg. ABPM provides valuable information supplementary to office BP in the evaluation of scenarios such as the following:

- Suspected white coat hypertension (BP measures higher in the office)

- Suspected masked hypertension (BP measures lower in the office)

- Suspected episodic hypertension

- Apparent treatment-resistant hypertension

- Hypotensive symptoms with antihypertensive medication treatment

- Autonomic dysfunction

- Possible nondipping (<10% nocturnal decrease in BP, which is associated with increased risk for cardiovascular events). Presence of nondipping can be evaluated in patients at high risk for future cardiovascular events, such as in those with CKD, diabetes with microvascular complications, and history of previous myocardial infarction or stroke.

ABPM is clinically helpful in these scenarios and is a better prognosticator of both end-organ damage (such as left ventricular hypertrophy) and hard outcomes (such as cardiovascular death) compared with office or home BP measurements.

Home Blood Pressure Monitoring

Home BP monitoring refers to the measurement of BP at home by the patient, often by using an electronic BP device. Observational data show that home systolic and diastolic BP readings are more predictive of cardiovascular death than office readings, but less predictive than ABPM average readings. The advantage of home BP monitoring over ABPM is that home monitoring is more readily available, less expensive, and less time consuming in that the patient does not have to come to the office to have the device put on and then return the device after the 24-hour period of monitoring. In addition, home BP monitoring encourages patients to play an active role

in their own BP management and be more aware of the need for adherence to lifestyle modifications and antihypertensive medications. However, unlike ABPM, which provides information regarding continuous BP measurements during awake and asleep periods as well as during ambulatory and exertion periods, home BP measurements can only be taken during awake hours and when the patient is at rest. Home BP monitoring can provide additional information ancillary to office BP in the following ways:

- Assess response to lifestyle modifications or treatment with antihypertensive medications

- Improve patient adherence

- Evaluate for white coat and masked hypertension

Several issues should be considered to ensure accuracy of home BP measurements. First, upper arm cuffs are preferred over newer devices that measure BP more distally, such as at the wrist, given that systolic BP is higher and diastolic lower in distal arteries, and finger measurements are generally not accurate. Second, education should be given regarding the proper use of the device, frequency and timing of measurements, and avoidance of self-adjustment of antihypertensive medications based on home BP. The patient should be instructed to sit in a comfortable position with legs uncrossed and back supported, and to place the left arm raised and supported to the level of the heart. The cuff should be wrapped snuggly around the upper part of the bare arm, and BP should be measured after at least 5 minutes of rest. BP readings and times of measurement should be recorded and a running list brought to office visits for evaluation and to assist with hypertension management. The device should be brought to the office initially and periodically to validate accuracy of readings. Those with home self-measured BP averaging ≥130/80 mm Hg are considered hypertensive.

KEY POINTS

- Repeat blood pressure measurements using proper technique are necessary before making clinical decisions regarding management.

- Ambulatory blood pressure monitoring can be used to evaluate for white coat, masked, episodic, or treatment-resistant hypertension; hypotensive symptoms with antihypertensive medication treatment; autonomic dysfunction; and dipping status.

- Home blood pressure monitoring can be used to assess response to lifestyle modifications or treatment, improve patient adherence, and evaluate for white coat or masked hypertension.

Definitions

The 2017 high BP guideline from the American College of Cardiology (ACC), the American Heart Association (AHA), and nine other organizations provides new BP definitions and recommendations (http://hyper.ahajournals.org/). This guideline is an update to the Seventh Report of the Joint National Committee on Prevention, Detection, Evaluation, and Treatment of High Blood Pressure (JNC 7). The new definitions of BP are listed in **Table 11**.

> **KEY POINT**
>
> - According to the 2017 high blood pressure guideline from the American College of Cardiology, the American Heart Association, and nine other organizations, hypertension is defined as blood pressure ≥130/80 mm Hg.

Screening and Diagnosis

The U.S. Preventive Services Task Force (USPSTF) recommends screening for hypertension in adults ≥18 years of age to identify those at increased risk for cardiovascular disease from hypertension and to begin early interventions to decrease this risk. Adults aged 18 to 39 years with a BP <130/85 mm Hg and without cardiovascular risk factors should be rescreened every 3 to 5 years. Those aged ≥40 years and persons at increased risk for hypertension (for example, those who have BP that is 130-139/85-89 mm Hg, are overweight, or are black) should be screened annually.

A diagnosis of hypertension (BP ≥130/80 mm Hg) should be based on an average of two or more elevated systolic and/or diastolic BP measurements obtained on two or more occasions. Out-of-office automated monitoring or self-monitoring of BP measurements is recommended to confirm hypertension diagnosis. Compared with a single measurement, multiple measurements over time have better positive predictive values for hypertension diagnosis. More recent evidence regarding the prevalence of white coat and masked hypertension suggests that confirmation of elevated BP with 24-hour ABPM (≥125/75 mm Hg) or self-measured home BP monitoring (≥130/80 mm Hg) may be prudent for hypertension diagnosis.

> **KEY POINTS**
>
> - The U.S. Preventive Services Task Force recommends screening for hypertension in adults ≥18 years of age to identify those at increased risk for cardiovascular disease from hypertension and to begin early interventions to decrease this risk.
> - A diagnosis of hypertension should be based on an average of two or more elevated systolic and/or diastolic blood pressure measurements obtained on two or more occasions; obtaining measurements outside of the clinical setting for diagnostic confirmation is recommended before starting treatment.

HVC

Evaluation of the Patient with Newly Diagnosed Hypertension

Initial evaluation of a patient with newly diagnosed hypertension includes a complete history, physical examination, and screening laboratory studies to address the following:

- Establish whether a familial pattern of hypertension is present.
- Rule out secondary, potentially reversible, causes.
- Identify and eliminate modifiable factors that can elevate BP.
- Assess for the presence of other cardiovascular risk factors.
- Assess for end-organ damage.
- Identify potential barriers to lifestyle modification for lowering BP.

History

A complete history should be elicited to identify a personal history of the following: stroke or myocardial infarction, thyroid disease, kidney disease, obstructive sleep apnea, and additional cardiovascular risk factors. Family history should be explored for a genetic pattern of hypertension and premature history of cardiovascular disease.

A complete review of the systems is warranted, especially to elicit the presence of episodic palpitations, headaches, or

TABLE 11.	Definitions of Blood Pressure for Adults		
Definitions[a]	Office-Based Readings (mm Hg)[a]	24-Hour Ambulatory Readings (mm Hg)[b]	Self-Recorded Readings (mm Hg)[b]
Normal	<120/80	<115/75	<120/80
Elevated Blood Pressure	120-129/<80	—	—
Hypertension, Stage 1	130-139/80-89	≥125/75	≥130/80
Hypertension, Stage 2	≥140/90	≥130/80	≥135/85
White Coat Hypertension	≥130/80	<125/75	<130/80
Masked Hypertension	<130/80	≥125/75	≥130/80

[a]Based on Whelton PK, Carey RM, Aronow WS, Casey DE Jr, Collins KJ, Dennison Himmelfarb C, et al. 2017 ACC/AHA/AAPA/ABC/ACPM/AGS/APhA/ASH/ASPC/NMA/PCNA guideline for the prevention, detection, evaluation, and management of high blood pressure in adults: a report of the American College of Cardiology/American Heart Association Task Force on Clinical Practice Guidelines. J Am Coll Cardiol. 2018;71:e127-e248. [PMID: 29146535]

[b]The corresponding thresholds of 24-hour ambulatory and self-recorded home blood pressure readings are provided as a guide and should be interpreted with caution, given that they are based on European, Australian, and Asian populations, with few available data in U.S. populations.

sweating (which may suggest pheochromocytoma); visual changes (to assess end-organ damage); or gross hematuria (which may suggest underlying kidney glomerular disease). Behavioral and psychosocial contributors to hypertension should also be explored, including a sedentary routine, illicit drug use, excessive alcohol, tobacco smoking, high dietary sodium intake, and emotional stress.

A complete list of prescription and nonprescription medications, including complementary and alternative medications (herbals) and illicit drugs, is of utmost importance because many medications can result in reversible BP elevations (**Table 12**). If the patient is taking any drugs that may result in BP elevation, the drug should be discontinued and BP remeasured in 1 month.

Physical Examination

Physical examination should focus on the following:

- Measure BP accurately in both arms.
- Measure body weight and calculate BMI to ascertain cardiovascular risk.
- Recognize target organ damage: eye examination (retinopathy or papilledema); volume status (elevated jugular venous pressure or lower extremity edema suggesting heart failure or CKD); peripheral vascular examination (unequal pulses in all extremities, carotid or abdominal bruits suggesting vascular disease); cardiac examination (laterally displaced point of maximal impulse or S_4 gallop suggestive of left ventricular hypertrophy).
- Identify abnormalities that suggest potential secondary causes (tachycardia for pheochromocytoma; abdominal bruit for renovascular hypertension; enlarged thyroid gland suggestive of thyroid disease; violaceous abdominal striae or "buffalo hump" fat pad suggesting Cushing syndrome).

Testing

Initial testing is performed to identify common secondary causes, assess for other cardiovascular risk factors, and detect end-organ damage.

- Baseline electrocardiography (ECG) to assess for left ventricular hypertrophy (end-organ damage) or previous silent myocardial infarction.
- Blood laboratory studies: complete blood count, serum creatinine, estimated glomerular filtration rate (GFR), serum sodium, potassium, calcium, bicarbonate, fasting glucose, lipid panel, thyroid-stimulating hormone.
- Urinalysis with microscopic examination; in addition, urine albumin-creatinine ratio in patients with diabetes mellitus and in those with a high clinical suspicion for underlying CKD, such as a positive family history or presence of other end-organ damage (left ventricular hypertrophy on ECG).

TABLE 12. Drugs That Can Raise Blood Pressure	
Drug/Drug Class	**Potential Mechanisms**
Prescription Drugs	
Antidepressants: monoamine oxidase inhibitors; selective serotonin reuptake inhibitors; serotonin-norepinephrine reuptake inhibitors	Adrenergic stimulation
Calcineurin inhibitors: cyclosporine A; tacrolimus	Vasoconstriction; sympathetic excitation; sodium retention
Contraceptives: estrogens; progesterones	Sodium retention; increased renin-angiotensin system activity
Glucocorticoids	Sodium retention; weight gain
Erythropoietin-stimulating agents	Vasoconstriction
NSAIDs	Sodium retention
Sympathomimetics (methylphenidate)	Adrenergic stimulation
Vascular endothelial growth factor antagonists	Endothelial dysfunction; vasoconstriction
Nonprescription Drugs	
Anabolic steroids	Sodium retention
Caffeine	Adrenergic stimulation
Ethanol	Adrenergic stimulation
Glycyrrhizic acid (in some licorice, cough drops, chewing tobacco)	Mineralocorticoid activity; sodium retention
Herbal supplements: ephedra; 1,3-dimethylamine; synephrine; N-methylamine; *Citrus aurantium*; *Caulophyllum thalictroides*	Sympathomimetic
Illicit drugs: amphetamines; cocaine; 3,4-methylenedioxymethamphetamine (ecstasy)	Sympathomimetic
NSAIDs	Sodium retention
Sympathomimetic nonprescription drugs: decongestants (phenylephrine, pseudoephedrine); appetite suppressants; vigilance enhancers	Sympathomimetic

- Echocardiography is not routinely recommended but may be helpful in suspected white coat hypertension in which presence of left ventricular hypertrophy would necessitate treatment with antihypertensive medication, even in the absence of elevated home BP. Echocardiography may also be used to detect hypertrophy in the presence of left bundle branch block on ECG or to assess baseline wall function in persons with a known history of ischemic heart disease.

More extensive diagnostic testing can be pursued if the history, physical examination, or initial testing raises suspicion for secondary causes (**Table 13**).

KEY POINTS

- Initial evaluation of patients with newly diagnosed hypertension includes a complete history, physical examination, and screening laboratory studies to assess for a familial pattern, secondary causes, other cardio-vascular risk factors, end-organ damage, and modifiable lifestyle factors.
- Baseline electrocardiography is appropriate for all patients with newly diagnosed hypertension.

Primary Hypertension
Pathogenesis

Ninety percent of patients with hypertension are identified as having primary (essential) hypertension, in which no secondary underlying etiology can be found. The pathogenesis is still not completely understood, but potential mechanisms include abnormal kidney sodium handling, increased activity of the renin-angiotensin system, and elevated sympathetic tone.

In general, hypertension is a complex polygenic disorder in which many genes or combinations may influence BP. Many genetic variants affect the distal tubular sodium transport and may result in excess sodium retention, leading to hypertension. Genetic polymorphisms involving oxidative stress, mediators of vascular smooth muscle tone, and vasoactive mechanisms have also been implicated. However, associated genetic variants have only small effects, such that the collective effect of all identified BP loci account for only about 3.5% of BP variability. Monogenic forms, in which single gene mutations explain the underlying pathophysiology of hypertension, are less common and include such diseases as glucocorticoid-remediable aldosteronism, Liddle disease, and Gordon syndrome.

TABLE 13. Secondary Causes of Hypertension	
Underlying Cause	**Diagnostic Testing**
Kidney disease	Serum creatinine; estimated glomerular filtration rate; urinalysis with microscopic examination; urine albumin-creatinine ratio; kidney ultrasonography
Renovascular disease	Renal duplex Doppler ultrasonography; CT or MR angiography; renal artery angiography
Obstructive sleep apnea	Polysomnography
Pheochromocytoma	Plasma fractionated metanephrines; 24-hour urine metanephrines and catecholamines
Hypo- or hyperthyroidism	Thyroid-stimulating hormone; free thyroxine
Primary hyperparathyroidism	Intact parathyroid hormone; serum calcium and phosphorus
Gordon syndrome (pseudohypoaldosteronism type II)	Clinical diagnosis; family history; aldosterone and renin levels; electrolytes
Aortic coarctation	Blood pressure measurements in arms and legs; CT or MR angiography; transthoracic echocardiography
Conditions Associated with Hypokalemia	**Diagnostic Testing**
High aldosterone conditions: Primary hyperaldosteronism: adrenal adenoma (rarely carcinoma or ectopic); bilateral adrenal hyperplasia Familial hyperaldosteronism type I (glucocorticoid-remediable aldosteronism; >50% normokalemic), type II, or type III Secondary hyperaldosteronism: renal artery stenosis; renin-secreting tumor	Serum sodium and potassium concentrations; plasma aldosterone concentration/plasma renin activity ratio; saline suppression test; CT imaging; adrenal vein sampling; genetic testing
Cushing syndrome	Dexamethasone suppression test; 24-hour urine cortisol excretion; salivary cortisol
Congenital adrenal hyperplasia	Clinical diagnosis
Apparent mineralocorticoid excess	Clinical diagnosis; aldosterone and renin levels; electrolytes
Liddle syndrome	Clinical diagnosis; family history; aldosterone and renin levels; electrolytes

Dietary factors have been implicated as contributors to hypertension development. Populations with low sodium intake have lower BP than those with high intake. Habitual high sodium intake along with low potassium intake seen in a modern diet is a critical factor contributing to the worldwide high prevalence of hypertension. This is especially true for those with salt sensitivity, common in black patients, older adults, and those with CKD or diabetes mellitus, in which an increase in sodium intake leads to a disproportionate increase in BP.

Positive correlations are also found between BP and physical inactivity, being overweight or obese, excess alcohol intake, hyperuricemia, and insulin resistance.

KEY POINT

- Habitual high sodium intake along with low potassium intake is a critical factor contributing to the worldwide high prevalence of hypertension.

Management
General Approach
Treatment recommendations for specific populations are elaborated upon in their respective sections. Importantly, consideration must be given to individual patient characteristics and circumstances to tailor management.

The 2017 ACC/AHA BP guideline provides treatment recommendations, including the following:

- Nonpharmacologic therapy is recommended for those with elevated BP (systolic BP between 120-129 mm Hg and diastolic BP <80 mm Hg) or stage 1 hypertension (systolic BP between 130-139 mm Hg or diastolic BP between 80-89 mm Hg) and a 10-year cardiovascular risk of <10%.

- Nonpharmacologic and drug treatment is recommended for those with BP ≥130/80 mm Hg and clinical cardiovascular disease or a 10-year cardiovascular risk ≥10% to a BP goal of <130/80 mm Hg.

- Nonpharmacologic and drug treatment is recommended for those with no cardiovascular disease and a 10-year cardiovascular risk of <10% for stage 2 hypertension (≥140/90 mm Hg).

- Adults with stage 2 hypertension and an average BP that is 20/10 mm Hg above their BP target should be treated with a combination of two first-line antihypertensive drugs of different classes.

- The target systolic BP goal for noninstitutionalized, ambulatory community-dwelling patients who are ≥65 years of age is <130 mm Hg.

- The target BP for patients with hypertension and diabetes mellitus is <130/80 mm Hg.

- The target BP for patients with hypertension and CKD is <130/80 mm Hg.

Lifestyle Modifications
Lifestyle modifications and cardiovascular risk factors should be addressed in all patients with elevated BP or hypertension, even if pharmacologic treatment is necessary. Several non-pharmacologic interventions have been shown to have efficacy in reducing BP (**Table 14**). The best evidence for BP-lowering effects in individuals with elevated BP or hypertension exists for weight loss, the Dietary Approaches to Stop Hypertension (DASH) diet, and dietary sodium reduction. Of the lifestyle interventions tested in clinical trials, weight reduction was most efficacious, followed by sodium reduction. Although difficult to achieve, a combination of lifestyle modifications (such as DASH combined with a low sodium diet alone or in combination with weight loss) had BP-lowering effects greater than or equal to those of single-drug therapy in hypertensive patients. Other nonpharmacologic interventions supported by evidence include potassium supplementation (preferably in dietary modification), increased physical activity, and moderation in alcohol consumption. Controlled trials of an increase in magnesium or calcium intake revealed less robust BP-lowering effects. Regardless of BP effects, tobacco cessation should be encouraged given that smoking is a significant risk factor for cardiovascular disease.

Based on the level of evidence for behavioral therapies, transcendental meditation, yoga, and biofeedback had modest, mixed, or no consistent BP-lowering effects. More data

TABLE 14.	Efficacy of Lifestyle Modifications for Reducing Blood Pressure	
Approach	**Recommendation**	**Effect on Systolic Blood Pressure**
Reduce weight	BMI <25	5 to 10 mm Hg reduction per 10-kg (22-lb) weight loss
Reduce dietary sodium	1500 to 2400 mg/d	2 to 8 mm Hg reduction
Consume DASH (Dietary Approaches to Stop Hypertension) diet	Fruits; vegetables; low-fat dairy; whole grains; legumes; low saturated fat and sodium; high potassium, magnesium, and calcium	8 to 14 mm Hg reduction
Increase potassium intake	4700 mg/d	Variable reductions
Moderate alcohol consumption	Men: ≤2 drinks per day; women: ≤1 drink per day	2 to 4 mm Hg reduction
Exercise	30 min/d, most days (not consistently independent of weight loss)	4 to 9 mm Hg reduction
Alternative approaches	Device-guided breathing; yoga; meditation; biofeedback; acupuncture	Variable reductions

support efficacy of device-guided breathing than acupuncture among the noninvasive procedures and devices that were evaluated.

It is imperative to tailor lifestyle modifications to the individual patient while considering patient needs, patient support systems and resources, and readiness for behavioral change.

KEY POINTS

- The 2017 high blood pressure guideline from the American College of Cardiology, the American Heart Association, and nine other organizations recommends a blood pressure goal of <130/80 mm Hg in most adult patient populations.

- Lifestyle modifications (weight loss, diet, dietary sodium reduction) and cardiovascular risk factors should be addressed in all patients with elevated blood pressure and hypertension.

Pharmacologic Therapy

Clinical trials data suggest that antihypertensive medication therapy can be associated with up to a 40% reduction in stroke, 25% reduction in myocardial infarction, and 50% reduction in heart failure. In addition to lifestyle modification, treatment with antihypertensive medications should be initiated in patients with stage 1 hypertension and clinical cardiovascular disease or a 10-year cardiovascular risk ≥10% and in all patients with stage 2 hypertension.

Clinical trial evidence reveals that lowering BP is more important than the class of antihypertensive drug used to achieve control. Head-to-head trials of antihypertensive medications revealed comparable effects on cardiovascular outcomes, except that for preventing heart failure, initial therapy with a thiazide diuretic was more effective than a calcium channel blocker (CCB) or ACE inhibitor, and an ACE inhibitor was more effective than a CCB. The primary agents recommended are those that were shown to reduce clinical events and include a thiazide diuretic, CCB, ACE inhibitor, or angiotensin receptor blocker (ARB) for hypertension in the general nonblack population, including those with diabetes. In black patients, initial antihypertensive therapy should include a thiazide diuretic or a CCB (see Specific Populations, Black Patients).

There are not enough good quality head-to-head randomized trials comparing other antihypertensive classes (β-blockers, central- or peripheral-acting α-blockers, vasodilators, aldosterone receptor antagonists, or loop diuretics) to the four drug classes mentioned. Therefore, these drug classes are not recommended as first-line therapy but can be used in specific populations (β-blockers for post–myocardial infarction or heart failure; aldosterone receptor blockers for heart failure; loop diuretics for advanced CKD) or as add-on therapy for resistant hypertension.

See **Table 15** for more information on frequently used antihypertensive medications.

Diuretics

Initial antihypertensive treatment may include thiazide diuretics, which act by inhibiting the sodium-chloride-cotransporter in the distal renal tubule. Although hydrochlorothiazide is the most commonly used thiazide diuretic, chlorthalidone is

TABLE 15. Frequently Used Antihypertensive Medications	
Class/Agent	**Common Side Effects/Contraindications**
Thiazide diuretics (e.g., hydrochlorothiazide; chlorthalidone)	Hypokalemia; hyponatremia; hyperlipidemia; hyperuricemia; hyperglycemia. Avoid in gout unless patient is on urate-lowering therapy.
ACE inhibitors (e.g., captopril; lisinopril; enalapril; benazepril)	Hyperkalemia; cough. Avoid use with angiotensin receptor blockers or direct renin inhibitors. Avoid in pregnancy.
Angiotensin receptor blockers (e.g., candesartan; losartan; valsartan; irbesartan)	Hyperkalemia. Avoid use with ACE inhibitors or direct renin inhibitors. Avoid in pregnancy.
Calcium channel blockers	
Dihydropyridines (e.g., amlodipine; felodipine; nifedipine)	Pedal edema; headache; flushing.
Non-dihydropyridines (e.g., diltiazem; verapamil)	Constipation. Avoid in HFrEF. Avoid routine use with β-blockers (heart block, bradycardia). Drug interactions (*CYP3A4* major substrate and moderate inhibitor).
β-Blockers (e.g., atenolol; metoprolol tartrate; metoprolol succinate; labetalol)	Fatigue; bronchospasm; sexual dysfunction; hyperglycemia.
Potassium channel openers (vasodilators) (e.g., hydralazine; minoxidil)	Edema. Hydralazine: lupus-like syndrome. Minoxidil: hypertrichosis.
α-Blockers (e.g., prazosin)	Orthostatic hypotension; dizziness.
Central α-agonists (e.g., clonidine, oral or patch)	Fatigue; depression; rebound hypertension.
Potassium-sparing diuretics (e.g., spironolactone; amiloride; eplerenone)	Hyperkalemia. Avoid if GFR <45 mL/min/1.73 m². Spironolactone: gynecomastia.

GFR = glomerular filtration rate; HFrEF = heart failure with reduced ejection fraction.

preferred due to a prolonged half-life, which allows once-daily dosing, and evidence from trials demonstrating efficacy in reducing cardiovascular events. Loop diuretics are preferred in patients with symptomatic heart failure or CKD with an estimated GFR <30 mL/min/1.73 m² (see Kidney Disease, Management).

Suboptimal BP therapy in patients with difficult-to-control hypertension is frequently the result of not including a diuretic medication, which ensures that extracellular volume expansion is prevented or treated. This is particularly important in sodium-retentive, edematous conditions such as heart failure, liver cirrhosis, or CKD. Even in the absence of edematous conditions, persistent intravascular volume expansion without apparent edema can still contribute to hypertension that appears resistant to treatment. In addition, diuretic medication should be prescribed in adequate doses, with dosing frequency tailored appropriately to the diuretic half-life. For example, loop diuretics such as furosemide should be dosed at least twice to three times daily, and higher doses should be used in patients with low GFR.

Potassium-sparing diuretics, such as aldosterone receptor antagonists (spironolactone or eplerenone) or epithelial sodium channel blockers (amiloride), are weaker diuretics. These are often used in liver cirrhosis, heart failure, or resistant hypertension. Caution and close monitoring are advised when these medications are prescribed concomitantly with other drug classes that also raise the serum potassium, such as ACE inhibitors, ARBs, or direct renin inhibitors, and in patients with reduced GFR.

Calcium Channel Blockers

There are two classes of CCBs: dihydropyridines (amlodipine, felodipine, nifedipine) and nondihydropyridines (diltiazem, verapamil). No data support the use of one class over the other for hypertension management, although long-acting dihydropyridines are usually chosen. Nondihydropyridines have more pronounced cardiac effects such as diminished cardiac contractility (negative inotropy) and atrioventricular nodal blockade, and caution should be taken in prescribing these medications concomitantly with β-blockers or in patients with heart failure with severely reduced ejection fraction, sick sinus syndrome, or second- or third-degree atrioventricular block. Additionally, short-acting nifedipine was associated with mortality if used immediately after acute myocardial infarction due to profound hypotension and sympathetic activation. Finally, there may be an increased risk for myopathy if a CCB (especially nondihydropyridines) is used concomitantly with a high-dose statin.

Renin-Angiotensin System Agents

Renin-angiotensin system (RAS) agents are ACE inhibitors, ARBs, and direct renin inhibitors (such as aliskiren). Clinical trials reported similar efficacy of ACE inhibitors and ARBs on reducing BP, progression of albuminuria and CKD, and risk for cardiovascular events. Therefore, neither agent is preferred over the other.

Dry cough is a side effect of ACE inhibitors but is generally not reported with ARBs. Angioedema, a life-threatening condition, is a complication of both ACE inhibitors and renin inhibitors. Patients with a compelling indication for RAS inhibition who develop angioedema can be treated with an ARB with very careful monitoring, given a low but possible risk for occurrence. There are less outcomes data on the effects of aliskiren, although similar BP-lowering effect is expected. RAS agents should not be used in combination, and they are contraindicated in pregnancy.

Combination Therapy

Combination therapy with more than one drug class (separately or as a single-dose pill) may be necessary to control BP. The 2017 ACC/AHA BP guideline recommends combination therapy with two first-line antihypertensive drugs of different classes for adults with stage 2 hypertension and an average BP of 20/10 mm Hg above their BP target (typically ≥150/90 mm Hg). There are no definitive recommendations for best drug combinations, but some data suggest an ACE inhibitor/CCB combination may be more efficacious than an ACE inhibitor/thiazide diuretic combination. Using a thiazide diuretic/CCB combination is also an option.

Combined use of any RAS drug classes (ACE inhibitors, ARBs, and direct renin inhibitors) is not recommended; several clinical trials (ONTARGET, NEPHRON-D, ALTITUDE) have revealed more adverse events with these combinations (hyperkalemia, hypotension, AKI), without additional cardiovascular or renal benefits.

Assessment of Efficacy and Medication Titration

Adherence and response to treatment should be assessed 4 weeks after treatment initiation or sooner, based on the urgency for BP lowering. Further assessments are necessitated until target is achieved. Three strategies are possible for dose titration:

1. Maximize the first medication dose before adding a second.

2. Add a second medication before reaching the maximum dose of the first.

3. Start with two medication classes separately or as fixed-dose combinations.

There are no randomized controlled trials comparing these strategies; therefore, the strategy should be tailored to the individual patient, dose-related side effects, and adherence patterns. Generally, there is diminishing return in BP lowering if dose is titrated up from 50% to 100% of maximum. Also, it is unlikely that increasing the dose from 50% to 100% of maximum will result in an additional >5 mm Hg BP reduction; an additional agent may therefore need to be added. Finally, titration to maximum doses may more commonly result in side effects and reduce adherence.

- In addition to lifestyle modification, pharmacologic therapy should be initiated in patients with stage 1 hypertension and clinical cardiovascular disease or a 10-year cardiovascular risk ≥10% and in all patients with stage 2 hypertension.

- A thiazide diuretic, calcium channel blocker, ACE inhibitor, or angiotensin receptor blocker is recommended as initial therapy for hypertension in the general nonblack population, including those with diabetes mellitus.

- Combination therapy with two first-line antihypertensive drugs of different classes is recommended for adults with stage 2 hypertension and an average blood pressure (BP) that is 20/10 mm Hg above their BP target.

White Coat Hypertension

White coat hypertension refers to elevated BP measured in the office, but out-of-office BP averages that are not elevated (see Table 11). In adults with untreated systolic BP >130 mm Hg but <160 mm Hg or diastolic BP >80 mm Hg but <100 mm Hg, it is reasonable to screen for white coat hypertension using either daytime ABPM or home BP monitoring. Before white coat hypertension is diagnosed, the reliability of out-of-office measurements must be confirmed; for example, the patient's home BP monitor should be calibrated against the office sphygmomanometer or, preferably, BP should be measured by ABPM.

The prevalence of white coat hypertension is approximately 13% and as high as 35% in some hypertensive populations. The risk for conversion of white coat hypertension to sustained hypertension is estimated to be about 1% to 5% per year by ABPM or home BP monitoring. Incidence of conversion is higher with older age, obesity, or black race. Additionally, such patients may have a slightly higher cardiovascular risk compared with normotensive patients, but a lower risk than in those with masked or sustained hypertension. Optimal management of such patients is uncertain. A 3-month trial of lifestyle modifications is suggested in those with suspected white coat hypertension. If this does not result in a decrease of daytime ABPM or home BP to <130/80 mm Hg, then initiation of an antihypertensive drug should be considered. Screening echocardiography may also be considered to evaluate for left ventricular hypertrophy, the presence of which necessitates treatment with antihypertensives.

- Lifestyle modifications and careful monitoring should be considered for patients with white coat hypertension due to increased risk for future development of hypertension and slightly higher cardiovascular risk compared with normotensive patients.

Masked Hypertension

Masked hypertension is defined as BP that is normal in the office but elevated in the ambulatory setting (see Table 11). It is associated with an increased prevalence of target organ damage and risk of cardiovascular disease, stroke, and mortality compared with normotension. In adults with elevated office BP (120-129/<80 mm Hg) but not meeting the criteria for hypertension or with end-organ damage such as left ventricular hypertrophy, screening for masked hypertension with daytime ABPM or home BP is reasonable.

The prevalence of masked hypertension varies from 10% to 26% in population-based surveys and from 14% to 30% in normotensive clinic populations. A 3-month trial of lifestyle modifications should be considered in suspected cases of masked hypertension. Antihypertensive treatment should be initiated if daytime ABPM or home BP is still ≥130/80 mm Hg.

- Masked hypertension is associated with an increased risk for sustained hypertension and cardiovascular disease; after a 3-month trial of lifestyle modifications, antihypertensive medication should be initiated if daytime ambulatory or home blood pressure is still ≥130/80 mm Hg.

Resistant Hypertension

Resistant hypertension is defined as BP that remains above goal despite concurrent use of three antihypertensive agents of different classes, or BP at goal but requiring four or more medications. One of these medications must be a diuretic to make the diagnosis. A prevalence of 2% to 10% is reported in the general population, but can be as high as 40% in patients with CKD. Risk factors include older age, male sex, black race, diabetes, and higher BMI.

Before the diagnosis is made, a systematic approach to BP control should include ensuring accuracy of BP readings, optimizing medication selection and dosing, and addressing potential secondary and reversible causes of hypertension. The importance of out-of-office BP measurements (home or ABPM) as a part of evaluation to rule out white coat hypertension and to confirm resistance is increasingly recognized. Behaviors that could lead to high BP, including excessive sodium consumption, should be reviewed, and use of recreational drugs and prescription or nonprescription medications (such as complementary and alternative medications) that may exacerbate hypertension should be excluded. Adherence to antihypertensive medications, including correct frequency and dosage, should be confirmed, and potential reasons for nonadherence, such as medication side effects, should be addressed.

The cornerstone of management includes a low sodium diet and treatment with an appropriate diuretic with attention to dosage and dosing frequency (see Diuretics). Patients should be treated with a combination of medications from different classes: a RAS blocker (either an ACE inhibitor, an ARB, or a direct renin inhibitor), a calcium antagonist, a diuretic, and possibly a β-blocker. Recent trials support the efficacy of adding a low-dose aldosterone receptor antagonist (spironolactone or eplerenone) for treatment of resistant hypertension. If additional agents are needed for BP control or the patient is intolerant of the aforementioned agents, then vasodilators (hydralazine or minoxidil), α-blockers (doxazosin, prazosin) or central sympathetic agonists (clonidine) can be added.

> **KEY POINTS**
>
> - Resistant hypertension is defined as blood pressure (BP) that remains above goal despite the concurrent use of three antihypertensive agents of different classes, or BP at goal but requires four or more medications; one of the medications must be a diuretic to make the diagnosis.
> - Management of resistant hypertension includes accurate out-of-office blood pressure (BP) measurement, addressing behaviors that contribute to high BP, avoiding drugs that exacerbate hypertension, reducing dietary sodium, and ensuring appropriate diuretic dose and frequency.

Secondary Hypertension

In about 10% of adults with hypertension, a specific and remediable cause can be identified for hypertension. Diagnostic testing for secondary causes of hypertension can be pursued if a high clinical suspicion exists following history, physical examination, and initial laboratory testing (see Table 13). Factors that raise pretest probability for secondary hypertension include hypertension onset at <30 years of age, abrupt-onset or worsening BP if previously well controlled, drug resistance, clinical features indicating a secondary process, presence of target organ damage disproportionate to hypertension duration or severity, diastolic hypertension onset in those aged ≥65 years, and unprovoked or excessive hypokalemia.

Kidney Disease
Pathophysiology and Epidemiology

Hypertension develops in the setting of both AKI and CKD. Underlying parenchymal kidney disease is an important cause of hypertension, and up to 85% of patients with CKD have high BP. Hypertension prevalence increases with GFR decline. Additionally, chronic uncontrolled hypertension is a leading cause of CKD and of CKD progression to ESKD. BP elevation in glomerular disease is primarily attributed to fluid overload, as evidenced by suppression of the RAS and increased release of atrial natriuretic peptide. In acute vascular diseases affecting the kidney (vasculitis or scleroderma renal crisis), elevated BP is thought to result from ischemia-induced activation of the RAS. Endothelial vascular injury, increased sympathetic tone, and impaired nitric oxide synthesis are also implicated.

Clinical Manifestations

Underlying kidney disease is suggested by an elevated serum creatinine concentration and/or an abnormal urinalysis or albuminuria. Patients can present with other evidence of hypertension end-organ damage (such as left ventricular hypertrophy) and edema, but the absence of either does not exclude kidney disease as hypertension etiology.

Diagnosis

Initial evaluation of hypertension in all patients includes assessment of serum creatinine and estimated GFR, urinalysis with microscopic examination to exclude hematuria and/or proteinuria, and urine albumin-creatinine ratio in those with diabetes mellitus or family history of kidney disease. Abnormalities in any of these tests can signify underlying kidney disease. In those with a normal serum creatinine but a high suspicion for certain kidney diseases, such as a positive family history of autosomal dominant polycystic disease, kidney ultrasonography can be undertaken.

Management

The 2017 ACC/AHA BP guideline recommends a BP target of <130/80 mm Hg for patients with hypertension and CKD. An ACE inhibitor or an ARB is a preferred drug for treatment of hypertension for patients with stage G3 CKD or higher or for those with stage G1 or G2 CKD with albuminuria (albumin-creatinine ratio ≥300 mg/g).

Kidney function and serum potassium should be reassessed 2 to 3 weeks after medication initiation. An increase in serum creatinine of 25% to 30% is acceptable, but the dose may need to be lowered or medication discontinued if more severe decline in kidney function is observed; in such cases, bilateral renovascular disease should also be considered.

Given that sodium retention and volume overload are major contributory factors in the hypertension of CKD, dietary sodium restriction to <2000 mg/d and addition of a diuretic are both essential for control of BP, especially in advanced CKD. The following factors addressing appropriate dose and dosing interval for diuretics should be considered:

- Higher doses of diuretics are required in patients with CKD due to decreased GFR.
- Thiazide diuretics may be less effective if the estimated GFR is <30 mL/min/1.73 m^2; although there are no head-to-head trials, it seems preferable to use chlorthalidone instead of hydrochlorothiazide in patients with CKD due to a longer half-life.
- For an estimated GFR <20 to 30 mL/min/1.73 m^2, a loop diuretic can be used effectively, with more frequent dosing interval (for example, furosemide should be dosed at least two to three times daily).
- The combination of a thiazide and a loop diuretic can be used to augment diuresis, with careful monitoring.
- Volume overload refractory to medical management in those with stage G5 CKD (estimated GFR <15 mL/min/1.73 m^2) may necessitate dialysis.

Renovascular Hypertension

Pathophysiology and Epidemiology

Prevalence of renovascular hypertension is higher in white than black populations. Pathogenesis involves renal hypoperfusion as a result of renal artery stenosis, with subsequent release of renin and angiotensin resulting in systemic vasoconstriction, sodium retention, and hypertension. Disease can be unilateral or bilateral. Parenchymal kidney damage with loss of kidney function can occur.

There are two types of renovascular disease: (1) atherosclerotic renovascular disease, which usually occurs in patients >45 years of age, especially in those with diffuse atherosclerosis, but can also be isolated to the kidney; and (2) fibromuscular dysplasia, a nonatherosclerotic disorder that usually affects the mid and distal portions of the renal artery and usually occurs in young persons, particularly women.

Clinical Manifestations

Patients with atherosclerotic renovascular disease often have other manifestations of atherosclerosis, including the presence of coronary artery, cerebrovascular, or peripheral vascular disease. Bruits may be auscultated, especially a systolic-diastolic abdominal bruit that lateralizes to one side. Clinical suspicion should be high in patients who present with onset of severe hypertension after age 55 years, recurrent flash pulmonary edema, refractory heart failure, AKI after initiation of an ACE inhibitor/ARB, or AKI after control of BP to target. Asymmetry in kidney sizes of >1.5 cm on imaging or the presence of a unilateral small kidney ≤9 cm also increases likelihood of renovascular disease.

Abrupt onset of hypertension at an age <35 years suggests fibromuscular dysplasia.

Diagnosis

Routine testing for renovascular disease may not change management because recent data suggest that medical therapy may be as beneficial as invasive procedures, especially for those with atherosclerotic renovascular disease. However, in young patients with resistant hypertension and a high clinical suspicion for fibromuscular dysplasia, renal artery imaging may be considered. Plasma renin activity, captopril renal scintigraphy, and selective renal vein renin measurements are no longer recommended as diagnostic tests given the availability of more sensitive and specific imaging tests.

Renal duplex Doppler ultrasonography is a reasonable imaging modality if performed by experienced sonographers. MR or CT angiography have higher diagnostic utility but are potentially harmful in patients with severe CKD given the risk for contrast nephropathy and gadolinium-induced nephrogenic systemic fibrosis. A stenosis >75% in one or both renal arteries or >50% with post-stenotic dilatation suggests the diagnosis. Renal intra-arterial angiography is the gold standard and can be considered if other noninvasive tests are negative, clinical suspicion is high, and an invasive procedure is being considered. It is not recommended as a routine test due to adverse risks, such as contrast nephropathy and cholesterol emboli.

Management

Three large randomized trials (STAR, ASTRAL, and CORAL) failed to show that renal artery angioplasty confers additional benefit above optimal medical therapy in patients with atherosclerotic renovascular disease and stable kidney function. Medical therapy in those suspected of having atherosclerotic renovascular disease includes treatment of underlying cardiovascular risk factors (such as hypercholesterolemia) and an ACE inhibitor or ARB. Patients who may benefit from percutaneous angioplasty and stenting or surgical intervention include those who present with a short hypertension duration; are refractory to medical therapy; have severe hypertension or recurrent acute flash pulmonary edema; have AKI following treatment with an ACE inhibitor or ARB; or have progressive impaired kidney function thought to result from bilateral renovascular disease or unilateral stenosis affecting a solitary functioning kidney. Patients with advanced CKD or with proteinuria >1000 mg/24 h are less likely to benefit from revascularization.

In young persons with fibromuscular dysplasia, studies have suggested that angioplasty alone may improve BP and even cure hypertension.

Primary Hyperaldosteronism

A triad of resistant hypertension, metabolic alkalosis, and hypokalemia (including in patients treated with low-dose thiazide diuretics) should raise suspicion for primary aldosteronism (see Table 13). Primary hyperaldosteronism, in which aldosterone production cannot be suppressed with sodium loading, is the most common cause of secondary hypertension in middle-aged adults and an important cause of resistant hypertension. Screening for primary hyperaldosteronism is recommended if any of the following are present: resistant hypertension, hypokalemia (spontaneous or substantial, if diuretic induced), incidentally discovered adrenal mass, family history of early-onset hypertension, or stroke at age <40 years. Calculation of plasma aldosterone concentration (PAC)/plasma renin activity (PRA) ratio is used for screening, with a very high ratio of PAC/PRA suggestive of the diagnosis. Confirmatory diagnostic testing is needed with a saline suppression test.

PAC and PRA are usually suppressed in other disorders with hypokalemia and hypertension, including Cushing syndrome, syndrome of apparent mineralocorticoid excess, familial hyperaldosteronism type I (glucocorticoid-remediable aldosteronism), and Liddle syndrome (see Table 13). Renal artery stenosis and renin-secreting tumors generate high PRA and, therefore, lower PAC, with subsequent lowering of the PAC/PRA ratio, to usually <10. See MKSAP 18 Endocrinology and Metabolism for details.

Pheochromocytomas

Pheochromocytomas are rare catecholamine-secreting neoplasms of the adrenal medulla or sympathetic ganglia that occur in <0.2% of patients with hypertension. Presence of the

CONT.

following characteristics raises clinical suspicion and may prompt testing: resistant hypertension; hypertension onset that is new or at a young age; paroxysmal hypertension; episodic tachycardia, headaches, and sweating; history of familial syndromes; adrenal adenoma found incidentally on imaging with or without hypertension; or pressor response during invasive procedures or anesthesia. Diagnostic tests include plasma fractionated metanephrines and 24-hour urine metanephrines and catecholamines. Positive test results should be followed by imaging to locate the tumor. Definitive treatment is surgical resection. See MKSAP 18 Endocrinology and Metabolism for details. H

KEY POINTS

- The 2017 high blood pressure guideline from the American College of Cardiology, the American Heart Association, and nine other organizations recommends a target blood pressure of <130/80 mm Hg in patients with hypertension and chronic kidney disease.

- Treatment of hypertension in patients with chronic kidney disease includes an ACE inhibitor or angiotensin receptor blocker, dietary sodium restriction to <2000 mg/d, and addition of a diuretic as needed to control intravascular volume.

- Medical therapy for renovascular disease, including treatment of underlying cardiovascular risk factors and use of an ACE inhibitor or angiotensin receptor blocker, may be as beneficial as invasive procedures.

- Primary hyperaldosteronism is the most common cause of secondary hypertension in middle-aged adults and an important cause of resistant hypertension; the plasma aldosterone concentration/plasma renin activity ratio is used for screening.

Hypertensive Urgency

Hypertensive urgency is defined as severely elevated BP—often a systolic BP ≥180 mm Hg and/or diastolic BP ≥110 mm Hg—in a patient without obvious signs or symptoms of acute or impending change in target organ damage or dysfunction. Patients are often asymptomatic or present with a mild headache in an ambulatory setting. The most important aspect of initial management is a focused history and physical examination to exclude the presence of acute end-organ damage in the setting of severely elevated BP, which would raise concern for hypertensive emergency. Referral to an emergency department may be required for further diagnostic testing to rule out target organ damage. See MKSAP 18 Pulmonary and Critical Care Medicine for information on hypertensive emergencies.

Management is very challenging and includes the assessment of imminent risk of cardiovascular events from severe hypertension versus risk of adverse sequelae from rapid BP reduction. These may include AKI, myocardial infarction, or

stroke resulting from decreased perfusion to organs and limited time for autoregulation to maintain perfusion. Therefore, recommendations regarding the rapidity of BP lowering in this setting are controversial and not based on strong evidence. Generally, systolic BP may be lowered in patients with imminent risk of target organ damage but without a compelling condition (aortic dissection, preeclampsia, or pheochromocytoma crisis) by no more than 25% within the first hour, then to <160/100 mm Hg within the next 2 to 6 hours, then cautiously to target during the following 24 to 48 hours. Choice of antihypertensive medication should be tailored to the specific patient. If there is concern for imminent end-organ damage, faster-acting antihypertensive agents, such as oral clonidine, can be given to lower BP. Several hours of observation in the ambulatory setting may be required to ensure that the patient remains asymptomatic and that BP is decreasing before discharge. In patients in whom hypertensive urgency developed because of medication nonadherence, antihypertensive medications can be resumed slowly and in a stepwise fashion, with care not to drop the BP precipitously. Close follow-up of such patients is necessary, and further management can include home monitoring of BP.

KEY POINTS

- Hypertensive urgency is defined as severely elevated blood pressure (BP)—often a systolic BP ≥180 mm Hg and/or diastolic BP ≥110 mm Hg—in a patient without obvious signs or symptoms of acute end-organ damage.

- Management of hypertensive urgency in patients with imminent risk of target organ damage but without a compelling condition includes lowering the systolic blood pressure by no more than 25% within the first hour, then to <160/100 mm Hg within the next 2 to 6 hours, then cautiously to target during the following 24 to 48 hours.

Specific Populations
Women

Hypertension prevalence is lower in women <50 years of age compared with men, but prevalence increases with older age and eventually becomes similar in both sexes. Women, particularly if premenopausal, are at a lower risk than men for hypertension complications, such as coronary artery disease, stroke, and left ventricular hypertrophy. Clinical trials suggest that women derive similar relative benefits from antihypertensive treatment as men, and recommendations for BP targets and agents are the same.

Women of childbearing age who anticipate pregnancy should not be prescribed RAS agents (ACE inhibitors, ARBs, or direct renin inhibitors) because of the risk for urogenital developmental abnormalities; these agents are contraindicated in pregnant women. Instead, transition to methyldopa, nifedipine, and/or labetalol during pregnancy is a reasonable choice. See The Kidney in Pregnancy for more information.

Oral contraceptives may be associated with modest increases in BP, which usually resolve with discontinuation; women prescribed these medications should be monitored. Hormone replacement therapy consists of much lower estrogen doses and is not associated with elevated BP.

Patients with Diabetes Mellitus

The 2017 ACC/AHA BP guideline recommends a BP goal of <130/80 mm Hg for patients with diabetes. First-line therapy in nonblack patients with diabetes includes a thiazide diuretic, CCB, ACE inhibitor, or ARB; ACE inhibitors or ARBs are reasonable choices in the presence of albuminuria. In black patients with diabetes, a thiazide diuretic or CCB is recommended as initial therapy.

The American Diabetes Association (ADA) recommends that most patients with diabetes and hypertension should be treated to a BP goal of 140/90 mm Hg; lower systolic and diastolic BP targets, such as 130/80 mm Hg, may be appropriate for individuals at high risk of cardiovascular disease if they can be achieved without undue treatment burden. The ADA also recommends an ACE inhibitor or ARB, at the maximum tolerated dose indicated for BP treatment, as first-line treatment for hypertension in patients with diabetes and albuminuria.

Black Patients

Although hypertension is more prevalent in black patients and correlates with a higher risk for cardiovascular and kidney outcomes, current recommendations for target BP are similar in black patients to those in other racial groups. The difference in management is with regard to the agent used. In general, ACE inhibitors are less efficacious in lowering BP in black patients than are CCBs. Additionally, a landmark trial (ALLHAT) revealed that in black patients, a thiazide diuretic was more effective in improving cardiovascular outcomes compared with an ACE inhibitor, and there was a higher risk of stroke with use of an ACE inhibitor as initial therapy compared with a CCB. Therefore, in the absence of CKD or heart failure, initial antihypertensive treatment should include a thiazide diuretic or CCB in black patients. If CKD is present, initial or add-on therapy should include an ACE inhibitor or ARB, especially in those with proteinuria, as illustrated by the AASK study. Choice of antihypertensive medication in patients with heart failure should be in accordance with appropriate guidelines.

Older Patients

Prevalence of hypertension increases with age and is as high as 60% to 80% in patients >65 years of age. A wide pulse pressure and isolated systolic hypertension (>160 mm Hg with diastolic <90 mm Hg) are common.

According to the 2017 ACC/AHA BP guideline, the target systolic BP goal for noninstitutionalized, ambulatory community-dwelling patients who are ≥65 years of age is <130 mm Hg. In those with a high burden of comorbidity and limited life expectancy, clinical judgement, patient preference, and an assessment of risk-benefit ratio should be considered for decisions about the intensity of BP control and antihypertensive medication choice.

On the other hand, a 2017 guideline from the American College of Physicians and American Academy of Family Physicians (http://annals.org/aim/article/2598413/pharmacologic-treatment-hypertension-adultsaged-60-years-older-higher-versus) addressed the treatment of hypertension in patients ≥60 years of age, including three recommendations:

- Initiate treatment in patients ≥60 years of age with a systolic BP persistently ≥150 mm Hg to achieve a target systolic BP <150 mm Hg to reduce the risk for mortality, stroke, and cardiac events.

- Consider initiating or intensifying pharmacologic treatment in patients ≥60 years of age with a history of stroke or transient ischemic attack to achieve a target systolic BP <140 mm Hg to reduce the risk for recurrent stroke.

- Consider initiating or intensifying pharmacologic treatment in some patients ≥60 years of age at high cardiovascular risk, based on individualized assessment, to achieve a target systolic BP <140 mm Hg to reduce the risk for stroke or cardiac events.

Regarding antihypertensive class, nonblack older patients without CKD can be treated with a thiazide diuretic, CCB, or ACE inhibitor or ARB, similar to patients <65 years of age. Care must be taken in initiating antihypertensive medications at lower doses with close monitoring of BP and attention to adverse events, given that older patients are more prone to drug-drug interactions, hyponatremia from thiazide diuretics, and orthostatic hypotension when treated with diuretics, vasodilators, α-blockers, and central-acting drugs (such as clonidine).

KEY POINTS

- Women of childbearing age who anticipate pregnancy should not be prescribed renin-angiotensin system agents because of the risk for urogenital developmental abnormalities; these agents are contraindicated in pregnant women.

- In the absence of chronic kidney disease, first-line therapy of hypertension in nonblack patients with diabetes is similar to treatment of patients without diabetes: a thiazide diuretic, calcium channel blocker, ACE inhibitor, or angiotensin receptor blocker.

- Initial antihypertensive treatment for black patients with or without diabetes mellitus includes a thiazide diuretic or calcium channel blocker.

- The 2017 ACC/AHA BP guideline recommends a target systolic BP goal of <130 mm Hg for noninstitutionalized, ambulatory community-dwelling patients who are ≥65 years, whereas the American College of Physicians and American Academy of Family Physicians recommend a target systolic BP goal of <150 mm Hg in patients ≥60 years of age.

Chronic Tubulointerstitial Nephritis

Epidemiology and Pathophysiology

Tubulointerstitial nephritis (TIN) is characterized by damage to the renal tubules and interstitium, resulting in tubulointerstitial edema and progressive fibrosis and tubular atrophy. TIN can be acute or chronic. Acute interstitial nephritis is commonly due to allergic drug reactions or infection and can cause acute kidney injury within days to weeks. It is characterized by inflammation of the renal interstitium and tubules, which is generally reversible after the offending drug is removed or the underlying disease is treated (see Acute Kidney Injury). Chronic TIN (CTIN) causes a slow decline in kidney function over months and years and is characterized by interstitial scarring, fibrosis, and tubular atrophy. Acute interstitial nephritis can progress to CTIN over time. CTIN can also develop in the setting of chronic primary glomerular disease, vascular diseases, and ischemia secondary to atherosclerosis and hypertension. Causes of CTIN are listed in **Table 16**.

Diagnosis and Evaluation

CTIN is often asymptomatic until severe loss of kidney function occurs. Presenting symptoms include polyuria and nocturia due to renal concentrating defects.

A careful history with a review of medications should be performed to determine the cause of CTIN (see Table 16). A thorough physical examination may provide clues to the diagnosis and may reveal hypertension, but often no characteristic findings exist. Urinalysis may be normal or demonstrate pyuria and/or proteinuria <1500 mg/24 h. See **Table 17** for other laboratory manifestations of CTIN. Kidney ultrasound may show small kidneys. Kidney biopsy may be necessary to establish a definitive diagnosis.

KEY POINTS

- Chronic tubulointerstitial nephritis is characterized by interstitial scarring, fibrosis, and tubular atrophy and results in a slow decline in kidney function over months and years.
- Features of chronic tubulointerstitial nephritis include polyuria and nocturia due to renal concentrating defects; hypertension; and a urinalysis that is normal or demonstrates pyuria and/or proteinuria <1500 mg/24 h.

Causes

See Table 16 for a list of causes of CTIN.

Immunologic Diseases

Sjögren Syndrome

Kidney involvement in Sjögren syndrome may include interstitial nephritis, distal (type 1) renal tubular acidosis (RTA), and glomerulonephritis. Nephrolithiasis, nephrocalcinosis, and progressive kidney disease may also occur.

Sarcoidosis

Kidney involvement in sarcoidosis is common and can manifest as nephrocalcinosis from hypercalcemia and hypercalciuria, obstructive uropathy, and TIN due to granulomatous interstitial nephritis. Urine findings of TIN include impaired urine concentration, mild proteinuria, and sterile pyuria. Kidney recovery is usually incomplete.

Systemic Lupus Erythematosus

The TIN that may occur in systemic lupus erythematosus is often associated with concurrent glomerular disease but can also be the only manifestation of lupus nephritis. The severity of TIN is a useful predictor of hypertension, progressive kidney disease, and kidney failure.

IgG4-Related Disease

IgG4-related disease can be associated with a TIN with an abundant IgG4-positive plasma cell interstitial infiltration. Other laboratory findings include decreased serum complement levels and peripheral eosinophilia.

Infections

Infections associated with acute interstitial nephritis and CTIN include bacterial (such as brucellosis and tuberculosis), viral, fungal, and parasitic infections.

In immunosuppressed patients with transplanted organs, BK polyoma virus can cause interstitial nephritis. Diagnosis of BK virus nephropathy can be difficult to distinguish from acute cellular rejection. The most important treatment intervention is to decrease immunosuppressive therapy.

Chronic pyelonephritis resulting from chronic infections or vesicoureteral reflux is a common cause of CTIN. Patients can present with fever, chills, dysuria, flank or back pain, and hypertension. Kidney manifestations include distal tubular dysfunction, pyuria, and leukocyte casts. Persistent chronic pyelonephritis can progress to localized xanthogranulomatous pyelonephritis, which is characterized by a destructive mass that invades the renal parenchyma and is associated with urinary tract obstruction, infection, nephrolithiasis, diabetes mellitus, and/or immunosuppression.

Malignancy

Lymphoproliferative disorders such as lymphoma and leukemia can infiltrate the kidney, causing TIN. Presenting features include proteinuria, sterile pyuria, and enlarged kidneys. Plasma cell dyscrasias such as multiple myeloma can cause TIN in the form of myeloma cast nephropathy, Fanconi syndrome, or interstitial light chain deposition.

TABLE 16. Causes of Chronic Tubulointerstitial Nephritis
Immunologic Diseases
Anti-tubular basement membrane antibody-mediated tubulointerstitial nephritis
Sarcoidosis
Sjögren syndrome
Systemic lupus erythematosus
IgG4-related disease
Tubulointerstitial nephritis with uveitis[a]
Toxic Causes
Balkan endemic nephropathy/aristolochic acid nephropathy (urologic evaluation is indicated due to increased risk of transitional cell carcinoma)
Heavy metal nephropathy (e.g., lead, cadmium, mercury, arsenic, bismuth, chromium, copper, gold, iron, uranium)
Hereditary Tubulointerstitial Nephritis
Medullary cystic kidney disease
Mitochondrial disorders
Nephronophthisis
Infection-Related Causes
Polyoma BK virus (most commonly post–kidney transplantation)
Brucellosis
Cytomegalovirus
Epstein-Barr virus
Hantavirus
HIV
Hepatitis B virus
Fungal infections
Legionella species
Mycobacterium tuberculosis
Toxoplasmosis
Chronic pyelonephritis
Malignancy-Related Causes
Leukemia
Lymphoma
Malignancy-associated monoclonal gammopathies (e.g., multiple myeloma, plasmacytoma)
Medication-Induced Causes
Analgesic nephropathy (e.g., acetaminophen, aspirin, caffeine, or NSAID combinations)
Sodium phosphate (phosphate nephropathy)
Orlistat; high doses of vitamin C (oxalate nephropathy)
Calcineurin inhibitors (cyclosporine, tacrolimus)
Lithium
Cyclooxygenase-2 inhibitors (celecoxib)
NSAIDs
Proton pump inhibitors (esomeprazole, lansoprazole, omeprazole, pantoprazole, rabeprazole)
H$_2$ blockers (famotidine, ranitidine, nizatidine, cimetidine)
Allopurinol
HIV medications (indinavir, abacavir, tenofovir)

(Continued on the next page)

TABLE 16. Causes of Chronic Tubulointerstitial Nephritis *(Continued)*

Medication-Induced Causes

Diuretics (triamterene, furosemide, thiazides)

Anticonvulsants (e.g., phenytoin, carbamazepine, phenobarbital, valproate)

5-Aminosalicylates (mesalamine)

Antibiotics (cephalosporins, fluoroquinolones, penicillins, rifampin, sulfonamides)

Antineoplastics (cisplatin, carboplatin, cyclophosphamide, ifosfamide, nitrosoureas)

Prolonged exposure to any medication that can cause acute interstitial nephritis

Secondary Tubulointerstitial Injury Due to Glomerular and Vascular Disorders

Hypertensive nephrosclerosis

Urinary Tract Obstruction

Obstructive uropathy

Nephrolithiasis

Reflux disease

[a]Tubulointerstitial nephritis with uveitis is an uncommon immune-mediated syndrome with the combination of tubulointerstitial nephritis and uveitis associated with autoimmune disorders, including hypoparathyroidism, thyroid disease, IgG4-related disease, and rheumatoid arthritis.

TABLE 17. Laboratory Manifestations of Chronic Tubulointerstitial Nephritis

Abnormality[a]	Causes
Decline in GFR	Obstruction of tubules; damage to microvasculature; interstitial fibrosis and sclerosis of glomeruli
Proximal tubular damage (Fanconi syndrome)	Incomplete absorption and kidney wasting of glucose, phosphate, uric acid, bicarbonate, and amino acids
Normal anion gap metabolic acidosis	Proximal and distal RTA; decreased ammonia production
Polyuria and isosthenuria	Decreased concentrating and diluting ability
Proteinuria	Decreased tubular protein reabsorption (usually <1500 mg/24 h)
Hyperkalemia	Defect in potassium secretion (type 4 [hyperkalemic] distal RTA)
Hypokalemia	Defect in potassium reabsorption (type 1 [hypokalemic] distal RTA)
Anemia	Injury to erythropoietin-producing cells in the kidney

GFR = glomerular filtration rate; RTA = renal tubular acidosis.

[a]The degree of these abnormalities depends on the extent and location of injury.

Medications
Analgesics
Analgesic nephropathy is a chronic progressive TIN thought to be due to the long-term use of combinations of phenacetin (banned since 1983) with aspirin, caffeine, acetaminophen, or NSAIDs. It can also occur with the individual drugs. When severe, analgesic nephropathy is associated with renal papillary necrosis, which manifests as gross hematuria, flank pain, and, occasionally, obstruction and infection.

Patients with analgesic nephropathy are typically women over the age of 45 years with a history of heavy analgesic use, low back pain or chronic musculoskeletal pain, and kidney disease with low-grade proteinuria, sterile pyuria, and anemia. CT may demonstrate microcalcifications at the papillary tips.

Calcineurin Inhibitors
The calcineurin inhibitors cyclosporine and tacrolimus can cause CTIN, in part via renal vasoconstriction. In kidney transplant recipients, cyclosporine- or tacrolimus-induced CTIN can be similar to chronic rejection. Clinical features of calcineurin inhibitor–induced TIN include hypertension and metabolic abnormalities from tubular dysfunction, including hyperkalemia, hyperuricemia, metabolic acidosis from type 4 (hyperkalemic distal) RTA, hypophosphatemia, hypomagnesemia, and hypercalciuria. Thrombotic microangiopathy might further contribute to both acute and chronic nephrotoxicity. Risk factors for CTIN are duration of exposure and cumulative dose.

Lithium
Lithium causes several kidney disorders, including distal tubular dysfunction (type 1 hypokalemic distal RTA), nephrogenic diabetes insipidus, and CTIN. CTIN from long-term lithium use can occur in up to 15% to 20% of patients. Risk factors for CTIN include advanced age, duration of lithium exposure, the cumulative dose, and repeated episodes of lithium toxicity with high serum levels. Lithium nephropathy is characterized by cystic dilation of the distal tubules with formation of microcysts. Kidney dysfunction can progress to end-stage kidney disease even with discontinuation of lithium. Amiloride can attenuate lithium-induced nephrogenic diabetes insipidus by blocking distal tubular reabsorption of lithium.

Antineoplastic Agents
Multiple chemotherapy agents can cause TIN, including cisplatin, carboplatin, cyclophosphamide, ifosfamide, and nitrosoureas (particularly streptozotocin and semustine). Newer

biologic agents such as immune checkpoint inhibitors have also been implicated.

Lead

Lead can result in tubular dysfunction and CTIN. Occupational exposure to lead occurs from welding, smelting, the battery industry, and mining. Toxicity may also develop after months to years of exposure to lead in water, soil, paint, or food products. Lead nephropathy should be considered in any patient with a history of lead exposure, hypertension, gout, and progressive kidney disease. Gout is common because lead reduces urine excretion of uric acid. The clinical diagnosis of lead nephropathy is based on history of exposure, evidence of kidney dysfunction, and blood lead levels. Levels may be normal if high-level lead exposure has abated.

Hyperuricemia

Both acute and chronic uric acid nephropathy can cause TIN from deposition of uric acid in renal tubules and interstitium. Clinical findings include elevated serum creatinine, bland urine sediment, mild proteinuria, and elevated serum urate levels. Kidney biopsy is necessary for definitive diagnosis.

Obstruction

Obstructive uropathy from prostate disease, malignancy, nephrolithiasis, pelvic radiation, medications such as methysergide, and retroperitoneal fibrosis can cause CTIN and progressive kidney dysfunction. RTA, hyperkalemia, and mild proteinuria are common.

KEY POINT

- Causes of chronic tubulointerstitial nephritis include various immunologic diseases, infections, malignancy, medications, lead, hyperuricemia, and obstruction.

Management

Management of acute and chronic TIN involves treating the underlying cause: discontinuing offending agents, administering immunosuppressive therapy for immunologic or drug-related allergic causes, treating infection and malignancy, and relieving obstruction. Treatment of lead nephropathy consists of EDTA chelation therapy or oral succimer, which can slow the progression of chronic kidney disease. In patients with CTIN and progressive kidney disease, management includes control of blood pressure and treatment of proteinuria and metabolic abnormalities (see Chronic Kidney Disease).

KEY POINT

- Management of chronic tubulointerstitial nephritis involves treating the underlying cause: discontinuing offending agents, administering immunosuppressive therapy for immunologic or drug-related allergic causes, treating infection and malignancy, and relieving obstruction.

Glomerular Diseases

Epidemiology and Pathophysiology

Glomerular diseases are the third leading cause of end-stage kidney disease (ESKD) in the United States, accounting for approximately 10,000 incident cases of ESKD per year and trailing only diabetes mellitus and hypertension. The term *glomerular disease* encompasses a wide array of conditions with etiologies that span autoimmune disease, malignancy-associated conditions, sequelae of infection, genetic mutations, and medication toxicities. These diseases are classified as either primary (idiopathic), in which the glomerular injury is an intrinsic process generally limited to the kidney, or secondary, in which the glomerular lesion is the result of a systemic disease with kidney involvement as one of many possible manifestations.

The normal, noninflamed glomerulus forms a tight barrier, largely due to the slit diaphragms that connect podocyte (visceral epithelial cell) foot processes on the outside surface of the glomerular basement membrane (**Figure 11**). When healthy, this filtration barrier prevents passage of blood and protein into the urinary filtrate. Glomerular diseases involve injury of the glomerular filter with subsequent passage of protein (proteinuria) and, in the setting of glomerulonephritis, blood (hematuria) into the urine. These urinary abnormalities are the earliest manifestation of a glomerular lesion. If the injury responsible for the hematuria and proteinuria goes unchecked, the result is scarring of the glomerular filters (glomerulosclerosis) with subsequent decline in kidney function that manifests as elevated serum creatinine.

Most etiologies of glomerular disease are diagnosed via kidney biopsy. No formal guidelines exist for the indications to perform a kidney biopsy in any age group. The decision to pursue a kidney biopsy should be individualized for each patient, but, in general, a kidney biopsy appears justified for

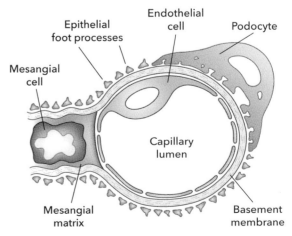

FIGURE 11. The podocyte, a visceral epithelial cell, sits on the outside surface of the glomerular basement membrane.

patients with two or more of the following four findings: hematuria, proteinuria >1000 mg/24 h, reduced kidney function (glomerular filtration rate <60 mL/min/1.73 m²), and/or positive serologies for systemic diseases with known potential for kidney involvement (for example, hepatitis B or C virus infection, systemic lupus erythematosus, and ANCA seropositivity).

Clinical Manifestations of Glomerular Disease

The two main categories of glomerular disease are the nephrotic and nephritic syndromes, each of which has a distinct clinical presentation.

The Nephrotic Syndrome

Clinical manifestations of the nephrotic syndrome stem from ongoing loss of protein, principally albumin, into the urine. This urinary loss of albumin causes hypoalbuminemia; in response, the liver increases its production of several proteins, including cholesterols, leading to hyperlipidemia. The resulting hallmark features of the nephrotic syndrome include the following:

- Urine protein excretion >3500 mg/24 h or a urine protein-creatinine ratio >3500 mg/g (nephrotic-range proteinuria)

- Hypoalbuminemia (usually <3.0 g/dL [30 g/L])

- Hypercholesterolemia

- Edema

Edema is typically most severe in the lower extremities. Many patients report periorbital edema upon awakening. Severe fluid retention can lead to pulmonary edema, pulmonary effusions, and anasarca. Despite avid salt and water retention, hypertension occurs only in a minority of patients.

Two explanations have been proposed for the edema seen in the nephrotic syndrome. The "underfill hypothesis" argues that low serum albumin concentrations lead to a reduction in intravascular oncotic pressure and a resultant shift of plasma from the capillary lumen to the interstitium. Further, the consequent intravascular depletion activates the renin-angiotensin system, which promotes salt and water retention throughout the nephron, exacerbating the edema. In contrast, the "overfill hypothesis" argues that sodium is primarily retained at the collecting duct, triggered by the abnormally filtered proteins themselves. Both hypotheses may be correct, and both provide a rationale for edema management in patients with the nephrotic syndrome. First, resolution of edema is only attainable long term by remission of proteinuria; lending support to the overfill hypothesis, edema will often subside when proteinuria has fallen but before albumin has returned to normal range. Second, diuretics are crucial to control the symptoms of edema, blocking the reabsorption of sodium (and water) at various points in the nephron.

The nephrotic syndrome is a hypercoagulable state due to urinary losses of protein. In addition to albuminuria, patients with the nephrotic syndrome lose in their urine a number of low-molecular-weight anticoagulants (for example, antithrombin III, protein S) and fibrinolytics (for example, plasminogen). Hepatic overproduction of proteins, as an intrinsic response to hypoalbuminemia, leads not only to hyperlipidemia but also to increased levels of procoagulants (for example, factor V, factor VIII, fibrinogen). As a result, patients with the nephrotic syndrome are at increased risk for lower extremity, pulmonary, and renal vein thrombosis. Clots are most often seen in patients with membranous glomerulopathy, but any patient with nephrotic-range proteinuria and significant hypoalbuminemia (usually <2.5 g/dL [25 g/L]) should be considered at risk.

Severe albuminuria should be treated with renin-angiotensin system blocking drugs to control blood pressure and reduce proteinuria. Hyperlipidemia should be treated with cholesterol-lowering medications. Edema should be managed with diuretics and dietary sodium restriction. This combination of renin-angiotensin system blocking drugs, cholesterol-lowering medications, and diuretics is generally considered conservative therapy for most forms of glomerular disease. A general strategy for edema management in a newly diagnosed patient with the nephrotic syndrome is to start with a loop diuretic, with a goal weight loss of 1 to 2 kg (2.2-4.4 lb) per week. In severe cases of edema when loop diuretics have been maximally uptitrated and weight loss/edema control is insufficient, it is often necessary to add a second diuretic (a thiazide diuretic and/or potassium-sparing diuretic) that works distal to the loop of Henle. In patients taking high doses of loop diuretics, increased delivery of salt and water to the distal portions of the nephron can lead to hypertrophy of these segments and overabsorption of sodium, undermining the effects of the loop diuretic.

The Nephritic Syndrome

The nephritic syndrome, also termed glomerulonephritis, can present as a number of clinical variants. Common features are hematuria (microscopic or macroscopic) and proteinuria, with the more severe variants typically including hypertension, edema, and kidney dysfunction (elevated serum creatinine). The glomerular hematuria seen in the nephritic syndrome can be distinguished from other causes of urinary tract bleeding by the presence of either dysmorphic erythrocytes (resulting from passage through a damaged glomerular basement membrane) or erythrocyte casts on urine microscopy (see Clinical Evaluation of Kidney Function).

The mildest forms of the nephritic syndrome are asymptomatic, microscopic hematuria with or without proteinuria, often discovered on routine laboratory assessment. Recurrent gross hematuria, in which macroscopic hematuria occurs several days after an upper respiratory infection or physical exertion, is a classic presentation of IgA nephropathy, particularly in younger patients. This nephritic presentation also usually follows a benign clinical course without associated chronic kidney disease.

On the other hand, the term *acute glomerulonephritis* is used to denote the more classical nephritic syndrome presentation, with variable degrees of kidney dysfunction, hypertension, edema, proteinuria, and hematuria. The most severe form of the nephritic syndrome is termed *rapidly progressive glomerulonephritis*, in which patients experience a rapid decline of kidney function over days or weeks that will progress to ESKD if untreated.

Conditions Associated With the Nephrotic Syndrome

Focal Segmental Glomerulosclerosis

Epidemiology and Pathophysiology

Focal segmental glomerulosclerosis (FSGS) is the most common form of the nephrotic syndrome in black patients and, in certain parts of the world, has replaced membranous glomerulopathy as the leading cause of the nephrotic syndrome in white patients. The prevalence of FSGS in the United States is more than 20,000 patients, with a yearly incidence of approximately 5000 newly diagnosed cases per year. In the United States, FSGS currently accounts for up to 40% of primary nephrotic syndromes in adults. Worldwide, the incidence of FSGS has been estimated at nearly 1 in 100,000 people per year.

FSGS stems from abnormalities in the podocyte. Podocyte detachment and death lead to the segmental sclerosis that is the hallmark histopathology of FSGS. The podocyte injury in FSGS, in turn, can stem from immunologic, genetic, and/or hyperfiltration causes. Immunologic injury is considered the main pathogenic mechanism behind primary forms of FSGS, with leukocytes producing a soluble circulating factor that directly targets podocytes. This mechanism is supported by cases of FSGS recurring almost immediately after kidney transplantation and responding briskly to plasmapheresis, although to date definitive identification of such a circulating factor has yet to occur. Identified genetic causes of FSGS are chiefly mutations in podocyte-specific proteins (for example, nephrin, podocin, formin). These mutations are more commonly found in infants, young (<25 years of age) patients who do not respond to glucocorticoid therapy, and patients with a family history of ESKD. Individuals of African ancestry carry approximately a five times higher risk of FSGS than those of

European descent, likely mediated in large part by variants in the *APOL1* gene (see Genetic Disorders and Kidney Disease). The third major cause of podocyte injury, hyperfiltration, causes a large proportion of secondary FSGS cases. This hyperfiltration form of FSGS is seen classically in obese patients but also can manifest in patients with a history of premature birth or solitary kidney. Finally, a drug-induced FSGS can occur as a rare complication of some commonly used treatments, including lithium, interferon, and pamidronate.

Clinical Manifestations

All patients with FSGS have proteinuria. Primary forms of FSGS usually present with nephrotic-range proteinuria and can be accompanied by the full nephrotic syndrome, including severe edema, whereas secondary forms typically have asymptomatic subnephrotic proteinuria. Any form of FSGS can present with reduced glomerular filtration rate, particularly when diagnosed late in the disease course.

Diagnosis

FSGS is diagnosed by kidney biopsy. On light microscopy, glomerulosclerosis (scarring of glomeruli) is seen in a focal (<50%) and segmental (affecting a portion but not the entirety of individual glomeruli) distribution (**Figure 12**). Histologic variants of FSGS include classic (or "not otherwise specified") FSGS, perihilar variant, glomerular tip lesion variant, cellular variant, and collapsing variant. The collapsing variant is often resistant to treatment and therefore carries the worst long-term prognosis, whereas the tip lesion usually responds to glucocorticoids and is unlikely to progress to ESKD.

Treatment and Prognosis

For all patients with FSGS, conservative therapy includes renin-angiotensin system blocking drugs to control proteinuria,

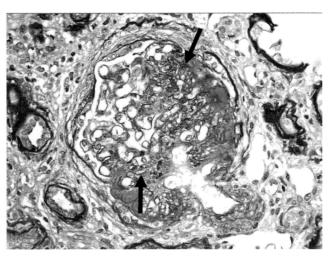

FIGURE 12. Light microscopy in focal segmental glomerulosclerosis shows scarring (*arrows*) in some, but not all, glomeruli in a segmental distribution, as demonstrated by this glomerulus.

Courtesy of Glen Markowitz, MD.

cholesterol-lowering medication, and edema management. Such conservative therapy measures suffice for FSGS patients with subnephrotic proteinuria.

When nephrotic-range proteinuria is present and if a primary form of FSGS is suspected, high-dose glucocorticoids remain the mainstay of initial therapy. Other immunosuppressants, including calcineurin inhibitors, mycophenolate mofetil, alkylating agents, and rituximab, have been reported to provide some benefit as second-line agents for patients who either do not respond to glucocorticoids or whose proteinuria relapses when glucocorticoids are tapered off.

Approximately 50% of patients with FSGS progress to ESKD within 10 years of diagnosis; this poor prognosis is rooted in low rates of treatment response.

Membranous Glomerulopathy
Epidemiology and Pathophysiology
Membranous glomerulopathy (membranous nephropathy) is a leading cause of the nephrotic syndrome in white adults. Epidemiology has remained constant over the past several decades. Disease occurs at an approximate rate of 1 case per 100,000 persons per year, with a peak incidence between 30 and 50 years of age. Approximately 75% of cases are considered primary; the remaining 25% are considered secondary to systemic diseases such as systemic lupus erythematosus, hepatitis B virus infection, and solid tumors.

In the past decade, target antigens and their associated autoantibodies responsible for the development of primary membranous glomerulopathy cases have been identified. The M-type phospholipase A2 receptor (PLA2R) is the specific podocyte antigen responsible for eliciting immune complex formation with circulating autoantibodies in most primary cases. Anti-PLA2R antibodies are detected in approximately 75% of primary cases and are rarely found in secondary forms. Additional alternative podocyte autoantigens have been reported in patients with primary membranous glomerulopathy, potentially filling in the missing gaps in PLA2R antibody–negative disease. Membranous glomerulopathy occurs when circulating antibodies permeate the glomerular basement membrane and, in the subepithelial space, form immune complexes with epitopes on podocyte membranes.

Clinical Manifestations
Patients typically describe slowly progressive edema, and laboratory testing reveals proteinuria, hypoalbuminemia, and hyperlipidemia, most often with preserved kidney function. Patients with membranous glomerulopathy are particularly prone to thrombotic complications. These clots include lower extremity, pulmonary, and renal vein thromboses; they can occur in up to 25% of patients and are most likely to occur within the first 2 years of diagnosis. The risk of clotting increases when serum albumin is <2.8 g/dL (28 g/L) and is highest when serum albumin is <2.2 g/dL (22 g/L).

Diagnosis
The diagnosis of membranous glomerulopathy is traditionally made by kidney biopsy, although FDA approval of serologic testing for anti-PLA2R antibodies in 2015 has introduced the possibility of diagnosing the disease noninvasively.

The hallmark biopsy finding is the presence of subepithelial immune deposits that alter the glomerular capillary wall, classically accompanied by intervening "spikes" of glomerular basement membrane extending between the immune deposits in more advanced cases. In addition to serologic testing for anti-PLA2R antibodies, the biopsy can be stained for the PLA2R antigen, which typically yields a higher sensitivity (>80%) than antibody testing in the serum. This testing is used not to make a diagnosis of membranous glomerulopathy but to help distinguish primary from secondary forms of the disease. Such a distinction is crucial because secondary forms are expected to remit if the underlying systemic disease responsible for the lesion is successfully treated. Notably, in patients with membranous glomerulopathy aged 65 years and older, malignancies have been detected in up to 25% within 1 year of their biopsy diagnosis. Therefore, age- and sex-appropriate cancer screening is recommended for all patients at the time of their diagnosis, even those with PLA2R positivity.

Treatment and Prognosis
Patients with newly diagnosed primary forms of membranous glomerulopathy are usually observed for 6 to 12 months on conservative therapy (renin-angiotensin system blockade, cholesterol-lowering medication, and edema management) before initiating a course of immunosuppression for patients with persistent nephrotic-range proteinuria. The observation period allows patients a chance to achieve spontaneous remission, which occurs in approximately 30% within 1 to 2 years of diagnosis. Patients who remain nephrotic have the option of two first-line immunosuppressive regimens: (1) a combination of glucocorticoids and alkylating agents, which achieves remission in approximately 75% to 80% of patients within 12 months, or (2) calcineurin inhibitors (cyclosporine or tacrolimus), which have reported remission rates of 70% to 75% in the first year of therapy. Relapse rates are higher in patients treated with calcineurin inhibitors than alkylating agents. Recent reports also suggest that rituximab may have efficacy in membranous glomerulopathy. Treatment of secondary forms of membranous glomerulopathy should be aimed at the underlying systemic disease or etiology (for example, resection of a tumor in malignancy-associated membranous glomerulopathy, treatment of hepatitis B in viral-associated membranous glomerulopathy).

Progression to ESKD depends on remission of proteinuria: The 10-year incidence of ESKD in patients who undergo complete or partial remission of proteinuria ranges from 0 to 10%, compared with a >50% incidence of ESKD in patients who maintain nephrotic-range proteinuria.

Minimal Change Glomerulopathy

Epidemiology and Pathophysiology

Minimal change glomerulopathy (MCG; also known as minimal change disease) is the most common cause of the nephrotic syndrome in children (>90% of cases). For this reason, unless clinical and serologic evidence suggests the presence of a disease other than MCG, a kidney biopsy is not performed in children with the nephrotic syndrome unless they do not respond to glucocorticoid therapy. In adults, biopsy series have shown that MCG is the cause of up to 10% to 15% of cases of the nephrotic syndrome, with a greater representation in older patients (≥65 years of age) and elderly patients (≥80 years of age).

The pathophysiology of MCG is not well understood. Similar to FSGS, MCG is a podocytopathy; the presumed model of injury is immunologic, in which a circulating factor (produced by B or T cells) alters podocyte function, resulting in massive proteinuria. The rapid response of most cases (>90%) of MCG to nonspecific immunosuppression (usually glucocorticoids) fits this model of a circulating factor-inducing disease. Most cases of MCG are primary, but the disease is associated with various conditions, including malignancies (Hodgkin lymphoma, non-Hodgkin lymphoma, thymoma), medications (NSAIDs, lithium), infections (strongyloides, syphilis, mycoplasma, ehrlichiosis), and atopy (pollen, dairy products).

Clinical Manifestations

The classic presentation of MCG is sudden-onset nephrotic syndrome. Microscopic hematuria is present in 10% to 30% of adult cases. Up to 25% of adults with MCG may also have acute kidney injury (AKI), more commonly occurring in older patients with hypertension, low serum albumin levels, and heavy proteinuria.

Diagnosis

MCG is diagnosed with kidney biopsy demonstrating normal glomerular histology on light microscopy, negative immunofluorescence staining for immunoglobulin and complement proteins, and complete effacement of the podocyte foot processes on electron microscopy.

Treatment and Prognosis

The 2012 Kidney Disease: Improving Global Outcomes (KDIGO) Clinical Practice Guideline for Glomerulonephritis recommends glucocorticoids as first-line therapy for children and adults with MCG, with remission achieved in more than 90% of children and 80% to 90% of adults. Time-to-response is prolonged in adults compared with children, and adults are not considered to have glucocorticoid-resistant disease until they have not responded to 16 weeks of glucocorticoid therapy. After an initial course of glucocorticoids, patients are subdivided into categories: glucocorticoid-sensitive MCG, glucocorticoid-dependent MCG, infrequently relapsing MCG, frequently relapsing MCG, and glucocorticoid-resistant MCG. Treatment of glucocorticoid-dependent, frequently relapsing, and glucocorticoid-resistant MCG has included calcineurin inhibitors, mycophenolate mofetil, alkylating agents, and rituximab, with variable results.

Diabetic Nephropathy

Epidemiology and Pathophysiology

Diabetes mellitus is the leading cause of chronic kidney disease (CKD) and ESKD worldwide. In the United States, diabetes accounts for over 50,000 new cases of ESKD requiring dialysis each year. Diabetic nephropathy, defined as clinical evidence of kidney injury in response to chronic, long-standing hyperglycemia, has a 10% incidence over 25 years among patients with type 1 diabetes and a 12% incidence over 25 years among patients with type 2 diabetes.

Advanced glycation end products are felt to be the primary mediator of injury in diabetic nephropathy, activating signaling cascades that promote mesangial cell synthesis of profibrogenic cytokines, including platelet-derived growth factor and transforming growth factor β.

Clinical Manifestations

Diabetic nephropathy manifests initially as moderately increased albuminuria (microalbuminuria). Over time, progressive proteinuria is followed by a decline in glomerular filtration rate, with progression to later stages of CKD and ESKD. When proteinuria is severe, it is typically accompanied by hypoalbuminemia, and many patients present with edema befitting a classic picture of the nephrotic syndrome.

Kidney disease due to diabetes is often accompanied by extrarenal microvascular complications of diabetes, including retinopathy and peripheral neuropathy, as well as macrovascular complications, such as peripheral vascular disease, coronary artery disease, and stroke.

Diagnosis

The American Diabetes Association recommends yearly assessment of albuminuria in patients with type 2 diabetes, and assessment after 5 years of disease in patients with type 1 diabetes. The diagnosis of diabetic nephropathy is usually made clinically in the presence of hallmark features: proteinuric CKD in a patient with long-standing diabetes and evidence of other (microvascular and/or macrovascular) complications of disease. If the clinical presentation is not entirely consistent with diabetic nephropathy, a kidney biopsy is performed. The biopsy finding of nodular mesangial sclerosis with glomerular and tubular basement thickening, in the absence of immune deposits, is the classic description of diabetic nephropathy.

Treatment and Prognosis

The cornerstone of treatment of diabetic nephropathy involves glycemic control and blood pressure control. Blockade of the renin-angiotensin system with an ACE inhibitor or angiotensin receptor blocker (ARB) is recommended, typically to the maximal tolerated dose, because these agents both reduce blood pressure and levels of

CONT.

proteinuria, which, along with glycemic control, are the most important modifiable risk factors for progression of diabetic nephropathy to ESKD. Combined use of any two of the three renin-angiotensin system drug classes (ACE inhibitor, ARB, and direct renin inhibitor) is not recommended given the results of several clinical trials that revealed more adverse events with these combinations (hyperkalemia, hypotension, AKI), without additional cardiovascular or renal benefits. Combining ACE inhibitors or ARBs with mineralocorticoid receptors (spironolactone or eplerenone) has been shown in small studies to be a safe and effective antiproteinuric strategy in diabetic nephropathy, but the risk for hyperkalemia should be considered.

The 2017 high blood pressure guideline from the American College of Cardiology (ACC), the American Heart Association (AHA), and nine other organizations recommends a blood pressure target of <130/80 mm Hg for patients with hypertension and diabetes mellitus and/or CKD. The American Diabetes Association recommends that most patients with diabetes and hypertension should be treated to a systolic blood pressure goal of <140 mm Hg and a diastolic blood pressure goal of <90 mm Hg; lower systolic and diastolic blood pressure targets, such as 130/80 mm Hg, may be appropriate for individuals at high risk of cardiovascular disease, if they can be achieved without undue treatment burden. H

KEY POINTS

- Initial treatment of focal segmental glomerulosclerosis is high-dose glucocorticoids; other immunosuppressants (calcineurin inhibitors, mycophenolate mofetil, alkylating agents, rituximab) may provide some benefit for patients who do not respond to glucocorticoids or relapse when glucocorticoids are tapered off.

- Newly diagnosed primary membranous glomerulopathy is typically treated with conservative therapy for 6 to 12 months before initiating immunosuppression for patients with persistent nephrotic-range proteinuria.

- Minimal change glomerulopathy (MCG) is initially treated with glucocorticoids; treatment options for glucocorticoid-dependent, frequently relapsing, and glucocorticoid-resistant MCG include calcineurin inhibitors, mycophenolate mofetil, alkylating agents, or rituximab.

- The American Diabetes Association recommends yearly assessment of albuminuria in patients with type 2 diabetes mellitus, and assessment after 5 years of disease in patients with type 1 diabetes mellitus.

- The cornerstone of treatment of diabetic nephropathy involves glycemic control and renin-angiotensin system blockade using either an ACE inhibitor or an angiotensin receptor blocker.

Conditions Associated With the Nephritic Syndrome
Rapidly Progressive Glomerulonephritis
Epidemiology and Pathophysiology
Rapidly progressive glomerulonephritis (RPGN; also known as crescentic glomerulonephritis) is not a specific disease; rather, RPGN is a clinical entity that can be caused by multiple diseases and manifests as (1) at least a 50% decline in glomerular filtration rate over a short period (usually days to weeks) with (2) pathology findings of extensive glomerular crescents (**Figure 13**). Crescents signal focal rupture of the glomerular capillary walls, the most severe glomerular damage that can be seen on light microscopy. This rupture allows accumulation of fibrin and fibronectin in the urinary space, where they activate de-differentiated glomerular parietal epithelial cells to proliferate, surround, and compress the glomerular tuft.

Clinical Manifestations
RPGN typically presents with macroscopic or microscopic hematuria, erythrocyte casts, varying ranges of proteinuria, and AKI that can lead rapidly to dialysis dependence.

Diagnosis
The diagnosis of all forms of glomerulonephritis is traditionally made by kidney biopsy, which can distinguish among the three major categories of glomerulonephritis (**Table 18**) and their associated etiologies. Serologic testing (for example, ANCA, anti–glomerular basement membrane antibodies, antinuclear antibodies) aids in the diagnosis. An alternative classification scheme for glomerulonephritis is based on low versus normal complement levels (**Table 19**). Although any form of glomerulonephritis can display an aggressive disease course that would fit the definition of an RPGN, the most common etiologies seen in RPGN cases are ANCA-associated

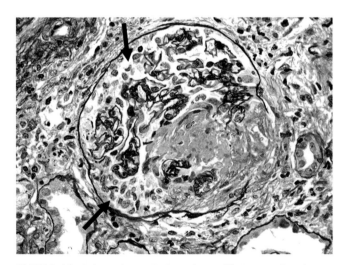

FIGURE 13. A glomerular crescent (*arrows*), named for its moon-shaped appearance, signals focal rupture of the glomerular capillary walls.

Courtesy of Glen Markowitz, MD.

TABLE 18. Categorization of Glomerulonephritis Based on Immunofluorescence Microscopy Findings

Immunofluorescence Staining Pattern		
Granular	**Pauci-immune**	**Linear**
Lupus nephritis	ANCA-associated GN	Anti-GBM antibody disease
Infection-related GN		
IgA nephropathy		
MPGN		
Cryoglobulinemic GN		

GBM = glomerular basement membrane; GN = glomerulonephritis; MPGN = membranoproliferative glomerulonephritis.

TABLE 19. Categorization of Glomerulonephritis Based on Serum Complement Levels

Low Serum C3 and/or C4 Levels	Normal Serum C3 and C4 Levels
Lupus nephritis	IgA nephropathy
Infection-related GN	ANCA-associated GN
MPGN	Anti-GBM antibody disease
Cryoglobulinemic GN	

GBM = glomerular basement membrane; GN = glomerulonephritis; MPGN = membranoproliferative glomerulonephritis.

glomerulonephritis, lupus nephritis, and anti–glomerular basement membrane glomerulonephritis.

Treatment and Prognosis

Treatment is based on the specific etiology of RPGN. If untreated, RPGN is expected to progress to dialysis dependence in a matter of days to weeks. If treated early, lesions can often be reversed, although CKD is often a lingering consequence.

Anti–Glomerular Basement Membrane Antibody Disease

Epidemiology and Pathophysiology

Anti–glomerular basement membrane (anti-GBM) antibody disease is a rare form of RPGN with an incidence of less than one case per million per year. Anti-GBM antibody disease accounts for about 20% of RPGN cases in adults. The lesion is more frequently seen in white patients and has a bimodal age and gender distribution, with peak incidences in young men in the second and third decades of life and in older women in the sixth and seventh decades of life. More than half of patients with anti-GBM antibody disease present with RPGN and pulmonary hemorrhage. About one third of patients present with isolated glomerulonephritis. Notably, up to one third of patients have concurrent circulating ANCA (usually antimyeloperoxidase [MPO]) antibodies.

Circulating anti-GBM antibodies target the alpha-3 chain of type IV collagen. When anti-GBM antibodies bind rapidly and tightly to the GBM, they incite an intense inflammatory response that translates to the typically fulminant nature of this disease.

Clinical Manifestations

The presentation of anti-GBM antibody disease is similar to that of other forms of RPGN previously described, with macroscopic or microscopic hematuria, erythrocyte casts, varying ranges of proteinuria, and usually moderate to severe AKI. Lung involvement (Goodpasture syndrome) occurs in >50% of patients; hemoptysis can be a presenting symptom, although shortness of breath or cough should also raise suspicion for a pulmonary-renal syndrome even in the absence of hemoptysis.

Diagnosis

Kidney biopsy in anti-GBM disease shows a crescentic glomerulonephritis on light microscopy and pathognomonic linear staining for IgG along the glomerular capillaries, indicative of antibodies directed against the GBM. Serologic testing for anti-GBM antibodies is performed at the time of diagnosis. The serologic test is done by indirect immunofluorescence or direct enzyme-linked immunoassay (ELISA), with sensitivity ranging from 60% to 100%; therefore, a kidney biopsy to confirm diagnosis is recommended unless contraindicated. Even with a renal biopsy diagnosis, antibody levels should be measured because their titers can be followed to assess efficacy of therapy.

Treatment and Prognosis

Outcomes in anti-GBM disease are based largely on the degree of AKI at the time of diagnosis and treatment. In an oft-cited series, patients with anti-GBM disease who presented with serum creatinine <5.65 mg/dL (500 μmol/L) had, at 10 years, a <5% overall mortality and a <20% risk for ESKD. In contrast, patients who presented with dialysis-dependent kidney failure had a 35% mortality rate within the first year of diagnosis, and only 8% were able to be taken off dialysis during this time. Treatment for anti-GBM disease consists of plasmapheresis, pulse glucocorticoids (high doses of intravenous glucocorticoids over a short period of time) followed by oral prednisone, and cyclophosphamide.

ANCA-Associated Glomerulonephritis

See MKSAP 18 Rheumatology for more information on ANCA-associated vasculitis.

Epidemiology and Pathophysiology

ANCA-associated glomerulonephritis (pauci-immune crescentic glomerulonephritis) accounts for more than half of all RPGN cases and has a particularly high prevalence in patients >65 years of age presenting with AKI and active urinary sediment. ANCA are autoantibodies that target proteins within neutrophil granules and monocyte lysosomes. There are two types of vasculitis-associated ANCA: p-ANCA (perinuclear) is directed against the neutrophil enzyme myeloperoxidase (MPO), and c-ANCA (cytoplasmic) is directed against the neutrophil proteinase 3 (PR3).

Clinical Manifestations

Most patients with ANCA-associated glomerulonephritis report a vasculitic prodrome of malaise, arthralgia, myalgia, and flu-like symptoms that can include fever. Kidney involvement can produce dark brown (tea-colored) urine, and laboratory studies will confirm the presence of hematuria, proteinuria, and AKI. Lung and sinus involvement often occurs in ANCA-associated glomerulonephritis, with patients reporting hemoptysis and/or epistaxis.

Diagnosis

Serologic testing for ANCA using enzyme-linked immunosorbent assay is usually performed at the time of presentation if RPGN is suspected. Light microscopy of the kidney biopsy shows a crescentic glomerulonephritis, but immunofluorescence shows a paucity or absence of immune-type deposits. Foci of necrosis or cellular crescents are highlighted by immunofluorescence staining for fibrinogen.

Treatment and Prognosis

The initial treatment of organ-threatening disease is an area of ongoing controversy. Typical induction therapy consists of glucocorticoids combined with either cyclophosphamide or rituximab. Plasmapheresis is reserved for patients with evidence of alveolar hemorrhage or severe kidney failure. Other induction options include cyclophosphamide or rituximab-based therapies. After remission is induced, maintenance therapy is usually continued for at least 12 to 24 months using rituximab, azathioprine, or mycophenolate mofetil.

Patients with c-ANCA/anti-PR3 have a significantly higher rate of relapse than patients with p-ANCA/anti-MPO, particularly if there is a history of lung or sinus involvement. ANCA-associated glomerulonephritis is associated with an approximately 20% mortality rate within the first year of diagnosis and results in ESKD in up to 25% of surviving patients within the first 4 years after diagnosis.

KEY POINTS

- Rapidly progressive glomerulonephritis can be caused by multiple diseases; it is characterized by at least a 50% decline in glomerular filtration rate over a short period with pathology findings of extensive glomerular crescents.

- More than half of patients with anti–glomerular basement membrane antibody disease have lung involvement manifesting as hemoptysis, shortness of breath, or cough.

- Treatment of anti–glomerular basement membrane antibody disease consists of plasmapheresis, pulse glucocorticoids followed by oral prednisone, and cyclophosphamide.

- ANCA-associated glomerulonephritis is characterized by a prodrome of malaise, arthralgia, myalgia, and flu-like symptoms; dark brown (tea-colored) urine, hematuria, proteinuria, acute kidney injury, hemoptysis, and epistaxis may occur.

Immune Complex–Mediated Glomerulonephritis

The glomerulonephritides with granular immunofluorescence microscopy staining patterns all fall under the umbrella category of immune complex–mediated glomerulonephritis, with antigen-antibody complexes depositing in the kidney at various locations and in various patterns (see Table 18). Immune complex deposition activates the classic complement pathway as a co-player in glomerular inflammation, injury, and, if unchecked, scarring. For this reason, most immune complex–mediated glomerulonephritides are associated with low levels of C3 and/or C4 (see Table 19). IgA nephropathy, which usually presents with normal C3 and C4 levels, is an exception due to the chronic, gradual nature of the disease; complement consumption is at a rate slow enough for hepatic production to replace complement proteins. In rare hyper-acute cases of IgA nephropathy that fulfill criteria for RPGN, however, complement levels are usually depressed.

IgA Nephropathy
Epidemiology and Pathophysiology

IgA nephropathy (IgAN) is the most common primary glomerular disease worldwide, diagnosed in up to 10% of all kidney biopsies done in the United States and approximately one third of all kidney biopsies in Asian countries, where the disease is the leading cause of ESKD. In contrast, IgAN is very rare among patients of African ancestry. IgAN can be diagnosed at any age, particularly because a significant subgroup of patients is asymptomatic, but is most commonly diagnosed in youth or early adulthood, with a 2:1 male-to-female ratio. In the United States, the overall incidence of IgAN is estimated at 2.5 cases per 100,000 person-years, with a prevalence of approximately 80,000 individuals.

In IgAN, there is defect in IgA1-producing cells leading to hypogalactosylation of the hinge region of IgA1. Blood levels of galactose-deficient IgA1 (Gd-IgA1) are elevated in patients with IgAN. Patients then develop antibodies directed against Gd-IgA1 to form immune complexes that accumulate in the glomerular mesangium.

Clinical Manifestations

IgAN can present with any of the manifestations of the nephritic syndrome. The mildest presentation, seen in up to one third of patients, is asymptomatic microscopic hematuria with or without proteinuria, usually discovered incidentally as part of a routine examination. Recurrent gross hematuria, in which macroscopic hematuria occurs in the setting of an upper respiratory infection (synpharyngitic hematuria) is a common presentation in younger patients; it usually portends a benign clinical course with recurrent episodes of gross hematuria without progression to CKD. IgAN can also present as an acute glomerulonephritis or an even more aggressive RPGN, with variable degrees of AKI, hypertension, edema, proteinuria, and hematuria.

Diagnosis

The diagnosis of IgAN may be suspected clinically but can only be made by kidney biopsy showing dominant mesangial immune-deposits of IgA with C3, and occasionally IgG or IgM. In some centers, patients with microscopic hematuria, normal kidney function, and proteinuria <500 mg/24 h are given an empiric diagnosis of IgAN without a biopsy because the disease course is expected to be mild in these cases. In other centers, patients with microscopic hematuria that is deemed to be glomerular in origin (that is, presence of dysmorphic erythrocytes or erythrocyte casts in the urine sediment) elicits a biopsy regardless of kidney function or proteinuria.

Treatment and Prognosis

There are no current standard care therapies for IgAN other than conservative, nonimmunomodulatory therapies. Antiproteinuric therapy using an ACE inhibitor or ARB is a hallmark for treating IgAN; it is usually coupled with lipid-lowering therapy and fish oil, although the efficacy of the latter two as specific IgAN therapies is unproven. The use of immunosuppression in IgAN remains controversial. In the United States, it is common for most patients with IgAN who progress to ESKD to have done so despite long-term renin-angiotensin system blockade and at least one course of immunosuppressive therapy.

Approximately one third of patients with IgAN will have a benign long-term course, with continued microscopic hematuria but little to no proteinuria and no evidence of kidney dysfunction. The disease progresses to CKD or ESKD in the remainder of patients, with up to 40% reaching ESKD within 15 years of diagnosis. The recent Oxford histopathology classification of IgAN provides evidence that advanced disease chronicity, manifesting as >50% tubular atrophy and interstitial fibrosis on kidney biopsy, is the most reliable predictor of progression to ESKD. Among clinical parameters, proteinuria ≥1000 mg/24 h has been shown to be a risk factor for progression.

IgA Vasculitis

IgA vasculitis (Henoch-Schönlein purpura) can present with the classic tetrad of rash, arthralgia, abdominal pain, and kidney disease. Considered a systemic version of IgAN, this vasculitis is often diagnosed empirically in the pediatric setting, because the differential diagnosis of vasculitis in children is extremely limited. In adults, the diagnosis should be confirmed with tissue biopsy (kidney or skin), because the presentation of IgA vasculitis can also fit with a non-IgA form of vasculitis. Skin biopsy is usually adequate to make the diagnosis when lesions less than 24 hours old in appearance are sampled. Kidney involvement in IgA vasculitis typically is more severe in adults than in children, with higher rates of AKI and the nephrotic syndrome. Treatment includes glucocorticoids and, in cases of associated RPGN, cyclophosphamide.

See MKSAP 18 Rheumatology for more information.

Lupus Nephritis

See MKSAP 18 Rheumatology for more information on systemic lupus erythematosus.

Epidemiology and Pathophysiology

Kidney involvement in systemic lupus erythematosus (SLE), generally termed lupus nephritis (LN), is a major contributor to SLE-associated morbidity and mortality. Up to 50% of patients with SLE will have clinically evident kidney disease at presentation; during follow-up, kidney involvement occurs in up to 75% of patients. LN has been shown to affect clinical outcomes in SLE both directly via target organ damage and indirectly through complications of therapy.

The immune deposits that incite LN are primarily complexes of anti–double-stranded DNA antibodies directed against nucleosomal antigens. A smaller fraction of autoantibodies can also bind directly to chromatin in the glomerular basement membrane (GBM) and mesangium. These immune complexes, when deposited in the mesangium and subendothelial space, are proximal to the GBM and are in communication with the systemic circulation. Subsequent activation of the classical complement pathway, triggered by the DNA/anti-DNA antibody complex formation, generates the potent chemoattractants, C3a and C5a, which elicit an influx of neutrophils and mononuclear cells. The pattern on light microscopy is a proliferative glomerulonephritis that can be mesangial (class II), focal endocapillary (class III), or diffuse endocapillary (class IV) (**Table 20**). Endocapillary proliferation refers to an increased number of inflammatory cells within glomerular capillary lumina, causing luminal narrowing or obliteration. Immune complex deposits in the subepithelial space can also activate complement but only locally; C3a and C5a are separated from the circulation by the GBM, and hence no influx of inflammatory cells occurs into this space. The injury in this class V LN (membranous) is limited to the glomerular epithelial cells, the primary clinical manifestation is proteinuria, and the histologic pattern on light microscopy is similar to primary membranous nephropathy.

Clinical Manifestations

Typically, patients with SLE initially present with evidence of non–kidney organ involvement (malar rash, arthritis, oral ulcers). After a diagnosis of SLE is confirmed, evidence of kidney disease, if present, usually emerges within the first 3 years of diagnosis. Kidney involvement in SLE first manifests with proteinuria and/or microscopic hematuria on urinalysis; this eventually progresses to reduction in kidney function. Early in the course of disease, it is unusual for patients to present with decreased kidney function, except for very aggressive cases of LN that present as RPGN. The symptoms of kidney involvement tend to correlate with laboratory abnormalities. For example, patients with nephrotic-range proteinuria can present with edema. When kidney function is impaired, elevated blood pressure is a common clinical finding.

TABLE 20. Classification of Lupus Nephritis with Associated Presentation and Treatment Options

ISN/RPS Class	Biopsy Findings	Clinical Features	Treatment	
			Induction Phase	Maintenance Phase
Class I: minimal mesangial LN	No LM abnormalities; isolated mesangial IC deposits on IF and/or EM	Normal urine or microscopic hematuria	Conservative, nonimmunomodulatory therapy (e.g., RAS blockade)	Not applicable
Class II: mesangial proliferative LN	Mesangial hypercellularity or matrix expansion with mesangial IC deposits on IF and/or EM	Microscopic hematuria and/or low-grade proteinuria	Conservative, nonimmunomodulatory therapy (e.g., RAS blockade)	Not applicable
Class III: focal LN	<50% of glomeruli on LM display segmental (<50% of glomerular tuft) or global (>50% of glomerular tuft) endocapillary and/or extracapillary proliferation or sclerosis; mesangial and focal subendothelial IC deposits on IF and EM	Nephritic urine sediment and subnephrotic proteinuria	Pulse IV glucocorticoids followed by tapering doses of oral glucocorticoids *and* IV cyclophosphamide for 6 doses (high-dose monthly vs. low-dose bimonthly) *or* Mycophenolate mofetil for 6 months	Lowest tolerable amount of oral glucocorticoids *and* Mycophenolate mofetil (tapered down every 3-6 months assuming stable disease) *or* Azathioprine (tapered down every 3-6 months assuming stable disease)
Class IV: diffuse LN	≥50% of glomeruli on LM display endocapillary and/or extracapillary proliferation or sclerosis; class IV-S denotes that ≥50% of affected glomeruli have segmental lesions; class IV-G denotes that ≥50% of affected glomeruli have global lesions; mesangial and diffuse subendothelial IC deposits on IF and EM	Nephritic and nephrotic syndromes; hypertension; reduced kidney function	Pulse IV glucocorticoids followed by tapering doses of oral glucocorticoids *and* IV cyclophosphamide for 6 doses (high-dose monthly vs. low-dose bimonthly) *or* Mycophenolate mofetil for 6 months	Lowest tolerable amount of oral glucocorticoids *and* Mycophenolate mofetil (tapered down every 3-6 months assuming stable disease) *or* Azathioprine (tapered down every 3-6 months assuming stable disease)
Class V: membranous LN[a]	Diffuse thickening of the glomerular capillary walls on LM with subepithelial IC deposits on IF and EM, with or without mesangial IC deposits	Nephrotic syndrome	Pulse IV glucocorticoids followed by tapering doses of oral glucocorticoids *and* IV cyclophosphamide for 6 doses (high-dose monthly vs. low-dose bimonthly) *or* Cyclosporine *or* Tacrolimus *or* Mycophenolate mofetil for 6 months	Lowest tolerable amount of oral glucocorticoids *and* Mycophenolate mofetil (tapered down every 3-6 months assuming stable disease) *or* Azathioprine (tapered down every 3-6 months assuming stable disease)
Class VI: advanced sclerosing LN	>90% of glomeruli on LM are globally sclerosed with no residual activity	Advanced CKD or ESKD with varying degrees of hematuria and/or proteinuria	Conservative, nonimmunomodulatory therapy (e.g., RAS blockade) with preparation for renal replacement therapy	Not applicable

CKD = chronic kidney disease; EM = electron microscopy; ESKD = end-stage kidney disease; IC = immune complex; IF = immunofluorescence; ISN/RPS = International Society of Nephrology/Renal Pathology Society; IV = intravenous; LM = light microscopy; LN = lupus nephritis; RAS = renin-angiotensin system.

[a]Class V may coexist with class III or class IV, in which case both classes are diagnosed.

Diagnosis

The diagnosis of LN is suspected by changes in laboratory parameters (elevated serum creatinine, hematuria and/or proteinuria, low serum complements) but can only be made definitively by kidney biopsy. The classic pattern of LN is an immune complex–mediated glomerulonephritis with a varied pathology that includes six distinct classes of disease (see Table 20). On immunofluorescence microscopy, the glomerular deposits in LN stain dominantly for IgG with co-deposits of IgA, IgM, C3, and C1q in a "full house" pattern. On electron microscopy, tubuloreticular inclusions, which represent "interferon footprints" in the glomerular endothelial cell cytoplasm, are essentially pathognomonic for LN.

Treatment and Prognosis

The current approach to treating LN is guided by histologic findings with appropriate consideration of presenting clinical parameters and the degree of kidney function impairment (see Table 20). Important recent changes in the management of LN include the preferential use of mycophenolate mofetil over cyclophosphamide as induction therapy for LN classes III, IV, and V based on similar efficacy rates and a more favorable side-effect profile with mycophenolate mofetil (in particular, the non-impact on fertility of mycophenolate mofetil compared with cyclophosphamide in a young patient population with childbearing potential). The landmark ALMS trial showed only a 56% response rate in the mycophenolate arm (compared with a 53% response rate in the cyclophosphamide arm).

Up to 30% of patients with LN will progress to ESKD within 10 years of diagnosis, depending in large part on the response to the initial course of immunosuppression. Severity of disease at the time of diagnosis as well as black race, Hispanic ethnicity, and socioeconomic status have also been reported to influence outcomes in LN.

Infection-Related Glomerulonephritis

Epidemiology and Pathophysiology

Infection-related glomerulonephritis (IRGN) results from a recently resolved infection or an infection that is ongoing at the time of development of glomerulonephritis. IRGN is preferred to the formerly used term "postinfectious glomerulonephritis," which adequately described classic poststreptococcal glomerulonephritis but did not address the increasingly recognized forms of glomerulonephritis that are manifestations of ongoing infection and nonstreptococcal infectious agents. Diabetes is the most common comorbidity (malignancy, immunosuppression, AIDS, alcoholism, and injection drug use are other recognized comorbidities), and older age is a key risk factor. Patients over 65 years of age account for about one third of IRGN cases in the developed world.

The incidence of poststreptococcal glomerulonephritis has declined throughout most of the world due to improvements in infection control and sanitation. The entity, however, remains a health concern in developing countries: More than 450,000 cases of poststreptococcal glomerulonephritis occur worldwide annually, resulting in approximately 5000 deaths, with >95% of these cases in less developed countries. In industrialized countries, much of the burden of IRGN has shifted from children to adults, with a decrease in IRGN attributed to streptococcal infections and an increase in IRGN cases associated with *Staphylococcus aureus* and gram-negative bacteria.

In the classical view of the pathogenesis of IRGN, antibodies directed at bacterial antigens form immune complexes in the circulation that subsequently deposit in the glomerulus. Additionally, however, antibodies directed at bacterial antigens planted within glomeruli can result in *in situ* formation of glomerular immune complexes.

Clinical Manifestations

The variable presentation of IRGN ranges from asymptomatic microscopic hematuria to RPGN. Proteinuria is usually subnephrotic.

In classic poststreptococcal glomerulonephritis, symptomatic patients (typically children) present with an acute nephritic syndrome of hematuria, proteinuria, hypertension, edema, and, in some cases, kidney dysfunction. The urine sediment is active with dysmorphic erythrocytes, erythrocyte casts, and leukocyturia. Hypocomplementemia is very common, with decreased C3 in up to 90% of cases. There is usually a latent period (1 to 2 weeks after upper respiratory infections; 2 to 4 weeks after skin infections) between the resolution of the streptococcal infection and the onset of the nephritic syndrome. Serologic markers of a recent streptococcal infection, including elevated antistreptolysin O, antistreptokinase, antihyaluronidase, and antideoxyribonuclease B antibody levels, are often detected. In adults, most cases of IRGN are no longer poststreptococcal, and the glomerulonephritis often coexists with the triggering infection. Low complement levels may be absent in these peri-infectious cases.

Diagnosis

The diagnosis of IRGN can be made clinically in the appropriate setting (for example, classic nephritic presentation with low complements and clear evidence of a recent infection), although the only definitive way to make the diagnosis is by kidney biopsy. The most common finding on light microscopy is a proliferative glomerulonephritis with significant presence of infiltrating neutrophils. On electron microscopy, the classic finding in poststreptococcal glomerulonephritis is hump-shaped subepithelial electron dense deposits, although these are not required for the diagnosis of IRGN.

Treatment and Prognosis

Treatment is typically supportive and aimed at the infectious etiology, although in some cases with severe proliferative glomerulonephritis on biopsy, a trial of glucocorticoids is used.

In children, prognosis for complete recovery is excellent, and treatment usually is supportive and aimed at the infecting organism. The prognosis of the newly recognized forms of IRGN (for example, due to *S. aureus* and gram-negative organisms) in adults is different, with more patients developing severe kidney dysfunction and progressing to CKD and sometimes ESKD.

Membranoproliferative Glomerulonephritis

Epidemiology and Pathophysiology

Membranoproliferative glomerulonephritis (MPGN) is a rare form of chronic glomerulonephritis diagnosed primarily in children and young adults. The name stems from its pattern of glomerular injury. The entity is divided into immune-complex forms of MPGN (mediated by antigen-antibody interactions triggering the classical complement pathway) versus complement-mediated forms of MPGN (also termed C3 glomerulopathies, due to a hyperactive alternative complement pathway). An immune-complex MPGN, with or without cryoglobulinemia, is the classic form of kidney involvement seen in patients with hepatitis C virus infection. The alternative complement pathway abnormalities that drive the C3 glomerulopathies are either mutations in regulators (for example, complement factor H) or activators (for example, complement factor B) of the alternative pathway, or antibodies directed at regulator or activator complement proteins.

Clinical Manifestations

Although MPGN can rarely present as an acute and severe form of glomerulonephritis, the more common presentation is a chronic glomerulonephritis that initially manifests with microscopic hematuria and subnephrotic proteinuria. As disease progresses, proteinuria can reach nephrotic range, and kidney dysfunction ensues.

Diagnosis

The diagnosis of MPGN is made by kidney biopsy. The distinction between immune-complex and complement-mediated MPGN is based on immunofluorescence microscopy, in which the absence of immunoglobulin staining signals an antibody-independent manner of triggering complement and hence alternative pathway hyperactivity.

Treatment and Prognosis

Currently, treatment of MPGN is nonspecific and includes immunosuppression (for example, glucocorticoids) when nephrotic-range proteinuria and/or kidney dysfunction is present. The advent of complement-targeting therapies such as the C5 monoclonal antibody, eculizumab, may bring disease-specific therapy for the complement-mediated forms of MPGN.

The overall prognosis of MPGN as a chronic form of glomerulonephritis is poor, with >50% of patients progressing to ESKD within 15 years of diagnosis.

Cryoglobulinemia

Cryoglobulinemia can be associated with the nephritic syndrome. Of the three types of cryoglobulins, kidney involvement is typically due to type II cryoglobulins.

See MKSAP 18 Hematology and Oncology for details on cryoglobulinemia; MKSAP 18 Rheumatology for information on cryoglobulinemic vasculitis; and Kidney Manifestations of Deposition Diseases in MKSAP 18 Nephrology for information on kidney involvement in cryoglobulinemia.

Collagen Type IV–Related Nephropathies

Type IV collagen is an integral component of the glomerular basement membrane. Structural defects in this protein due to genetic variations can result in a hereditary form of glomerulonephritis, discussed in more detail in Genetic Disorders and Kidney Disease.

KEY POINTS

- Treatment of IgA nephropathy consists of conservative therapy using an ACE inhibitor or angiotensin receptor blocker.
- Kidney biopsy is required to diagnose and classify lupus nephritis, which guides therapy.
- Treatment of classes I and II lupus nephritis (LN) includes conservative therapy with an ACE inhibitor or angiotensin receptor blocker; classes III, IV, and V LN may require aggressive immunosuppressive therapy; and class VI LN may be treated with conservative therapy.
- Infection-related glomerulonephritis results from a recently resolved infection or an infection that is ongoing at the time of development of glomerulonephritis; in industrialized countries, clinical disease is seen more often in adults and is associated with *Staphylococcus aureus* and gram-negative bacteria.
- Treatment of membranoproliferative glomerulonephritis is nonspecific and includes immunosuppression when nephrotic-range proteinuria and/or kidney dysfunction is present.

Kidney Manifestations of Deposition Diseases

Overview

Various kidney diseases are associated with deposition of immunoglobulin (Ig) and non-Ig proteins. On electron microscopy, these deposits can be unstructured or organized into fibrils or tubules (**Figure 14**). Monoclonal Ig deposits may be caused by myeloma, Waldenström macroglobulinemia, or chronic lymphocytic leukemia, or by the clonal expansion of Ig-secreting cells that do not meet the strict definition of these disorders, which has been termed *monoclonal gammopathy of renal significance* (MGRS). The pathological findings associated with monoclonal Ig deposition can include proliferative glomerulonephritis, AL amyloid, type 1 cryoglobulinemia, and, occasionally, immunotactoid and fibrillary glomerulopathy. Polyclonal Ig deposits include

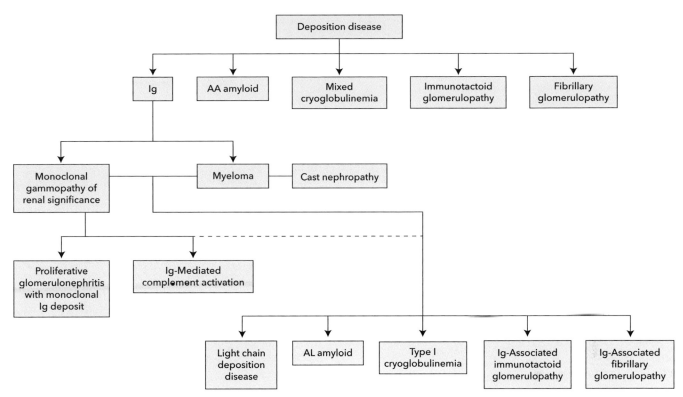

FIGURE 14. Deposition diseases can be divided into five major categories: immunoglobulin (Ig)-related disease, amyloid, cryoglobulinemia, immunotactoid glomerulopathy, and fibrillary glomerulopathy. Ig-related disease can be further divided into multiple myeloma and monoclonal gammopathy of renal significance (MGRS). Although some histopathological findings occur more commonly in either multiple myeloma (such as cast nephropathy) or MGRS, most have been reported in either disorder.

mixed cryoglobulinemia, whereas non-Ig proteins contribute to AA amyloid and to most cases of immunotactoid and fibrillary glomerulopathy.

Monoclonal Immunoglobulin–Associated Kidney Disease

A wide array of renal lesions can be caused by clonal expansion of Ig-secreting cells. If there are greater than 10% plasma cells on bone marrow biopsy or the presence of an extramedullary plasmacytoma, a diagnosis of multiple myeloma can be made. However, as noted above, paraproteinemia caused by clonal expansion of Ig-secreting cells that do not meet the strict definition of myeloma, Waldenström macroglobulinemia, or chronic lymphocytic leukemia can be associated with nephrotoxicity. Although some of the findings noted pathologically occur more frequently with either MGRS or myeloma, except for myeloma cast nephropathy seen exclusively with myeloma, all the renal lesions can occur in each of these disorders. Because filtered light chains are endocytosed by proximal tubule cells and are nephrotoxic, patients may present with proximal tubular dysfunction with Fanconi syndrome; common features include glycosuria, phosphaturia, and normal anion gap metabolic acidosis. Kidney function may be normal or abnormal.

Myeloma Cast Nephropathy

Myeloma cast nephropathy occurs in the presence of a markedly increased concentration of free light chains and is always associated with multiple myeloma. Light chains are freely filtered by the glomerulus and combine with secreted Tamm-Horsfall protein to form obstructing casts. These tubular casts have a characteristic fractured appearance on microscopic examination. Patients with cast nephropathy present with acute or slowly progressive kidney injury. Serum free light chains are extremely elevated. Treatment is aimed at reducing the concentration of free light chains using chemotherapy. Plasmapheresis may also be beneficial in selected patients.

Monoclonal Gammopathy of Renal Significance

Monoclonal gammopathy of renal significance (MGRS) is characterized by kidney damage caused by monoclonal Ig that is secreted by a B cell or plasma cell clone not meeting diagnostic criteria for multiple myeloma or a lymphoproliferative disorder. All pathological findings associated with the clonal expansion of Ig-secreting cells can be seen in both myeloma and MGRS. The underlying pathology is likely determined by the characteristics of the secreted protein. Entities associated with MGRS include proliferative glomerulonephritis with monoclonal Ig deposits (PGNMID), C3 glomerulopathy with monoclonal gammopathy, AL amyloid, type 1 cryoglobulinemia, fibrillary glomerulonephritis, and immunotactoid glomerulopathy.

Kidney manifestations of MGRS are usually caused by deposition of monoclonal Ig light chains. Patients can present with both nephrotic and subnephrotic proteinuria, hematuria, and elevated serum creatinine.

Kidney biopsy is necessary to make the diagnosis. In addition to evaluating for underlying myeloma and chronic lymphocytic leukemia, further testing may include serum and urine protein electrophoresis, immunofixation, measurement of free light chains, and bone marrow biopsy. Because treatment is aimed at eradication of the expanded clonal line, it is important that the care of patients with MGRS be coordinated with a myeloma specialist.

Amyloidosis

Amyloidosis is a disorder characterized by the fibrillary deposition of insoluble amyloid proteins that form β-pleated sheets, which exhibit green birefringence on polarizing microscopy when stained with Congo red. Amyloid fibrils are approximately 10 nm in diameter, as opposed to the larger microtubules seen in fibrillary glomerulonephritis and immunotactoid glomerulopathy. Although amyloid can be made up of numerous proteins, kidney disease is most commonly caused by AL amyloid or AA amyloid. AL amyloid is composed of monoclonal λ (most commonly) or κ light chains produced by either MGRS or myeloma; AA amyloid is formed by serum amyloid A protein, an acute phase reactant produced in various inflammatory diseases such as rheumatoid arthritis, inflammatory bowel disease, chronic osteomyelitis, and familial Mediterranean fever. Patients with renal amyloid frequently present with nephrotic-range proteinuria. Less commonly, amyloid can affect only the renal vasculature or tubular-interstitium and have minimal or no proteinuria. Treatment is aimed at the underlying disease.

Monoclonal Immunoglobulin Deposition Disease

Monoclonal light chains (usually κ) or heavy chains can be deposited in the kidney and manifest as proteinuria and kidney failure. Unlike AL amyloid, these proteins do not form β-pleated sheets and do not stain with Congo red. These deposits can be limited to the basement membrane, giving a microscopic appearance similar to that of diabetic nodular sclerosis (light chain deposition disease), or can activate complement and induce a proliferative glomerulonephritis (PGNMID). In some cases, an underlying plasma cell dyscrasia or lymphoproliferative disorder can be identified, but criteria for myeloma or chronic lymphocytic leukemia are often absent.

Cryoglobulinemia

Of the three types of cryoglobulinemia, kidney involvement occurs most frequently with type II (mixed Ig) cryoglobulinemia and is usually associated with hepatitis C virus infection. Patients can present with a nephritic picture: elevated serum creatinine, hypertension, proteinuria, and hematuria. Membranoproliferative glomerulonephritis is usually noted on biopsy. Occasionally, a rapidly progressive glomerulonephritis with crescent formation can occur. A palpable purpuric rash is frequently present on the lower extremities. Because hepatitis C is the predominant cause, treatment is aimed at eradication of the virus.

Fibrillary and Immunotactoid Glomerulopathy

Although rare, both fibrillary and immunotactoid glomerulopathy are becoming increasingly recognized causes of kidney disease. These diseases are caused by glomerular deposition of microtubular structures that are larger than amyloid (20 nm in fibrillary glomerulopathy and >30 nm in immunotactoid glomerulopathy) and do not stain with Congo red. Proteinuria, frequently in the nephrotic range, and hematuria are common. Although the pathogenesis of these entities is unknown, both have been associated with paraproteinemia. Treatment is usually unsuccessful, and kidney outcomes are poor.

KEY POINTS

- Patients with myeloma cast nephropathy present with acute or slowly progressive kidney injury and have extremely elevated serum free light chains; treatment is aimed at reducing the concentration of free light chains using chemotherapy.
- Diseases causing monoclonal gammopathy of renal significance can present with either nephrotic or subnephrotic proteinuria, hematuria, and elevated serum creatinine; kidney biopsy is necessary to make the diagnosis, and treatment is aimed at eradication of the expanded clonal line.
- Kidney disease in amyloidosis is most commonly caused by AL amyloid composed of monoclonal λ or κ light chains or AA amyloid formed by serum amyloid A protein; patients frequently present with nephrotic-range proteinuria, and treatment is aimed at the underlying disorder.
- Kidney involvement in cryoglobulinemia occurs most frequently with type II (mixed) cryoglobulins and is usually associated with hepatitis C virus infection; treatment is directed at eradication of hepatitis C virus.

Genetic Disorders and Kidney Disease

Genetic Cystic Kidney Disorders

Genetic cystic kidney disorders are categorized in **Table 21**.

Autosomal Dominant Polycystic Kidney Disease

Autosomal dominant polycystic kidney disease (ADPKD) is the leading genetic cause of end-stage kidney disease (ESKD) and the fourth leading cause of ESKD. ADPKD manifests as large kidneys with multiple kidney cysts (**Figure 15**). Genetic mutations in *PKD1* and *PKD2*, which encode for proteins that regulate differentiation and proliferation of renal tubular epithelial cells, account for approximately 85% and 15% of cases, respectively. More than 90% of mutations are inherited as an autosomal dominant trait, with spontaneous germline mutations accounting for the remaining cases.

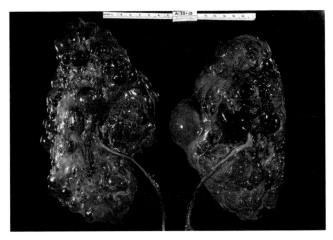

FIGURE 15. Autosomal dominant polycystic kidney disease with multiple bilateral cysts, which replace the normal smooth architecture of the kidneys and lead to markedly increased kidney size.

Image from the CDC Public Health Image Library.

Screening and Diagnosis

Ultrasonography is the most common and least costly screening method for ADPKD. Ultrasonography criteria for diagnosing ADPKD are based on the number of visible cysts, the patient's age, and a family history of ADPKD. Direct DNA sequencing of the *PKD1* and *PKD2* genes is increasingly used to confirm diagnosis or, in some cases, is performed in lieu of imaging. Gene linkage testing, which identifies DNA markers in several members of a family, can also be used in patients with a family history of ADPKD.

Clinical Manifestations

Early in the disease, there are generally no symptoms. Diagnosis is therefore often delayed in patients without a known family history of ADPKD. The first sign of ADPKD is often hypertension; other early signs and symptoms include hematuria (macroscopic or microscopic), pain or bloating in the back or abdomen, urinary tract infection, or kidney stones. In patients without a family history, these presentations usually lead to imaging studies that reveal ADPKD. CT or MRI may be used to evaluate for complications in patients with known ADPKD, such as bleeding into a cyst or a suspected kidney stone.

Extrarenal manifestations include hepatic cysts (detected in >80% of patients over their lifetime), mitral valve prolapse, inguinal and umbilical hernias, and intracranial aneurysms (detected in 5%-10% of patients, with a strong familial pattern).

Management

Patients with ADPKD have a >50% chance of progressing to ESKD by age 70 years. No disease-specific therapies currently exist; therefore, management is focused on controlling blood pressure and addressing complications of disease. Vasopressin blockade with tolvaptan in patients with ADPKD has been shown in two randomized clinical trials to delay the need for

TABLE 21.	Genetic Cystic Kidney Disorders		
Disorder	**Inheritance**	**Gene(s)**	**Features/Comments**
Autosomal dominant polycystic kidney disease	AD	PKD1 PKD2	Most common inherited kidney disorder (5% of ESKD cases); intracranial cerebral aneurysm; mitral valve prolapse; hepatic cysts; diverticulosis
Autosomal recessive polycystic kidney disease	AR	PKHD1	Causes ESKD in infancy or childhood; hepatic fibrosis; portal hypertension; homozygous mutations cause complete loss of function: severe cystic kidney disease, oligohydramnios, pulmonary hypoplasia, Potter syndrome (limb deformities, typical facial appearance, pulmonary hypoplasia)
Tuberous sclerosis complex	AD	TSC1 TSC2	Characterized by benign hamartomas; epilepsy, brain tumors, developmental delay, autism, and lung disease may also occur; renal angiomyolipomas are common; kidney cysts may develop
Nephronophthisis	AR	Multiple (13)	Most common genetic cause of ESKD detected in childhood/adolescence; interstitial fibrosis; renal medullary cysts; a renal concentrating defect and/or salt wasting; retinitis pigmentosa

AD = autosomal dominant; AR = autosomal recessive; ESKD = end-stage kidney disease.

dialysis from 6 to 9 years. However, tolvaptan carries an FDA-mandated safety warning about the possibility of irreversible liver injury, and it has not been approved by the FDA for use in ADPKD.

The Guidelines for the Management of Patients with Unruptured Intracranial Aneurysms from the American Heart Association/American Stroke Association recommend that patients with a history of ADPKD, particularly those with a family history of intracranial aneurysm, should be offered screening by CT angiography or MR angiography. This is a class I recommendation (should be performed because benefit greatly exceeds risk) based on level B evidence (data derived from a single randomized trial or nonrandomized studies).

Tuberous Sclerosis Complex

Tuberous sclerosis complex (TSC) is a genetic disorder with mutations in the tumor-suppressing genes *TSC1* or *TSC2* and resulting tumors in many organs, primarily in the brain, eyes, heart, kidney, skin, and lungs. Although TSC is most frequently diagnosed in the pediatric population, mild disease may escape detection until adulthood. Nearly 1 million people worldwide are estimated to have TSC, with approximately 50,000 in the United States.

Renal angiomyolipomas occur in 75% of patients with TSC and can be detected by CT, ultrasonography, or MRI. Renal cell carcinoma occurs in 1% to 2% of adults with TSC, and therefore screening with abdominal MRI is recommended every 1 to 3 years. Kidney cysts may also develop. The features of TSC that most strongly affect quality of life are generally associated with the brain: seizures, developmental delay, intellectual disability, and autism.

Therapy is rarely needed for the kidney manifestations of TSC. Surgery or related interventions (radiofrequency ablation, selective arterial embolization) may be required for large or hemorrhagic angiomyolipomas.

KEY POINTS

- Autosomal dominant polycystic kidney disease is characterized by large kidneys with multiple kidney cysts, hypertension, hematuria, pain or bloating in the back or abdomen, urinary tract infection, or kidney stones.
- No disease-specific therapies currently exist for autosomal dominant polycystic kidney disease; therefore, management is focused on controlling blood pressure and addressing complications of disease.
- Kidney manifestations of tuberous sclerosis complex include renal angiomyolipomas, renal cell carcinoma, and cysts; surgery or related interventions may be required for large or hemorrhagic angiomyolipomas.

Genetic Noncystic Kidney Disorders

Genetic noncystic kidney disorders are categorized in **Table 22**.

Collagen Type IV-Related Nephropathies

Type IV collagen is an integral component of the glomerular basement membrane (GBM). Structural defects in this protein, due to genetic variations, can result in manifestations spanning from GBM thinning to progressive glomerular injury.

Hereditary Nephritis

Hereditary nephritis (Alport syndrome) is a glomerular disease associated with sensorineural hearing loss and characteristic ocular findings that include corneal dystrophies, microcornea, arcus, iris atrophy, cataracts, spontaneous lens rupture, spherophakia, and anterior lenticonus. There are three genetic variants: X-linked (80%), autosomal recessive (15%), and autosomal dominant (5%). Females with the X-linked variant can be asymptomatic carriers or can develop kidney disease depending on activity of the X chromosome in somatic renal cells. The disease has a prevalence of 0.4% among U.S. adults.

Diagnosis has traditionally been made by kidney biopsy with electron microscopy; the hallmark finding is prominent thickening and lamellation of the GBM in a "basket-weave" appearance. In patients with a clearly documented family history and abnormal urinary findings, diagnosis is increasingly being made by genetic testing. Genetic testing is also the most reliable way to identify heterozygote carriers of type IV collagen mutations. Proteinuria, hypertension, and chronic kidney disease (CKD) usually progress to ESKD between the late teenage years and the fourth decade of life. Management is supportive, including blood pressure control via renin-angiotensin system blockade.

Thin Glomerular Basement Membrane Disease

Thin glomerular basement membrane disease (benign familial hematuria) is associated with type IV collagen variants causing GBM thinning, which results in hematuria without significant proteinuria or ensuing glomerulosclerosis. Up to 5% of the population may be affected. Although diagnosis can be made using electron microscopy of kidney biopsy material, thin glomerular basement membrane disease is usually a clinical diagnosis based on benign presentation and course (normal kidney function with microscopic hematuria and little or no proteinuria) and positive family history of similarly benign phenotype (family history of isolated hematuria without kidney failure). The disease has excellent long-term prognosis with rare progression to CKD. Management is supportive.

Fabry Disease

Fabry disease is an X-linked recessive inborn error of glycosphingolipid metabolism caused by deficiency of α-galactosidase A. The gene responsible for α-galactosidase is located on the long arm of the X chromosome, with almost 200 mutations identified. The enzyme deficiency leads to defective storage of sphingolipid and progressive endothelial

TABLE 22. Genetic Noncystic Kidney Disorders

Disorder	Inheritance	Gene(s)	Features/Comments
Autosomal dominant tubulointerstitial kidney disease (also called medullary cystic kidney disease or uromodulin-associated kidney disease)	AD	*UMOD; REN; MUC1; HNF1B*	Rare; medullary cysts may or may not be present; slow progression to ESKD; bland urine sediment; may be associated with gout and anemia
Collagen type IV–related nephropathies			
Hereditary nephritis (Alport syndrome)	X-linked	*COL4A5*	Sensorineural hearing loss; lenticonus (conical deformation of the lens)
	AD or AR	*COL4A3*	Similar phenotype as X-linked with some variability
	AD or AR	*COL4A4*	Similar to *COL4A3*
Thin glomerular basement membrane disease (benign familial hematuria)	Primarily AD	*COL4A3; COL4A4*	Microscopic or macroscopic hematuria
Hereditary nephrotic syndromes			
Congenital nephropathy (Finnish type)	AR	*NEPH1; NEPH2*	Severe perinatal nephrotic syndrome; ESKD; kidney transplantation is only treatment
Familial FSGS	AR or AD	*NEPH2; ACTN4; TRPC6; INF2; APOL1*	The nephrotic syndrome; ESKD; should be considered in FSGS patients who are infants, are young (<25 years) and steroid-resistant, or have family history of ESKD
Denys-Drash syndrome	AR	*WT1*	Cause of pediatric nephrotic syndrome; associated with urogenital abnormalities
Fabry disease	X-linked	*GLA*	Progressive kidney disease; premature coronary artery disease; severe neuropathic pain; telangiectasias; angiokeratomas
APOL1 nephropathy	AR	*APOL1*	High-risk genotypes present in ~13% of black persons; account for a large fraction of nondiabetic kidney disease in black persons

AD = autosomal dominant; *APOL1* = apolipoprotein 1; AR = autosomal recessive; ESKD = end-stage kidney disease; FSGS = focal segmental glomerulosclerosis.

accumulation, causing abnormalities in the skin, eye, kidney, heart, brain, and peripheral nervous system.

Fabry disease should be considered as a cause of CKD of unknown etiology in young adulthood. Diagnosis can be made by kidney biopsy but also can be made noninvasively with measurement of leukocyte enzymatic activity and subsequent genetic confirmation. Screening for the disease is recommended for family members of affected patients. Enzyme replacement therapy with recombinant human α-galactosidase A is available.

Apolipoprotein L1 Nephropathy

Black persons develop kidney failure at rates four to five times higher than white persons. Recently, genetic variants in the apolipoprotein L1 (*APOL1*) gene were discovered that explain a large fraction of this health disparity. Two risk alleles for kidney disease (G1 and G2) have been identified in the *APOL1* gene. The transmission of disease risk is consistent with recessive inheritance: The high-risk *APOL1* genotype can be G1/G1, G1/G2, or G2/G2. Approximately 12% to 15% of black persons inherit a high-risk *APOL1* genotype; this accounts for a large fraction of nondiabetic kidney disease in black persons. High-risk *APOL1* alleles are unusually prevalent possibly because they conferred a survival advantage in sub-Saharan Africa by

enhancing innate immunity against African trypanosomal disease (African sleeping sickness).

Persons with a high-risk *APOL1* genotype have an approximately 10-fold increased risk for focal segmental glomerulosclerosis, a 7-fold increased risk for hypertension-attributed ESKD, and, among those with HIV infection, a 29-fold increased risk for HIV-associated nephropathy. In addition, the *APOL1* risk genotype is associated with an increased risk for progression to CKD in other nondiabetic kidney diseases, including lupus nephritis and primary membranous nephropathy.

KEY POINTS

- Hereditary nephritis (Alport syndrome) is a glomerular disease associated with sensorineural hearing loss and characteristic ocular findings; proteinuria, hypertension, and chronic kidney disease usually progress to end-stage kidney disease between the late teenage years and the fourth decade of life.

- Thin glomerular basement membrane disease (benign familial hematuria) results in hematuria without significant proteinuria or ensuing glomerulosclerosis, with rare progression to chronic kidney disease.

(Continued)

- Fabry disease should be considered as a cause of chronic kidney disease of unknown etiology in young adulthood; treatment with recombinant human α-galactosidase A is available.

- High-risk *APOL1* genotype confers increased risk for chronic kidney disease in black persons, including an approximately 10-fold increased risk for focal segmental glomerulosclerosis, a 7-fold increased risk for hypertension-attributed end-stage kidney disease, and a 29-fold increased risk for HIV-associated nephropathy among those with HIV infection.

Acute Kidney Injury

Definition

Acute kidney injury (AKI) is characterized by a sudden decrease in kidney function resulting in an increase in serum creatinine concentration and the accumulation of nitrogenous excretory products over a course of hours to days. AKI is commonly accompanied by decreased urine output, fluid retention, metabolic acidosis, hyperkalemia, and hyperphosphatemia. The Kidney Disease: Improving Global Outcomes (KDIGO) Acute Kidney Injury Work Group definitions for AKI are described in **Table 23**. Multiple studies have shown a correlation between more severe stages of AKI and worse clinical outcomes.

AKI is associated with high morbidity, mortality, and health care costs. Patients with AKI have an increased risk for developing chronic kidney disease (CKD) and end-stage kidney disease (ESKD). Likewise, patients with pre-existing CKD are at an increased risk for developing acute-on-chronic kidney failure. Given its substantial morbidity and mortality, AKI care should be focused on prevention, early recognition and diagnosis, and management of complications.

TABLE 23. KDIGO Definition of Acute Kidney Injury[a]

Stage	Serum Creatinine Criteria	Urine Output Criteria
1	Increase in S_{Cr} to 1.5 to 1.9 times baseline within 7 days or ≥0.3 mg/dL (26.5 µmol/L) within 48 h	<0.5 mL/kg/h for 6 to 12 h
2	Increase in S_{Cr} to 2 to 2.9 times baseline	<0.5 mL/kg/h for ≥12 h
3	Increase in S_{Cr} to 3 times baseline or ≥4.0 mg/dL (356.6 µmol/L) or initiation of RRT or, in patients <18 years, a decrease in eGFR <35 mL/min/1.73 m²	<0.3 mL/kg/h for ≥24 h or anuria for ≥12 h

eGFR = estimated glomerular filtration rate; KDIGO = Kidney Disease: Improving Global Outcomes; RRT = renal replacement therapy; S_{Cr} = serum creatinine.

[a]The KDIGO definition is based on the RIFLE (Risk, Injury, Failure, Loss, and ESKD) and AKIN (Acute Kidney Injury Network) criteria.

- The Kidney Disease: Improving Global Outcomes (KDIGO) Acute Kidney Injury Work Group defines acute kidney injury by any of the following: increase in serum creatinine by ≥0.3 mg/dL (26.5 µmol/L) within 48 hours; an increase in serum creatinine to ≥1.5 times baseline over 7 days; or a urine volume <0.5 mL/kg/h for 6 hours.

Epidemiology and Pathophysiology

The reported incidence of AKI varies markedly depending on the definition of AKI applied and the patient population studied. The incidence of AKI based on the KDIGO definition is estimated to be 21% of all hospital admissions, with 11% requiring dialysis support. In the ICU, AKI affects >50% of patients. Mortality varies depending on the severity of AKI, underlying cause, and patient population. Critically ill patients with AKI in the context of multiorgan failure have been reported to have mortality rates >50%, especially when dialysis therapy is required.

AKI can be divided into prerenal, intrinsic, and postrenal causes (**Table 24**). Prerenal AKI (prerenal azotemia) is caused by decreased renal perfusion. The integrity of renal tissue is preserved, and tubular and glomerular function remains normal. Intrinsic AKI is caused by structural damage to the renal parenchyma. Postrenal AKI refers to AKI caused by urinary tract obstruction. Prerenal AKI and acute tubular necrosis (ATN) account for approximately 65% to 75% of AKI cases in hospitalized patients. **H**

- Prerenal acute kidney injury and acute tubular necrosis account for approximately 65% to 75% of acute kidney injury cases in hospitalized patients.

Clinical Manifestations

Patients with AKI can be asymptomatic until extreme loss of kidney function occurs, and patients with mild to moderate AKI are often diagnosed by laboratory studies only. Patients with AKI can also present with oliguria (urine output <500 mL/d or <0.3 mL/kg/h) or anuria (urine output <50 mL/d). Severe AKI can lead to symptoms from volume overload, electrolyte abnormalities, anemia, platelet dysfunction, and uremia. Uremic symptoms include nausea, vomiting, anorexia, weight loss, fatigue, muscle cramps, restless legs, mental status changes, pruritus, asterixis, seizures, and pericarditis. **H**

- Patients with acute kidney injury (AKI) can be asymptomatic until extreme loss of kidney function occurs; severe AKI can lead to symptoms from volume overload, electrolyte abnormalities, anemia, platelet dysfunction, and uremia.

TABLE 24. Causes of Acute Kidney Injury

Cause	Examples
Prerenal	
Volume depletion	Renal losses; GI fluid losses; hemorrhage; burns
Decreased cardiac output	Heart failure; massive pulmonary embolus; acute coronary syndrome
Systemic vasodilation	Sepsis; cirrhosis; anaphylaxis; anesthesia
Intrarenal vasoconstriction	Drugs (NSAIDs, COX-2 inhibitors, amphotericin B, calcineurin inhibitors, contrast agents); hypercalcemia; hepatorenal syndrome
Efferent arteriolar vasodilation	Renin inhibitors; ACE inhibitors; ARBs
Intrinsic	
Acute tubular necrosis	Ischemic: prolonged prerenal AKI; abdominal compartment syndrome
	Drug-induced: aminoglycosides; vancomycin; polymyxins; lithium; amphotericin B; pentamidine; cisplatin; foscarnet; tenofovir; cidofovir; carboplatin; ifosfamide; zoledronate; contrast agents; sucrose; immune globulins; mannitol; hydroxyethyl starch; dextran; NSAIDs; synthetic cannabinoids; amphetamines
	Pigment: rhabdomyolysis; intravascular hemolysis
Acute interstitial nephritis	Drug-induced: cephalosporins; penicillin; methicillin; fluoroquinolones; sulfonamides; rifampin; NSAIDs; COX-2 inhibitors; proton pump inhibitors; 5-aminosalicylates; indinavir; abacavir; allopurinol; phenytoin; triamterene; furosemide; thiazide diuretics; phenytoin; carbamazepine; Chinese herb nephropathy
	Infection: pyelonephritis; viral nephritides; leptospirosis; *Legionella*; *Mycobacterium tuberculosis*
	Autoimmune: Sjögren syndrome; sarcoidosis; SLE; TINU syndrome; IgG4-related disease
	Malignancy: lymphoma; leukemia; multiple myeloma
Acute glomerulonephritis	Infection-related glomerulonephritis; cryoglobulinemia; RPGN; IgA; lupus nephritis; renal vasculitis; anti-GBM antibody disease
Acute vascular syndromes	Macrovascular: renal artery occlusion; renal vein thrombosis; polyarteritis nodosa
	Microvascular:
	Disease-associated TMA: HUS; atypical HUS; TTP; HELLP; scleroderma renal crisis; hypertensive emergency
	Drug-induced TMA: quinine; cancer therapies (gemcitabine, mitomycin, bevacizumab, bortezomib, sunitinib); calcineurin inhibitors (cyclosporine, tacrolimus); drugs of abuse (cocaine, ecstasy, intravenous extended-release oxymorphone)
	Other drugs: clopidogrel; cyclosporine; tacrolimus; anti-angiogenesis drugs; interferon; mTOR inhibitors
	Atheroembolic disease
Intratubular obstruction	Paraprotein: myeloma
	Crystals: TLS; sulfonamides; triamterene; ciprofloxacin; ethylene glycol; acyclovir; indinavir; atazanavir; methotrexate; orlistat; large doses of vitamin C; sodium phosphate purgatives
Postrenal	
Upper tract obstruction	Nephrolithiasis; blood clots; external compression
Lower tract obstruction	BPH; neurogenic bladder; blood clots; cancer; urethral stricture

AKI = acute kidney injury; ARB = angiotensin receptor blocker; BPH = benign prostatic hyperplasia; COX = cyclooxygenase; GBM = glomerular basement membrane; GI = gastrointestinal; HELLP = hemolysis, elevated liver enzymes, and low platelets; HUS = hemolytic uremic syndrome; mTOR = mammalian target of rapamycin; RPGN = rapidly progressive glomerulonephritis; SLE = systemic lupus erythematosus; TINU = tubulointerstitial nephritis and uveitis; TLS = tumor lysis syndrome; TMA = thrombotic microangiopathy; TTP = thrombotic thrombocytopenic purpura.

Diagnosis

The diagnosis of AKI is based on increased levels of serum creatinine and blood urea nitrogen (BUN). The most reliable way to distinguish AKI from CKD is knowledge of previous serum creatinine levels; documentation of similarly elevated creatinine levels for ≥3 months suggests that the kidney failure is chronic. However, serum creatinine and BUN concentrations can be increased by multiple factors independent of kidney function, limiting their specificity for diagnosis of AKI

(Table 25). Furthermore, serum creatinine is not a sensitive marker of kidney injury in patients with sepsis, liver disease, muscle wasting, or fluid overload and does not provide any information regarding the cause of AKI. BUN can also be normal in patients with AKI who are malnourished or have liver disease. Moreover, the rise in serum creatinine is delayed 24 to 36 hours after the onset of injury and decline in glomerular filtration rate (GFR).

A thorough patient history, physical examination, and analysis of laboratory and image findings are necessary to

TABLE 25. Selected Examples of Causes of Elevated Blood Urea Nitrogen and Serum Creatinine Without Acute Kidney Injury

Elevated Blood Urea Nitrogen
Gastrointestinal bleeding
Protein loading, including albumin infusions
Catabolic steroids
Tetracycline antibiotics
Elevated Serum Creatinine
Medications that block creatinine secretion: cimetidine; trimethoprim; cobicistat; dolutegravir
Creatine ethyl ester (an aid for athletic performance and for muscle development for body builders)
Substances that interfere with creatinine assay: acetoacetate; cefoxitin; flucytosine

CONT.

identify the AKI as prerenal, intrinsic, or postrenal. The history focuses on identifying potential nephrotoxic medications (including over-the-counter medications, herbal products, and recreational drugs), recent exposure to iodinated contrast agents, predisposing conditions for AKI, and urinary obstructive symptoms (see Table 24). Physical examination focuses on volume status, signs of systemic illness that might impair kidney function, and evidence of urinary obstruction (such as a palpable bladder or flank pain). Laboratory evaluation includes BUN and creatinine concentrations, electrolytes, complete blood count, and assessment of the urine (urine indices, urinalysis, and microscopic evaluation of the urine sediment) (**Table 26**).

In patients with oliguria, the fractional excretion of sodium (FE_{Na}) can help distinguish between prerenal AKI and ATN. FE_{Na} measures the ratio of sodium excreted (urine sodium × volume) to sodium filtered (serum sodium × GFR) and is calculated as follows:

$$(U_{Sodium} \times P_{Creatinine})/(U_{Creatinine} \times P_{Sodium}) \times 100\%$$

In prerenal AKI, decreased renal perfusion increases sodium and water reabsorption, resulting in a decrease in urinary sodium excretion and $FE_{Na} <1\%$. However, $FE_{Na} <1\%$ can occur with other causes of AKI that are not prerenal but have intact tubular function: contrast nephropathy, pigment nephropathy, glomerulonephritis, and early obstruction. $FE_{Na} >2\%$ suggests impaired tubular ability to reabsorb sodium and is consistent with ATN. However, FE_{Na} may be >2% in patients with prerenal AKI who have urinary sodium loss due to diuretics, adrenal insufficiency, or from bicarbonaturia in severe metabolic alkalosis. FE_{Na} may also be >2% in prerenal patients with CKD as a result of impaired tubular function.

In the setting of diuretics, the fractional excretion of urea (FE_{Urea}) can be used to diagnose prerenal AKI, with $FE_{Urea} <35\%$ suggesting the diagnosis. FE_{Urea} is calculated as follows:

$$(U_{Urea} \times P_{Creatinine})/(U_{Creatinine} \times P_{Urea}) \times 100\%$$

Ultrasonography of the kidneys and bladder should be obtained for suspected urinary tract obstruction or when the underlying cause of AKI is unclear. Kidney size may help distinguish between AKI and CKD because diminished kidney size and cortical thinning suggest CKD. Kidney size can be normal in patients with CKD from infiltrative disorders such as diabetes mellitus, HIV-associated nephropathy, amyloidosis, or multiple myeloma. Kidney biopsy should be considered in patients with AKI from no apparent cause, suspected glomerulonephritis, or unexplained systemic disease. ■

TABLE 26. Diagnostic Findings in Acute Kidney Injury

Condition	BUN-Creatinine Ratio	Urine Osmolality (mOsm/kg H₂O)	Urine Sodium (mEq/L [mmol/L])	FE_{Na}	Urinalysis and Microscopy
Prerenal	>20:1	>500	<20	<1%	Specific gravity >1.020; normal or hyaline casts
Acute tubular necrosis	10-15:1	~300	>40	>2%ᵃ	Specific gravity ~1.010; pigmented granular (muddy brown) casts and tubular epithelial cells
Acute interstitial nephritis	Variable	Variable, ~300	Variable	Variable	Mild proteinuria; leukocytes; erythrocytes; leukocyte casts; eosinophiluria
Acute glomerulonephritis	Variable	Variable	Variable	Variable	Proteinuria; dysmorphic erythrocytes; erythrocyte casts
Intratubular obstruction	Variable	Variable	Variable	Variable	Crystalluria or Bence-Jones proteinuria
Acute vascular syndromes	Variable	Variable	Variable	Variable	Variable hematuria
Postrenal	Variable	Variable	Variable	Variable	Variable; bland

BUN = blood urea nitrogen; FE_{Na} = fractional excretion of sodium.

ᵃFE_{Na} can be low in contrast-induced nephropathy and pigment nephropathy.

- In patients with oliguria, the fractional excretion of sodium (FE_{Na}) can help distinguish between prerenal acute kidney injury (AKI) and acute tubular necrosis (ATN); FE_{Na} <1% indicates prerenal AKI, and FE_{Na} >2% is consistent with ATN.
- In the setting of diuretics, the fractional excretion of urea (FE_{Urea}) can be used to diagnose prerenal acute kidney injury, with FE_{Urea} <35% suggesting the diagnosis.
- Ultrasonography of the kidneys and bladder should be obtained for suspected urinary tract obstruction or when the underlying cause of acute kidney injury is unclear.

Causes

AKI can be divided into prerenal, intrinsic, and postrenal causes.

Prerenal Acute Kidney Injury

See Table 24 for the causes of prerenal AKI.

Prerenal AKI (prerenal azotemia) is caused by underperfusion of the kidney with a subsequent decrease in GFR, which is reversible with appropriate therapy. Renal hypoperfusion can occur due to intravascular volume depletion, decreased effective arterial circulation, renal vasoconstriction, and/or medications. Patients may have a history of acute hemorrhage, loss of gastrointestinal fluids, heart failure, decompensated liver disease, sepsis, or recent diuretic or NSAID use. Physical signs of hypovolemia include hypotension, tachycardia, orthostasis, and decreased skin turgor. Patients with heart failure or cirrhosis have physical examination findings supporting these conditions.

In prerenal AKI, the kidney responds by reabsorbing urea, sodium, and water, often resulting in a BUN-creatinine ratio >20:1; however, a normal BUN-creatinine ratio does not exclude prerenal AKI. Other laboratory values that support a diagnosis of prerenal AKI are listed in Table 26. Prerenal AKI due to hypovolemia can be distinguished from ATN by the renal response to a fluid challenge. If serum creatinine recovers to baseline with fluid repletion, the cause of AKI is likely to be prerenal.

Drug-induced prerenal AKI typically results from decreased blood flow to the kidney or intraglomerular hemodynamic alterations. Diuretics can cause prerenal AKI from volume depletion. Drugs affecting vasodilatation of the afferent arterioles or vasoconstriction of the efferent arterioles can cause prerenal AKI, especially in the setting of volume depletion, decreased effective arterial circulation, or CKD. NSAIDs, including cyclooxygenase-2 inhibitors, cause AKI by diminishing the renal vasodilatory effect of prostaglandins. ACE inhibitors and angiotensin receptor blockers (ARBs) prevent efferent vasoconstriction by inhibiting angiotensin II. Calcineurin inhibitors such as cyclosporine and tacrolimus can cause prerenal AKI from afferent and efferent vasoconstriction.

Management of prerenal AKI includes discontinuing nephrotoxins and increasing renal perfusion by treating the underlying cause, such as correcting volume deficits. If prerenal AKI is not recognized and treated in a timely fashion, prolonged renal hypoperfusion will result in ATN and progressive intrinsic kidney failure. H

- Prerenal acute kidney injury is caused by underperfusion of the kidney with a subsequent decrease in glomerular filtration rate, which is reversible with discontinuing nephrotoxins and treating the underlying cause.

Intrinsic Kidney Diseases

Intrinsic AKI occurs from structural damage to the renal tubules, interstitium, glomerulus, or vascular structures, or intratubular obstruction (see Table 24).

Acute Tubular Necrosis

ATN due to ischemia, nephrotoxins, and/or sepsis is the most common cause of AKI in hospitalized patients. A patient history of sepsis or nephrotoxin exposure along with assessment of hemodynamics and volume status can aid in the diagnosis. Laboratory values suggestive of ATN include a BUN-creatinine ratio <10 to 15:1, an FE_{Na} >2%, and a urine osmolality of approximately 300 mOsm/kg H_2O (see Table 26), reflecting the failure to maximally dilute or concentrate urine (isosthenuria). Urine sediment is characterized by many tubular epithelial cells and coarse granular (muddy brown) casts (**Figure 16**).

Unlike prerenal AKI, ATN does not rapidly improve with restoration of intravascular volume and blood flow to the kidneys. Treatment is supportive because no pharmacologic therapies exist. Complete or partial renal recovery can take days to weeks.

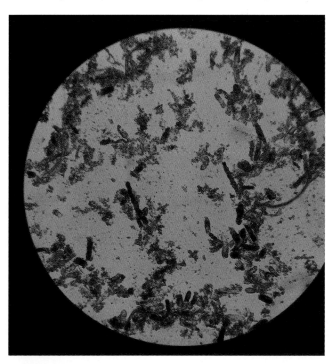

FIGURE 16. Urine sediment showing multiple coarse, granular (muddy brown) casts characteristic of acute tubular necrosis.

CONT.

Compared with oliguric ATN, patients with nonoliguric ATN are thought to have less severe kidney injury and a better renal prognosis. Patients with baseline CKD are less likely to recover kidney function compared with patients with baseline normal kidney function. Patients with severe ATN who require acute dialysis may recover kidney function or progress to dialysis-dependent ESKD.

Ischemic Acute Tubular Necrosis

Severe ischemia due to prolonged hypotension or prolonged prerenal state can cause ATN (see Table 24). The ischemic injury leads to cytokine release, oxygen-free radical and enzyme production, endothelial activation and leukocyte adhesion, activation of coagulation, and apoptosis. GFR declines due to renal vasoconstriction, tubular back leak of filtrate into the bloodstream, and tubular obstruction from sloughed cellular debris. Ischemic ATN is mostly reversible but can result in permanent kidney failure.

Normotensive ischemic ATN can occur without overt hypotension in conditions with impaired renal autoregulation. These conditions include older age, hypertension, atherosclerotic or renovascular disease, and CKD. Patients with hypertension can develop normotensive ischemic ATN if their blood pressure is decreased to a value lower than what they are accustomed to but within normal range. Management involves treating any potential volume deficits and decreasing antihypertensive medications to allow the blood pressure to increase to baseline levels.

Drug-Induced Acute Tubular Necrosis

Drug-induced ATN can be a consequence of prolonged hemodynamic alterations or direct tubular injury (see Table 24). The drugs associated with prerenal AKI can cause ATN from prolonged hypoperfusion. Early recognition and prompt discontinuation of the drug are essential for renal recovery. The risk of drug-induced ATN increases in the elderly and in patients with decreased effective arterial circulation, CKD, or concomitant nephrotoxin exposure.

Osmotic nephrosis is a form of tubular injury due to hyperosmolar substances such as sucrose-containing intravenous immunoglobulin, mannitol, hydroxyethyl starch, dextran, and contrast media. It is characterized by vacuolization and swelling of the renal proximal tubular cells with resultant tubular obstruction and damage.

Contrast agents can cause nonoliguric ATN primarily through renal vasoconstriction. The serum creatinine increases within 24 to 48 hours after contrast administration. Aminoglycosides cause nonoliguric ATN through direct tubular toxicity with an increase in serum creatinine occurring 5 to 7 days after initiation of therapy. Hypomagnesemia, hypokalemia, hypocalcemia, and hypophosphatemia can be seen. Cisplatin causes ATN through direct tubular toxicity, renal vasoconstriction, and inflammation. Hypomagnesemia with urinary magnesium wasting is common. Amphotericin B causes dose-related AKI through both renal vasoconstriction and direct tubular toxicity. It can be associated with potassium and magnesium wasting, metabolic acidosis due to type 1 (distal) renal tubular acidosis, and nephrogenic diabetes insipidus. Lipid-based preparations decrease the risk for nephrotoxicity. Vancomycin nephrotoxicity occurs in the setting of high trough levels (>15 mg/L), high vancomycin dose (≥4 g/d), prolonged duration of therapy, and/or concomitant nephrotoxic drugs (for example, an aminoglycoside or piperacillin-tazobactam). Certain types of synthetic cannabinoids used as recreational drugs have been associated with ATN.

Pigment Nephropathy

Heme pigment released from myoglobin or hemoglobin can cause AKI through intravascular volume depletion (seen in rhabdomyolysis), renal vasoconstriction, direct proximal tubular injury, and tubular obstruction. In rhabdomyolysis, myoglobin is released in the circulation from damaged skeletal muscle. Major causes of rhabdomyolysis include trauma, drugs and toxins, seizures, metabolic and electrolyte disorders, endocrinopathies (diabetic ketoacidosis, hyperglycemic hyperosmolar syndrome, hypothyroidism), and exercise. Rhabdomyolysis-induced AKI is more likely to occur with serum creatine kinase levels >5000 U/L. In addition to elevated serum creatine kinase and serum creatinine levels, hyperkalemia, hypocalcemia, hyperphosphatemia, hyperuricemia, metabolic acidosis, increased lactate dehydrogenase concentration, and increased aspartate and alanine aminotransferase levels can occur. Urinary findings include FE_{Na} <1% (due to renal vasoconstriction), myoglobinuria, pigmented (red) granular casts, and a positive urine dipstick for blood with absence of erythrocytes.

In addition to correcting the underlying cause, prevention and management of AKI involve aggressive intravenous isotonic fluid resuscitation aimed at maintaining urine output >200 to 300 mL/h. Limited studies suggest that alkalinization of the urine with intravenous bicarbonate to increase the urine pH >6.5 may prevent tubular cast formation. If urine alkalinization is used, it should be discontinued if the patient develops symptomatic hypocalcemia or alkalosis, or if urine pH does not increase to >6.5 after several hours. Dialysis may be necessary for severe electrolyte and acid-base abnormalities. Most patients have partial or complete renal recovery.

Heme pigment nephropathy is less common and occurs when large amounts of heme pigment are released into circulation due to intravascular hemolysis. Causes include glucose-6-phosphate dehydrogenase (G6PD) deficiency, drug reactions, hemolysis related to cardiopulmonary bypass circuits, transfusion of stored red blood cells, paroxysmal nocturnal hemoglobinuria, malaria, certain poisonings, and snakebites. In addition to elevated serum creatinine concentration, other laboratory abnormalities include anemia, increased lactate dehydrogenase, and decreased haptoglobin. Urinary findings include FE_{Na} <1%, hemoglobinuria, pigmented granular casts, and urine dipstick positive for blood with no erythrocytes. Both myoglobinuria and hemoglobinuria can cause tea-colored urine; however, only hemoglobin causes a reddish brown color of centrifuged serum

CONT. because it is too large to be effectively filtered in kidneys. Treatment of hemoglobinuria involves treating the underlying cause as well as volume repletion with intravenous fluids.

Acute Interstitial Nephritis

Acute interstitial nephritis (AIN) is a common cause of AKI characterized by inflammation and edema of the interstitium. The classic clinical presentation of fever, rash, and peripheral eosinophilia occurs in only 10% to 30% of patients with AIN. Urinary findings can include eosinophiluria by Hansel stain, leukocytes, erythrocytes, and leukocyte casts (see Table 26). Urine eosinophils are neither sensitive nor specific for AIN; AIN can still occur in their absence, and eosinophiluria can occur in other causes of AKI such as acute glomerulonephritis, atheroembolic disease, pyelonephritis, cystitis, and prostatitis.

Drug-induced AIN, especially due to antibiotics, is the most common cause of AIN and should be considered in any patient with AKI, a characteristic urinalysis, and history of any drug exposure. Other causes include infections, systemic diseases such as autoimmune disorders, and idiopathic cases (see Table 24). Typically, the serum creatinine gradually increases 7 to 10 days after drug exposure but can increase much sooner following repeat exposure of the drug.

Drug-induced AIN from NSAIDs, including selective cyclooxygenase-2 inhibitors, is usually not associated with fever, rash, or eosinophilia and develops 6 to 18 months after drug exposure. AIN from NSAIDs can be associated with the nephrotic syndrome due to minimal change glomerulopathy or membranous glomerulopathy. Proton pump inhibitors are also associated with AIN without fever, rash, and eosinophilia. The onset of AIN is variable but typically occurs 10 to 11 weeks after exposure. Proton pump inhibitors are thought to be a risk factor for the development of CKD.

Renal recovery from drug-induced AIN is usually complete if the drug is stopped immediately after the onset of kidney injury but may take weeks to several months. Irreversible interstitial fibrosis can develop after 2 weeks of continued exposure. Kidney biopsy should be considered if there is no improvement in kidney function after 5 to 7 days of drug discontinuation. Early glucocorticoid administration may limit damage associated with drug-induced AIN. ▣

Acute Glomerulonephritis

Acute glomerulonephritis with AKI results from immune-mediated damage to glomeruli. Urinary findings include proteinuria, dysmorphic erythrocytes, and erythrocyte casts (see Table 26). Constitutional signs and symptoms are often present. Serologic assays and kidney biopsy identify most causes. Early recognition is extremely important because, without treatment, it can be fatal and result in irreversible kidney damage. See Glomerular Diseases for more information.

Acute Vascular Syndromes

Macrovascular (large and medium vessel) or microvascular (small vessel) disease can cause AKI (see Table 24).

Examples of macrovascular disease include severe abdominal aortic disease, major renal artery occlusion, and renal vein thrombosis. Acute renal arterial occlusion and acute renal vein thrombosis cause acute renal infarction and present as abdominal or flank pain, elevated serum lactate dehydrogenase levels, and hematuria. Treatment usually consists of anticoagulation and supportive care.

AKI can also occur from polyarteritis nodosa, a systemic vasculitis that affects medium and occasionally small arteries at branching points. It causes microaneurysms that subsequently rupture, resulting in hemorrhage, thrombosis, and organ ischemia and infarction. AKI results from renovascular ischemic changes and renal artery vasculitis. See MKSAP 18 Rheumatology for more information.

Patients with atherosclerotic disease who undergo an invasive vascular procedure such as vascular surgery or angiography are at increased risk for atheroemboli-induced AKI (cholesterol emboli). Atheroembolic events can occur spontaneously or several days to weeks after manipulation of the aorta. Plaque rupture causes cholesterol embolization to distal small- and medium-sized arteries, resulting in ischemia with end-organ damage. In addition to the kidneys, atheroemboli can affect the arteries in the skin, muscle, gastrointestinal tract, liver, eyes, and central nervous system. Physical examination findings may include livedo reticularis (lacy network of bluish red vessels, usually seen on legs), Hollenhorst plaques on funduscopic examination (yellow refractile body within arteriole), ulcerations, and blue toes from ischemia (**Figure 17**). Laboratory findings can include low serum complements,

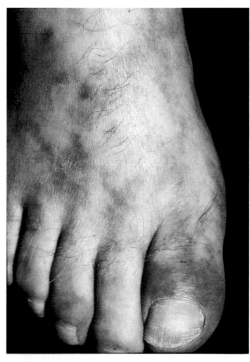

FIGURE 17. Blue toe syndrome presents as a cyanotic toe with necrosis of the skin caused by occlusion of the small vessels from cholesterol emboli, as seen in atheroembolic acute kidney injury.

peripheral eosinophilia, and eosinophiluria; urinalysis may be unremarkable or can have proteinuria, microscopic hematuria, or erythrocyte casts. Treatment of atheroemboli is supportive and consists of risk factor reduction: aspirin, statins, and hypertension management. The use of anticoagulants for treatment of cholesterol emboli is controversial because anticoagulants and thrombolytics can induce atheroemboli. Renal prognosis is poor.

AKI from microvascular disease can present as thrombotic microangiopathy (TMA) with microangiopathic hemolytic anemia, thrombocytopenia, and glomerular capillary thrombosis. Diseases that can lead to TMA include thrombotic thrombocytopenic purpura, hemolytic uremic syndrome, the HELLP (hemolysis, elevated liver enzymes, and low platelets) syndrome, hypertensive emergency, scleroderma renal crisis, complement-mediated TMA, and drug-induced TMA. Urine may show hematuria, erythrocyte casts, and/or proteinuria. Treatment of TMA is based on the underlying cause. Drug-induced TMA is treated by discontinuation of the drug.

Intratubular Obstruction

Intratubular obstruction can cause AKI through precipitation of either protein or crystals within the tubular lumen. Examples include monoclonal light chain deposition in multiple myeloma, calcium oxalate deposition from ethylene glycol ingestion, crystals from drugs, and uric acid from tumor lysis syndrome (see Table 24).

In multiple myeloma, AKI from light chain cast nephropathy is the most common type of kidney disease. Cast nephropathy is due to direct tubular toxicity and obstruction from the precipitation of filtered free light chains. See Kidney Manifestations of Deposition Diseases for more information.

Ethylene glycol intoxication causes AKI from intratubular precipitation of calcium oxalate crystals, which can be seen on urine microscopy. Ethylene glycol should be suspected in a patient with a history of ingestion and whose laboratory studies demonstrate an increased anion gap metabolic acidosis and osmolal gap. Treatment consists of supportive care, the antidote fomepizole, and hemodialysis if needed. Orlistat, a gastrointestinal lipase inhibitor used to induce clinically significant weight loss by fat malabsorption, has also been associated with intratubular calcium oxalate deposition and AKI. High doses of vitamin C, which is metabolized to oxalate, can also lead to AKI from calcium oxalate precipitation in the tubules.

Drugs associated with crystal-induced AKI are listed in Table 24. Urinary findings include hematuria, pyuria, and crystals. AKI is usually reversed after discontinuation of the drug. Predisposing factors include volume depletion, CKD, and changes in urine pH. Correction of volume depletion with intravenous fluids is critical for both the prevention and treatment of crystal-induced AKI. Bolus intravenous acyclovir can cause acyclovir crystal deposition in the tubules, which can be prevented by prior intravenous fluid administration and slow rate of drug infusion. Because crystals from sulfonamide antibiotics and methotrexate are more likely to form in acidic

urine, urinary alkalinization can prevent crystal deposition. Crystals from protease inhibitors can cause AKI from both crystal deposition and nephrolithiasis.

Acute phosphate nephropathy is a potentially irreversible cause of AKI due to phosphate-containing bowel preparations. A transient severe increase in serum phosphate in the setting of volume depletion causes acute and chronic tubular injury from tubular and interstitial precipitation of calcium phosphate crystals. AKI can present days to months after exposure. Predisposing factors include volume depletion, CKD, older age, NSAIDs, and hypertension treated with ACE inhibitors, ARBs, or diuretics. **H**

KEY POINTS

- Acute tubular necrosis due to ischemia, nephrotoxins, and/or sepsis is the most common cause of acute kidney injury in hospitalized patients; a history of sepsis or nephrotoxin exposure along with hemodynamic and volume status assessment can aid in the diagnosis.

- Drug-induced acute interstitial nephritis is associated with a gradual increase in serum creatinine 7 to 10 days after drug exposure; renal recovery is usually complete if the drug is stopped immediately after the onset of kidney injury.

- In atheroemboli-induced acute kidney injury, plaque rupture causes cholesterol embolization to distal small- and medium-sized arteries, resulting in ischemia with end-organ damage; treatment is supportive.

- Acute kidney injury from microvascular disease can present as thrombotic microangiopathy (TMA); conditions that can lead to TMA include thrombotic thrombocytopenic purpura, hemolytic uremic syndrome, the HELLP (hemolysis, elevated liver enzymes, and low platelets) syndrome, hypertensive emergency, scleroderma renal crisis, complement-mediated TMA, and drug-induced TMA.

- Intratubular obstruction causes of acute kidney injury include monoclonal light chain deposition in multiple myeloma; calcium oxalate deposition from ethylene glycol ingestion, orlistat, and high doses of vitamin C; crystals from drugs; and uric acid from tumor lysis syndrome.

Postrenal Disease

Postrenal AKI can occur from obstruction anywhere from the renal pelvis to the external urethral meatus (see Table 24). Upper urinary tract obstruction (at the level of the ureters or renal pelvis) must be bilateral or affect a single functioning kidney to cause AKI. Obstruction of urinary flow leads to hydronephrosis and eventual renal parenchymal damage. If postrenal AKI is not treated promptly, the obstruction can predispose the patient to urinary tract infections and urosepsis, and it can also lead to CKD and ESKD.

Postrenal AKI should be suspected in patients with a history of benign prostatic hyperplasia, diabetes, nephrolithiasis, pelvic malignancies, abdominal or pelvic surgeries, or retroperitoneal adenopathy. Patients can present with anuria, oliguria, polyuria, or normal urine output. Symptoms of lower tract obstruction include abdominal fullness or pain, urinary frequency, urgency, hesitancy, nocturia, overflow incontinence, and incomplete voiding. Acute nephrolithiasis may present with flank pain and hematuria. Urine chemistries can be variable with obstruction (see Table 26).

Lower urinary tract obstruction can be diagnosed by placement of a urinary catheter with return of a large volume of urine or an elevated postvoid residual volume by ultrasound. Ultrasonography can yield false-negative results in the early stages of hydronephrosis or obstruction from encasement of the ureter or kidney, as seen in retroperitoneal disease. Noncontrast CT is indicated for suspected nephrolithiasis. Treatment focuses on removing the obstruction. Renal prognosis depends upon the severity and duration of the obstruction. Renal recovery is generally good if the obstruction is relieved within 1 to 2 weeks. **H**

KEY POINT

- Postrenal acute kidney injury can occur from obstruction anywhere from the renal pelvis to the external urethral meatus; diagnosis can be made via ultrasonography or noncontrast CT, with generally good renal recovery if the obstruction is relieved within 1 to 2 weeks.

Specific Clinical Settings

Contrast-Induced Nephropathy

Contrast-induced nephropathy (CIN) is a common cause of reversible AKI in the hospital. CIN is defined as an increase in serum creatinine within 24 to 48 hours following contrast exposure. The pathogenesis is not completely understood, but CIN is thought to be due to ATN from contrast-induced vasoconstriction, decreased renal blood flow, medullary hypoxia, oxidative stress, and direct tubular cytotoxicity. AKI tends to be nonoliguric, with an FE_{Na} <1%. The urinary sediment may be bland or show classic ATN findings. Risk factors include CKD, diabetic nephropathy, conditions of decreased renal perfusion (heart failure, hypovolemia, hypotension), multiple myeloma, concomitant nephrotoxins, high contrast dose, hyperosmolar contrast, and intra-arterial contrast administration.

Preventive strategies for patients at high risk for CIN include minimizing the amount of contrast, using low or iso-osmolar contrast, discontinuing nephrotoxins, and administering either intravenous isotonic saline or sodium bicarbonate. A randomized controlled trial demonstrated that oral acetylcysteine was no more effective than placebo for the prevention of CIN. Statins have been shown in observational studies and several randomized controlled trials to prevent CIN by acting as stabilizers of the endothelium and free radical scavengers in a model of ischemic nephropathy. Further studies are

needed to establish their benefit. There is no role for prophylactic hemodialysis or hemofiltration following contrast exposure. Treatment of CIN is supportive.

Cardiorenal Syndrome

Cardiorenal syndrome (CRS) is a disorder of the heart and kidneys whereby acute or long-term dysfunction in one organ induces acute or long-term dysfunction in the other. CRS is characterized by the triad of concomitant decreased kidney function, diuretic-resistant heart failure with congestion, and worsening kidney function during heart failure therapy. The decreased kidney function in CRS is thought to be due to neurohumoral activation, increased intra-abdominal pressure leading to venous congestion and increased renal venous pressure, reduced renal perfusion, and right ventricular dysfunction. CRS can be classified into five types (**Table 27**).

Management is challenging because treatment directed toward improving cardiac function (diuretics, ACE inhibitor/ARB, vasodilators, and inotropes) can worsen kidney function. Ultrafiltration has been used for volume overload refractory to diuretics. Current evidence does not support the use of ultrafiltration over intensive diuretic management. Decreased kidney function in patients with heart failure is an independent risk factor for all-cause mortality.

Hepatorenal Syndrome

Hepatorenal syndrome (HRS) is a reversible functional kidney impairment that occurs in the setting of portal hypertension due to liver cirrhosis, severe alcoholic hepatitis, or acute liver failure. HRS is characterized by increased renal vasoconstriction and peripheral arterial vasodilation. Tubular function is preserved with the absence of significant hematuria and proteinuria, as well as lack of renal histological changes.

Type 1 HRS is a clinical diagnosis made after exclusion of other causes of kidney dysfunction. It is characterized by a rise in serum creatinine of at least 0.3 mg/dL (26.5 µmol/L) and/or ≥50% from baseline within 48 hours, bland urinalysis, and

TABLE 27.	Classification of Cardiorenal Syndrome
Type	**Definition**
Type 1	Acute worsening of cardiac function (acute heart failure; acute coronary syndrome; cardiogenic shock) leading to acute kidney injury
Type 2	Chronic abnormalities in cardiac function leading to progressive chronic kidney disease
Type 3	Acute worsening of kidney function leading to acute cardiac dysfunction
Type 4	Primary chronic kidney disease leading to cardiac injury (left ventricular remodeling and dysfunction; diastolic dysfunction; acute heart failure; acute coronary syndrome)
Type 5	Systemic condition (such as diabetes mellitus, sepsis, amyloidosis) causing both cardiac and kidney dysfunction

CONT.

normal findings on kidney ultrasound. It is also supported by a lack of improvement in kidney function after withdrawal of diuretics and 2 days of volume expansion with intravenous albumin. Often, patients also have low urine sodium, low FE_{Na}, and oliguria. Type 2 HRS is defined as a more gradual decline in kidney function associated with refractory ascites.

Patients with HRS have an overall poor prognosis without liver transplantation. General management includes discontinuing diuretics, restricting sodium, restricting water in hyponatremic patients, and searching for precipitating factors. Therapeutic interventions include treatment with vasoconstrictors and albumin, placement of a transjugular intrahepatic portosystemic shunt in select patients, renal replacement therapy, and liver transplant. Renal replacement therapy is usually reserved for patients with severe AKI who are liver transplant candidates.

Tumor Lysis Syndrome

Tumor lysis syndrome (TLS) is characterized by the rapid lysis of malignant cells leading to hyperuricemia, hyperkalemia, hyperphosphatemia, hypocalcemia, and AKI. TLS typically occurs after initiation of chemotherapy in hematologic malignancies with high cell turnover rate, rapid growth rate, or high tumor bulk (acute lymphoblastic leukemia, Burkitt lymphoma, acute myeloid leukemia); however, it can also occur spontaneously. AKI occurs from deposition of uric acid and/or calcium phosphate crystals in the renal tubules.

Management of TLS requires the initiation of preventive measures in high-risk patients prior to cytotoxic therapy, as well as the timely initiation of supportive care for patients who develop TLS. Treatment of established TLS includes intravenous hydration, urate-lowering therapy, management of hyperkalemia and hyperphosphatemia, and renal replacement therapy in refractory cases. Patients at risk for or presenting with TLS require aggressive volume expansion to achieve a urine output of at least 80 to 100 mL/m²/h. Urinary alkalinization is no longer recommended because the high urine pH can cause an increase in calcium phosphate crystal deposition. Allopurinol, a competitive inhibitor of xanthine oxidase, prevents the formation of new uric acid and is recommended as prophylaxis for patients at intermediate risk for TLS (those with highly chemotherapy-sensitive solid tumors); it has no effect on existing serum urate levels. Rasburicase, a recombinant urate oxidase that makes uric acid more soluble in urine with rapid reduction in serum urate levels, is given to patients at high risk of TLS or those with TLS. Rasburicase is contraindicated in patients with G6PD deficiency.

Abdominal Compartment Syndrome

Abdominal compartment syndrome is defined as a sustained intra-abdominal pressure (IAP) >20 mm Hg associated with at least one organ dysfunction. Abdominal compartment syndrome occurs in the setting of abdominal surgery, trauma, hemoperitoneum, retroperitoneal bleed, ascites, bowel obstruction, ileus,

and pancreatitis. It can also occur from capillary leak from massive fluid resuscitation or sepsis. Increasing IAP causes hypoperfusion and ischemia of the intestines and other peritoneal and retroperitoneal structures, leading to hemodynamic, respiratory, neurologic, and kidney impairment. Renal vein compression and renal artery vasoconstriction cause oliguric AKI.

Abdominal compartment syndrome is diagnosed by measuring IAP; measurement of bladder pressure with an indwelling catheter is the standard methodology. Management includes supportive therapy, abdominal compartment decompression, and correction of positive fluid balance.

KEY POINTS

- Preventive strategies for patients at high risk for contrast-induced nephropathy include minimizing the amount of contrast, using low or iso-osmolar contrast, discontinuing nephrotoxins, and administering intravenous isotonic saline or sodium bicarbonate.

- Cardiorenal syndrome is characterized by the triad of concomitant decreased kidney function, diuretic-resistant heart failure with congestion, and worsening kidney function during heart failure therapy.

- Hepatorenal syndrome occurs in the setting of portal hypertension due to liver cirrhosis, severe alcoholic hepatitis, or acute liver failure and is characterized by increased renal vasoconstriction and peripheral arterial vasodilation.

- Acute kidney injury in the setting of tumor lysis syndrome (TLS) occurs from deposition of uric acid and/or calcium phosphate crystals in the renal tubules; management of TLS requires preventive measures in high-risk patients prior to cytotoxic therapy, and timely supportive care for established TLS.

- Abdominal compartment syndrome is defined as a sustained intra-abdominal pressure >20 mm Hg associated with at least one organ dysfunction; in this setting, renal vein compression and renal artery vasoconstriction cause oliguric acute kidney injury.

Management

General Considerations

In most cases of AKI, treatment of the underlying medical condition and discontinuation of nephrotoxic medications lead to improvement in kidney function. No specific pharmacologic therapy is effective in established ATN. Supportive measures include optimizing hemodynamics and renal perfusion, preventing further kidney injury, treating AKI complications, and providing appropriate nutrition. Diuretics can be used for volume overload. Bicarbonate can be administered to correct metabolic acidosis. Dietary potassium, magnesium, and phosphate should be restricted. Phosphate binders may be required to prevent severe hyperphosphatemia. In patients with severe AKI, initiation of renal replacement therapy may be the only option.

Renal Replacement Therapy

Renal replacement therapy (RRT) is used to manage the urgent complications of severe AKI, including hyperkalemia, metabolic acidosis, volume overload refractory to diuretics, uremic manifestations, and dialyzable toxins. Options for RRT for AKI include intermittent hemodialysis (IHD), continuous renal replacement therapy (CRRT), "hybrid" therapies such as prolonged intermittent renal replacement therapy (PIRRT), and peritoneal dialysis (PD). IHD, CRRT, and PIRRT are extracorporeal therapies that require vascular access in the form of a large-bore, double-lumen central venous catheter; PD requires the placement of an intra-abdominal dialysis catheter.

IHD, typically delivered 3 to 6 times a week for 3 to 5 hours per session, allows for rapid correction of electrolyte disturbances and rapid removal of drugs or toxins. The main disadvantage of IHD is the risk for hypotension caused by the rapid solute and volume removal. Furthermore, rapid solute removal from the intravascular space can cause cerebral edema and increased intracranial pressure, limiting this therapy in patients with head trauma or hepatic encephalopathy. CRRT represents a variety of dialysis modalities developed specifically to manage critically ill patients with AKI who cannot tolerate IHD due to hemodynamic instability. CRRT is administered 24 hours a day and removes solutes and fluid much more slowly than IHD, resulting in better hemodynamic tolerance. PIRRT removes solutes and fluid more slowly than IHD but more quickly than CRRT and is administered 8 to 12 hours daily. PD is not as effective as the other forms of RRT but may be useful when the other types of RRT are unavailable or vascular access cannot be obtained.

Randomized clinical trials have not shown a survival benefit of CRRT over IHD or PIRRT for critically ill AKI patients. IHD is typically chosen for patients who are hemodynamically stable, whereas CRRT or PIRRT is chosen for patients who are unstable, are fluid overloaded, and/or have sepsis and multiorgan failure. IHD is favored in patients who need rapid solute removal, such as those with severe hyperkalemia or drug intoxications. CRRT is preferred in patients with cerebral edema because IHD may worsen neurologic status by compromising cerebral perfusion pressure. Transitions in therapy are common depending on the changing needs of the patient.

KEY POINTS

- In most cases of acute kidney injury, treatment of the underlying medical condition and discontinuation of nephrotoxic medications leads to improvement in kidney function.
- Renal replacement therapy is used to manage the urgent complications of severe acute kidney injury, including hyperkalemia, metabolic acidosis, volume overload refractory to diuretics, uremic manifestations, and dialyzable toxins.

Kidney Stones
Overview

Approximately 7% to 11% of the U.S. population will develop nephrolithiasis, and 50% will have recurrent disease. Risk factors for developing kidney stones include male gender, increased age, white race, obesity, diabetes mellitus, the metabolic syndrome, decreased fluid intake, chronic diarrheal states, and Roux-en-Y gastric bypass.

Clinical Manifestations

Although kidney stones may be asymptomatic and diagnosed as an incidental finding on imaging, the typical presentation is waxing and waning "colicky" flank pain that radiates to the groin. Stone movement may result in pain migration to the lateralized genitalia. The patient frequently finds it difficult to achieve a comfortable position. Nausea, vomiting, and dysuria may also be present. Microscopic hematuria is usually noted, although its absence does not exclude a stone.

Similar symptoms may be present with pyelonephritis and acute abdominal processes, which need to be considered. In addition, the ureteral passage of blood clots can mimic renal colic pain.

KEY POINT

- Kidney stones typically present with waxing and waning "colicky" flank pain that radiates to the groin; nausea, vomiting, and dysuria may also be present.

Diagnosis

Nephrolithiasis should be considered in all patients who present with flank pain. Costovertebral angle tenderness may be present. Microscopic examination of the urine for hematuria, leukocytes that may indicate infection, pH measurement, and crystals is mandatory but nonspecific. The presence of crystals may help to identify the type of stone. A complete blood count and complete metabolic panel should be obtained to exclude infection and acute kidney injury, and to screen for common metabolic causes of stone disease.

Definitive diagnosis is made with imaging. Noncontrast helical CT is the gold standard modality because of its high sensitivity and specificity. Although less sensitive than CT, kidney ultrasonography is less expensive, has no radiation exposure, and can be used in pregnant women or when CT is unavailable. Plain abdominal radiography has a low sensitivity and should not be ordered except to follow the stone burden in established disease.

KEY POINT

- Noncontrast helical CT is the gold standard modality to diagnose nephrolithiasis because of its high sensitivity and specificity; kidney ultrasonography, although less sensitive than CT, is less expensive and has no radiation exposure and can be used if CT is unavailable and in pregnant women.

Types of Kidney Stones

See **Table 28** for details on kidney stones and Table 3 in Clinical Evaluation of Kidney Function for images of crystals.

Calcium

Eighty percent of kidney stones contain calcium; most are composed of calcium oxalate, and the remainder are composed of calcium phosphate or a combination of the two.

Calcium oxalate stones are associated with hypercalciuria, hyperoxaluria, and hypocitraturia. Up to 50% of patients with recurrent stones have elevated 24-hour urine calcium levels. This increase may be secondary to elevated serum calcium as seen in hyperparathyroidism, sarcoidosis, or excessive vitamin D intake, but is more frequently idiopathic. Hyperoxaluria can be primary or can occur secondary to increased dietary oxalate intake; malabsorption syndrome due to the binding of gastrointestinal calcium to fatty acids, allowing for increased absorption of oxalate; decreased dietary calcium; and high vitamin C intake. Rous-en-Y gastric bypass surgery is associated with hyperoxaluria and an increase risk of stone formation. The weight loss drug orlistat, by inducing fat malabsorption, is also associated with hyperoxaluria and

the formation of calcium oxalate stones. Because citrate prevents calcium crystal formation, low urine levels are associated with increased stone formation. Citrate excretion is decreased in the presence of metabolic acidosis, as occurs with chronic diarrhea and distal renal tubular acidosis.

Calcium phosphate stones occur when there is persistently elevated urine pH and are therefore commonly associated with distal renal tubular acidosis and hyperparathyroidism. In addition, the use of carbonic anhydrase inhibitors such as acetazolamide or topiramate, by raising urine pH and decreasing citrate excretion, are associated with increased incidence of calcium phosphate stones. Imaging may reveal nephrocalcinosis.

Struvite

Struvite stones occur in the presence of urea-splitting bacteria such as *Proteus*, *Klebsiella*, or, less frequently, *Pseudomonas* species. These bacteria split urea into ammonium, which markedly increases urine pH and results in the precipitation of magnesium ammonium phosphate (struvite). The pH of the urine will be >7.5. Struvite stones commonly produce staghorn calculi (stones that bridge two or more renal calyces) and occur most frequently in older women with chronic urinary tract infections. Because struvite stones are large and grow rapidly, they do not pass into the ureter to cause pain typical of smaller stones. Signs and symptoms typically are related to the underlying infection. Because of their association with infections, there is significant morbidity and mortality associated with these stones.

Uric Acid

Uric acid stones (<10% of stones) develop in the presence of a persistently acidic urine, which decreases the solubility of uric acid. In addition, some individuals overproduce uric acid, resulting in increased urine uric acid; both gout and increased urine uric acid are associated with uric acid stones, but hyperuricosuria is not required for uric acid stone formation. Chronic diarrhea, resulting in metabolic acidosis and low urine volume, is a common cause of uric acid stones. The metabolic syndrome is also associated with uric acid stone formation. Uric stones are radiolucent but are visualized on ultrasound and CT.

Cystine

Cystine stones (1%-2% of stones) result from cystinuria, an autosomal recessive disease that presents at a young age. These stones are recognized by characteristic hexagonal crystals in the urine. They may also form staghorn calculi, and are less radio-opaque then calcium-containing stones. **H**

TABLE 28.	Kidney Stone Risk Factors and Therapy	
Stone Type	**Risk Factors**	**Therapy**
Calcium oxalate	Hypercalciuria; hyperoxaluria; hypocitraturia	Increase fluids
		Decrease sodium intake
		Thiazide diuretics
		Low oxalate diet
		Potassium citrate or bicarbonate
Calcium phosphate	Elevated urine pH; distal renal tubular acidosis; hyperparathyroidism	Increase fluids
		Decrease sodium intake
		Thiazide diuretics
		Treat hyperparathyroidism
		Potassium citrate or bicarbonate
Uric acid	Low urine pH; diarrhea; metabolic syndrome; gout; hyperuricosuria	Increase fluids
		Potassium citrate or bicarbonate
		Allopurinol
Struvite	Chronic urinary tract infections with urea-splitting organism	Treat infection
		Urologic intervention
Cystine	Cystinuria; low urine pH	Increase fluids
		Potassium citrate or bicarbonate
		Acetazolamide
		Penicillamine
		Tiopronin

KEY POINTS

- Eighty percent of kidney stones contain calcium; most are composed of calcium oxalate, which is associated with hypercalciuria, hyperoxaluria, and hypocitraturia.

(Continued)

- Struvite stones commonly produce staghorn calculi and occur most frequently in older women with chronic urinary infections; because of their association with infections, there is significant morbidity and mortality associated with these stones.

- Uric acid stones form in persistently acidic urine and are associated with chronic diarrhea, the metabolic syndrome, and gout.

- Cystine stones result from cystinuria, an autosomal recessive disease that presents at a young age; these stones produce characteristic hexagonal crystals in the urine.

Management

Acute management of symptomatic nephrolithiasis is aimed at pain management and facilitation of stone passage. Pain can be relieved by NSAIDs and opioids as needed. Stone passage decreases with size. Only 50% of stones >6 mm will pass, and stones >10 mm are extremely unlikely to pass spontaneously. Medications, including tamsulosin, nifedipine, silodosin, and tadalafil, appear to increase the rate of spontaneous passage for most stones and can be considered for stones <10 mm.

Urologic intervention is required in all patients with evidence of infection, acute kidney injury, intractable nausea or pain, and stones that fail to pass. This may necessitate shock wave lithotripsy, ureteroscopy with laser ablation, or percutaneous nephrolithotomy.

Patients should strain their urine to collect stone fragments for chemical analysis if the type of stone is unknown. In addition to the initial evaluation previously described, a 24-hour urine for measurement of volume, calcium, oxalate, citrate, uric acid, and sodium should be collected on all recurrent stone formers.

Increased fluid intake is the most important intervention to prevent recurrent disease regardless of stone composition. Urine output should be >2500 mL/d to decrease urine solute concentration.

Other interventions should be based on findings in the metabolic workup and stone analysis (see Table 28). If hypercalciuria is present, calcium excretion can be decreased by the use of thiazide diuretics. Because calcium excretion parallels sodium excretion, limiting sodium intake will also lower urine calcium. Unless excessive, dietary calcium should not be restricted because this will increase oxalate absorption. Oxalate excretion can be decreased by limiting foods high in oxalate such as nuts, cocoa, spinach, rhubarb, and beets. Potassium citrate or potassium bicarbonate will increase urinary citrate excretion. An additional benefit of potassium citrate is a decrease in renal calcium excretion, possibly related to preventing calcium release from bone.

In patients with uric acid stones, management consists of increasing the solubility of uric acid by alkalinizing the urine with potassium citrate or bicarbonate; allopurinol can be beneficial if uric acid excretion is elevated.

Urinary cystine excretion can be reduced by limiting sodium intake and by alkalizing the urine to a pH >7.0. If unsuccessful, additional interventions may be required.

Struvite stones typically require urologic intervention. Before any surgical procedure, it is important that active infection be treated with antibiotics to avert sepsis. To prevent recurrent stone formation, all stone fragments must be removed from the kidney. In patients unable to undergo surgery, the urease inhibitor acetohydroxamic acid may reduce urine alkalinity and decrease stone growth; however, this is best used as an adjunct to urologic intervention.

- Acute management of symptomatic nephrolithiasis includes pain management and facilitation of stone passage.

- Urologic intervention is required in all patients with evidence of infection, acute kidney injury, intractable nausea or pain, and stones that fail to pass.

- Increased fluid intake to >2500 mL/d is the most important intervention to prevent recurrent kidney stones, regardless of stone composition.

The Kidney in Pregnancy
Normal Physiologic Changes in Pregnancy

Pregnancy is a state of volume expansion and vasodilation. Sodium and water retention increase plasma volume, augmenting renal blood flow and increasing glomerular filtration rate (GFR) by up to 50%. With the GFR increase, serum creatinine levels decrease. Therefore, high normal serum creatinine levels may indicate significant kidney impairment. Despite the volume expansion, blood pressure begins to decrease in the first trimester and reaches the nadir in the second trimester due to peripheral vasodilation.

Proteinuria increases, with the upper limit of normal increasing from 100 mg/24 h (in nonpregnant) to approximately 200 mg/24 h. Values >300 mg/24 h are considered abnormal. Prepartum proteinuria may also worsen during pregnancy, making pregnancy-related changes difficult to distinguish from a flare of an underlying kidney disease or development of preeclampsia.

Due to increased renal vascular and interstitial volume, kidney size may increase by 1 to 1.5 cm. Physiologic hydronephrosis and hydroureter, due in part to external compression of the ureters, are common in pregnancy, increase as pregnancy advances, and may take weeks to resolve postpartum. The dilated collecting system can lead to urinary stasis, which increases the risk for pyelonephritis. Therefore, screening for asymptomatic bacteriuria at least once in early pregnancy is recommended, and treatment is indicated.

Respiratory alkalosis due to progesterone-induced hyperventilation commonly decreases P_{CO_2} to 27 to 32 mm Hg. Renal compensation results in serum bicarbonate levels between 18 and 20 mEq/L (18-20 mmol/L), with a serum pH of approximately 7.45.

Changes in antidiuretic hormone response to osmolality (reset osmostat) cause mild hyponatremia (decrease in serum sodium of 4-5 mEq/L [4-5 mmol/L]) with a decrease in serum osmolality by 8 to 10 mOsm/kg H_2O. No treatment is indicated. Rarely, transient gestational diabetes insipidus can develop due to excessive metabolism of antidiuretic hormone by placental vasopressinase.

KEY POINTS

- Pregnancy is associated with decreased blood pressure, increased glomerular filtration rate with decreased serum creatinine, and increased proteinuria.

- Dilatation of the urinary system during pregnancy increases the risk for pyelonephritis; therefore, screening for asymptomatic bacteriuria at least once in early pregnancy is recommended, and treatment is indicated.

Hypertension in Pregnancy

Chronic Hypertension

The American College of Obstetricians and Gynecologists (ACOG) defines chronic hypertension as a systolic blood pressure (BP) ≥140 mm Hg or diastolic BP ≥90 mm Hg starting before pregnancy or before 20 weeks of gestation or persists longer than 12 weeks postpartum. It is associated with worse maternal and fetal outcomes. Hypertension first recognized during pregnancy before 20 weeks' gestation usually indicates chronic hypertension. The lower BP measurements associated with physiologic changes of pregnancy can mask hypertension during the first trimester.

To avoid overtreatment of hypertension and associated fetal risk, the 2013 ACOG Taskforce on Hypertension in Pregnancy recommends treating persistent systolic BP ≥160 mm Hg or diastolic ≥105 mm Hg in women with chronic hypertension, and maintaining BP at 120-160/80-105 mm Hg. However, these goals remain controversial, with some suggesting lower targets. Antihypertensive treatment reduces the risk of progression to severe hypertension by 50% compared with placebo but has not been shown to prevent preeclampsia, preterm birth, being small for gestational age, or infant mortality. Any evidence of end-organ damage requires treatment, even with lower BPs. All antihypertensive medications cross the placenta; drug selection is based on safety profiles.

Renin-angiotensin system agents (ACE inhibitors, angiotensin receptor blockers, and direct renin inhibitors) are all contraindicated due to teratogenicity, even early in pregnancy, and should be stopped prior to conception. If conception has already occurred, they should be stopped immediately and the mother counseled regarding possible fetal effects.

First-line therapy includes methyldopa and labetalol, which have been used safely and extensively in pregnancy. Methyldopa monotherapy may be insufficient, in which case it can be replaced with labetalol. Calcium channel blockers can be added; nifedipine has been used most extensively. The β-blockers metoprolol and pindolol have also been used in pregnancy, but atenolol and propranolol may have adverse fetal effects. Diuretics must be used with caution because they may induce oligohydramnios if started during pregnancy.

Gestational Hypertension

Gestational hypertension first manifests after 20 weeks of pregnancy without proteinuria or other end-organ damage (features of preeclampsia) and resolves within 12 weeks of delivery. Preeclampsia occurs in approximately one third of cases. Hypertension persisting beyond 12 weeks postpartum is considered chronic hypertension. Gestational hypertension can recur in subsequent pregnancies and is associated with an approximately fourfold risk for development of chronic hypertension.

KEY POINTS

- Chronic hypertension precedes pregnancy or is present before 20 weeks' gestation.

- The 2013 American College of Obstetricians and Gynecologists Taskforce on Hypertension in Pregnancy recommends treating persistent systolic blood pressure (BP) ≥160 mm Hg or diastolic BP ≥105 mm Hg in women with chronic hypertension.

- Renin-angiotensin system agents (ACE inhibitors, angiotensin receptor blockers, and direct renin inhibitors) are contraindicated in pregnancy due to teratogenicity; they must be stopped prior to conception or stopped immediately if conception has already occurred.

- First-line therapy of chronic hypertension in pregnancy includes methyldopa and labetalol.

- Gestational hypertension first manifests after 20 weeks of pregnancy without proteinuria or other end-organ damage and resolves within 12 weeks of delivery.

Preeclampsia

Preeclampsia is defined by new-onset hypertension and proteinuria (≥300 mg/24 h from a timed collection or ≥300 mg/g by urine protein-creatinine ratio) that occurs after 20 weeks of pregnancy (**Table 29**). New-onset hypertension with new-onset end-organ damage (such as liver or kidney injury, pulmonary edema, cerebral or visual symptoms, or thrombocytopenia) is also diagnostic of preeclampsia. Severe preeclampsia is identified by persistent systolic BP >160 mm Hg or diastolic BP >110 mm Hg and end-organ damage. Eclampsia is the presence of seizures in context of preeclampsia without other cause. The HELLP (hemolysis, elevated liver enzymes, low platelets) syndrome is a life-threatening state complicating 10% to 20% of preeclampsia cases. Risk factors for preeclampsia include prior preeclampsia (with an approximate 20% recurrence rate), nulliparity, diabetes mellitus, advanced maternal age, multiple gestation, and family history.

The pathophysiology of preeclampsia is poorly understood. Abnormal placental vascular development and generalized endothelial dysfunction occur. Two angiogenic and antiangiogenic factors, soluble fms-like tyrosine kinase-1

TABLE 29. Diagnostic Criteria for Preeclampsia

Blood pressure	≥140 mm Hg systolic or ≥90 mm Hg diastolic on two occasions at least 4 hours apart after 20 weeks of gestation in a woman with a previously normal blood pressure
	≥160 mm Hg systolic or ≥110 mm Hg diastolic; hypertension can be confirmed within a short interval (minutes) to facilitate timely antihypertensive therapy
and	
Proteinuria	≥300 mg/24 h urine collection (or this amount extrapolated from a timed collection)
	or
	Urine protein-creatinine ratio ≥300 mg/g
	Dipstick reading of 1+ (used only if other quantitative methods are not available)
Or, in the absence of proteinuria, new-onset hypertension with the new onset of any of the following:	
Thrombocytopenia	Platelet count <100,000/µL (100 × 10⁹/L)
Kidney dysfunction	Serum creatinine concentrations >1.1 mg/dL (97.2 µmol/L) or a doubling of the serum creatinine concentration in the absence of other kidney disease
Impaired liver function	Elevated blood concentrations of liver aminotransaminases to twice the normal concentration
Pulmonary edema	—
Cerebral or visual symptoms	—

With permission from American College of Obstetricians and Gynecologists; Task Force on Hypertension in Pregnancy. Hypertension in pregnancy. Report of the American College of Obstetricians and Gynecologists' Task Force on Hypertension in Pregnancy. Obstet Gynecol. 2013;122(5):1122-31. [PMID: 24150027]

(sFlt-1) and soluble endoglin (sEng), are elevated in women with preeclampsia; their role in treatment and diagnosis continues to be elucidated.

Symptoms of preeclampsia include rapid weight gain due to edema, nausea, vomiting, abdominal pain (particularly concerning if in the right upper quadrant, signifying possible HELLP syndrome), headaches, altered mental status, and blurred vision. If untreated, preeclampsia ultimately leads to maternal end-organ damage and fetal growth retardation, and it may cause maternal and/or fetal death.

Low-dose (81 mg/d) aspirin started after 12 weeks of pregnancy reduces the rate of preeclampsia in women at high risk. Antihypertensive medications do not prevent preeclampsia but reduce complications of stroke, heart failure, and kidney injury. Most experts initiate treatment at BP >150–160/100–110 mm Hg, although there is no consensus.

Definitive treatment of preeclampsia is delivery. Maternal risk for complications diminishes in the hours after delivery, although proteinuria may take months to resolve. Maternal benefits must be weighed against neonatal risks for a preterm delivery, but severe preeclampsia is an indication for immediate delivery regardless of gestational age. Mild preeclampsia may be managed conservatively, with maternal and fetal monitoring and treatment of hypertension. In all cases, close attention to hypertension is recommended in the postpartum period.

KEY POINTS

- Preeclampsia is defined by new-onset hypertension and proteinuria that occurs after 20 weeks of pregnancy.
- Low-dose (81 mg/d) aspirin started after 12 weeks of pregnancy reduces rates of preeclampsia in women at high risk.
- Definitive treatment of preeclampsia is delivery.

Chronic Kidney Disease in Pregnancy

Chronic kidney disease (CKD) complicates management of pregnancy; the obstetric literature notes a serum creatinine cutoff of >1.4 mg/dL (124 µmol/L) as that at which complications are of most concern. Proteinuria may also increase risk, but reduced GFR has greater impact. Complications include preeclampsia, acute kidney injury, progression of CKD, end-stage kidney disease, preterm delivery, gestational hypertension, intrauterine growth retardation, and fetal loss. Preconception counseling regarding these risks is essential.

Pregnancy is uncommon in women receiving dialysis, which is frequently associated with infertility. Levels of β-human chorionic gonadotropin (β-hCG) may increase with dialysis in the absence of pregnancy; therefore, ultrasonography is usually necessary to confirm pregnancy. Pregnancy in the context of dialysis is associated with very high risk of preeclampsia and fetal loss, although live birth rates have improved to 60% to 80%. To optimize fetal outcomes, hemodialysis frequency and dose are increased to improve BP and volume status.

Pregnancy in women with kidney transplants is more common than in those receiving dialysis due to increased fertility after transplant. Outcomes are improved with better allograft function (serum creatinine <1.5 mg/dL [132.6 µmol/L]) and stable immunosuppression; transplant patients should await 1 to 2 years with a stable allograft before attempting conception. No immunosuppressive medication has been extensively studied in pregnancy, and all have some associated risk. Although calcineurin inhibitors (tacrolimus and cyclosporine) have been used safely, mycophenolate mofetil is teratogenic and needs to be replaced 3 to 6 months prior to conception with azathioprine, which has an extensive history of use in pregnancy. Sirolimus is contraindicated due to fetal toxicity. Glucocorticoids increase risk for pregnancy-induced hypertension and diabetes.

KEY POINTS

- Women with chronic kidney disease (CKD) have a greater risk for preeclampsia, acute kidney injury, progression of CKD, end-stage kidney disease, preterm delivery, gestational hypertension, intrauterine growth retardation, and fetal loss.

- Kidney transplant recipients should wait at least 1 to 2 years after transplantation with a stable allograft and stable immunosuppression before attempting conception.

- The immunosuppressive medications mycophenolate mofetil and sirolimus used in kidney transplant recipients are teratogenic and must be discontinued prior to attempting conception.

Chronic Kidney Disease
Definition and Staging

Chronic kidney disease (CKD) is defined as abnormal kidney structure or function present for >3 months. CKD is stratified into stages 1 to 5 based on the level of estimated glomerular filtration rate (eGFR). Stages G1 and G2 do not have reductions in eGFR and therefore are defined by the presence of anatomical defects or markers of kidney damage such as albuminuria, hematuria, or electrolyte abnormalities. Because albuminuria is associated with increased renal and cardiovascular morbidity and mortality, the Kidney Disease: Improving Global Outcomes (KDIGO) group further subdivides the eGFR-based kidney stages by degree of albuminuria (**Figure 18**). This dual eGFR and albuminuria staging algorithm provides a means for predicting which patients are at highest risk for developing progressive CKD into end-stage kidney disease (ESKD), defined as CKD stage G5 treated with chronic dialysis or kidney transplantation.

Epidemiology and Pathophysiology

CKD, defined by either albuminuria or eGFR <60 mL/min/1.73 m^2, affects approximately 15% of the U.S. adult population. About 50% of patients with prevalent CKD have stage G3 disease or worse; the other 50% have CKD due to the presence of albuminuria. The prevalence of CKD is heavily influenced by age and has increased severalfold in elderly persons over the past 20 years. The largest increase over time, as assessed by the National Health and Nutrition Examination Survey (NHANES), is in stage G3 disease. In the United States, the prevalence of

				Persistent albuminuria categories Description and range		
				A1	**A2**	**A3**
				Normal to mildly increased	Moderately increased	Severely increased
				<30 mg/g	30-300 mg/g	>300 mg/g
GFR categories (mL/min/1.73 m^2) Description and range	**G1**	Normal or high	≥90			
	G2	Mildly decreased	60-89			
	G3a	Mildly to moderately decreased	45-59			
	G3b	Moderately to severely decreased	30-44			
	G4	Severely decreased	15-29			
	G5	Kidney failure	<15			

Green: low risk (if no other markers of kidney disease, no CKD); Yellow: moderately increased risk; Orange: high risk; Red: very high risk.

FIGURE 18. The Kidney Disease: Improving Global Outcomes (KDIGO) chronic kidney disease staging system. Prognosis of chronic kidney disease by glomerular filtration rate and albuminuria category. CKD = chronic kidney disease; GFR = glomerular filtration rate.

CKD stage G3 or worse is 0.3% in those aged 20 to 39 years, 3.3% in those aged 40 to 59 years, and 22.6% in those aged ≥60 years. In contrast, the prevalence of albuminuria is less age dependent. Approximately 6% of persons aged 40 to 59 years have a urine albumin-creatinine ratio ≥30 mg/g, compared with 8.5% of those aged ≥60 years. Advanced CKD, defined by stages G4 or G5, is present in <1% of the population. Compared with men, women have a slightly higher prevalence of both eGFR <60 mL/min/1.73 m² (7.9% versus 6.4%) and albuminuria (10.9% versus 8.8%).

CKD results from various etiologies that cause chronic damage to the glomeruli, tubulointerstitium, or both. Glomerular damage is reflected by proteinuria or albuminuria. Although a large degree of tubulointerstitial damage (both chronic inflammation and fibrosis) can exist subclinically and thus go unnoticed, eventually the underlying structural abnormalities affect kidney function, and GFR falls below normal levels.

Not all patients with CKD progress to ESKD. The most important predictors of progression are the baseline level of eGFR and the degree of albuminuria/proteinuria. eGFR trajectory over time also adds prognostic value for ESKD and cardiovascular outcomes. Patients with diabetic CKD usually progress faster than those without diabetes. The rate of eGFR decline ranges between -3 and -6 mL/min/1.73 m² per year in patients who have type 2 diabetes with high albuminuria. Renal risk variants in the apolipoprotein L1 (*APOL1*) gene are prevalent in black persons and are associated with higher rates of ESKD and progression of CKD, regardless of diabetes status (see Genetic Disorders and Kidney Disease).

Screening

CKD is typically asymptomatic except in advanced stages (G4, G5). Controversy exists regarding screening patients for CKD. The U.S. Preventive Services Task Force (USPSTF) and the American College of Physicians recommend against screening for CKD in asymptomatic adults with or without risk factors for CKD. In contrast, the American Society of Nephrology advises screening all adults for CKD, including, but not limited to, those with a family history of kidney disease or adults with risk factors for CKD (diabetes, hypertension, or cardiovascular disease).

Clinical Manifestations

CKD is typically asymptomatic except in advanced stages (G4, G5). When eGFR falls below 30 mL/min/1.73 m², numerous alterations in metabolic pathways, including 1,25-dihydroxyvitamin D production and erythrocyte production, become altered due to the lack of nephron mass and loss of 1α-hydroxylase and erythropoietin synthesis. Moderate to severe CKD can also result in impaired ability to excrete salt and water, and may manifest as edema. CKD in a patient with nephrotic-range proteinuria may also result in edema or anasarca.

When CKD progresses to ESKD, several nonspecific ("uremic") symptoms can occur such as fatigue, nausea, loss of appetite, insomnia, irritability, difficulty concentrating, confusion, or pruritus. Uremia can also induce serositis, including pleuritis and pericarditis. However, a large proportion of patients with CKD stage G5 manifest few or only intermittent uremic symptoms, for unexplained reasons. Although rarely seen today due to increased awareness and the widespread availability of dialysis, patients who have prolonged uremia that is untreated with renal replacement therapy may develop "uremic frost," which appears as chalky whitish skin and is due to crystallized urea deposits and other nitrogenous waste products that evaporated from sweat (**Figure 19**).

Diagnosis

CKD may be clinically suspected, or it may be incidentally detected on a basic chemistry panel that includes serum creatinine. Initial assessment of GFR includes establishing eGFR based on serum creatinine using the Chronic Kidney Disease Epidemiology (CKD-EPI) Collaboration creatinine equation. If confirmation of GFR is required because of conditions that affect serum creatinine independent of GFR (such as extremes of muscle mass or diet), cystatin C should be measured to employ the CKD-EPI creatinine-cystatin equation, or GFR should be measured directly using a clearance procedure. Initial assessment of albuminuria includes a random urine albumin-creatinine ratio. If confirmation of albuminuria is required because of diurnal variation or conditions affecting creatinine excretion, the albumin excretion rate should be

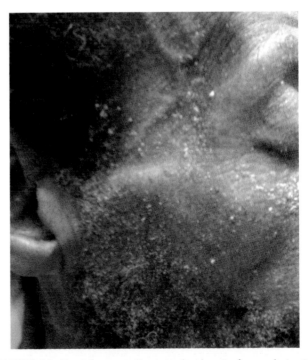

FIGURE 19. Uremic frost presenting as powdery deposits of urea and uric acid salts on the skin in a patient with untreated chronic kidney disease.

measured from a timed urine collection. See Clinical Evaluation of Kidney Function for more information.

Diagnosis of CKD requires a low eGFR confirmed at least 3 months after initial assessment, or persistent proteinuria or albuminuria. Kidney biopsy is used to determine the etiology of CKD when a glomerulonephritis, unexplained tubulointerstitial disease, or severe proteinuria is likely based upon clinical history, urine sediment, and laboratory results and/or antibody tests. Kidney biopsy is not indicated in the presence of shrunken kidneys (<9 cm), which generally indicate chronic irreversible disease. Occasionally, patients are noted to have "medical kidney disease" on imaging (such as ultrasound revealing hyperechoic kidneys). Urinalysis done for other nonspecific reasons may detect previously undiagnosed hematuria or proteinuria, which may suggest the presence of CKD and should prompt close observation or additional evaluation depending on the clinical scenario. There is currently a lack of evidence regarding the use of urinalysis as a routine screening test for CKD.

Patients who experience acute kidney injury (AKI) can have slow recovery; studies have demonstrated that kidney function can continue to recover for up to 1 year after an initial episode of AKI. Therefore, although diagnosis of CKD requires at least 3 months of persisting abnormalities in structure or function, a diagnosis of CKD after AKI may be premature in some patients between 3 and 12 months after the AKI episode.

KEY POINTS

- Chronic kidney disease is defined as abnormal kidney structure or function present for >3 months.

- Staging of chronic kidney disease is based on estimated glomerular filtration rate and albuminuria.

- The U.S. Preventive Services Task Force and the American College of Physicians recommend against screening for chronic kidney disease (CKD) in asymptomatic adults with or without risk factors for CKD, whereas the American Society of Nephrology advises screening all adults for CKD, including, but not limited to, those with a family history of kidney disease or adults with risk factors for CKD (diabetes, hypertension, or cardiovascular disease).

Complications and Management

According to KDIGO guidelines, referral to a nephrologist is indicated for evaluation and management of CKD in the presence of the following: AKI or an abrupt, sustained fall in GFR; GFR <30 mL/min/1.73 m^2; persistent albuminuria (>300 mg/g); progression of CKD; erythrocyte casts; >20 erythrocytes/hpf that is sustained and not readily explained; hypertension refractory to treatment with four or more antihypertensive agents; persistent abnormalities of serum potassium; recurrent or extensive nephrolithiasis; or hereditary kidney disease.

A kidney failure risk equation (KFRE) has been developed and validated. The KFRE uses four variables (age, sex, eGFR, and albuminuria) to predict 2-year and 5-year risk for ESKD in patients with CKD stages G3 to G5. The KFRE performs well across age, sex, race, and presence/absence of diabetes. The use of this equation is consistent with KDIGO guidelines, which recommend integration of risk prediction in the evaluation and management of CKD.

Cardiovascular Disease

Cardiovascular disease is the leading cause of death among patients with CKD. The risk for cardiovascular-related death in patients with CKD stages G3 and G4 is 4 to 5 times higher than the risk for progression to ESKD. Mortality risk increases with decreasing eGFR and increasing albuminuria. Unfortunately, many landmark clinical trials that guide the prevention or treatment of cardiovascular disease did not include patients with advanced CKD, and the findings may not be generalizable to patients with CKD. However, most post-hoc analyses of randomized controlled trials that had participants with some degree of CKD demonstrated efficacy regardless of baseline CKD status, including for interventions such as percutaneous coronary interventions. Thus, experts recommend against withholding otherwise efficacious therapies from those with CKD due to unsubstantiated concerns of lack of efficacy or harm. These also include coronary angiography or thrombolysis and/or platelet antagonists for patients with acute coronary syndromes or acute strokes and contrast-based CT studies for patients with high pretest probability of pulmonary embolism or aortic dissection.

Hypertension

Both KDIGO and the 2017 high blood pressure guideline from the American College of Cardiology (ACC), the American Heart Association (AHA), and nine other organizations recommend a blood pressure target of <130/80 mm Hg in patients with CKD.

An ACE inhibitor or an angiotensin receptor blocker is a preferred drug for treatment of hypertension for patients with stage G3 CKD or higher or for those with stage G1 or G2 CKD with albuminuria (albumin-creatinine ratio ≥300 mg/g). These medications may also slow the progression of CKD in some patients. Thiazide diuretics are a cornerstone of hypertension treatment but may lose efficacy with severe CKD. Loop diuretics therefore serve an important role in managing salt and water retention associated with proteinuria and CKD. Dietary sodium chloride restriction is essential for blood pressure control in most forms of CKD, and KDIGO recommends restricting sodium intake to <2000 mg/d.

See Hypertension for more information.

Dyslipidemia

Elevated LDL cholesterol and triglyceride levels with low HDL cholesterol levels are common among patients with CKD. Conflicting data exist on the effect of treating dyslipidemia in reducing proteinuria and in slowing the progression of CKD. Statins have been shown to reduce cardiovascular and all-cause mortality in patients with CKD, although large trials have failed to demonstrate a mortality benefit for statins in patients with dialysis-dependent ESKD (unless initiated pre-dialysis). KDIGO guidelines recommend treatment with a statin in all patients aged ≥50 years with non-dialysis-dependent CKD and in adults aged 18 to 49 years with non-dialysis-dependent CKD and any one of the following: coronary disease, diabetes mellitus, prior ischemic stroke, or a >10% estimated risk of coronary death or nonfatal myocardial infarction. Statins are also recommended for adult kidney transplant recipients.

Dyslipidemia associated with the nephrotic syndrome helps maintain plasma oncotic pressure but, over time, may hasten the progression of glomerular injury. Dyslipidemia in the nephrotic syndrome requires aggressive treatment to prevent atherosclerotic disease, especially in patients with existing cardiovascular risk factors and in younger patients to prevent premature cardiovascular disease. See Glomerular Diseases for more information on the nephrotic syndrome.

Coronary Artery Disease

There is a significantly increased prevalence of coronary artery disease (CAD) among patients with CKD compared with the general population. This is partly explained by the high prevalence of shared risk factors/comorbidities such as diabetes or hypertension. However, CKD is independently associated with CAD, and this association strengthens with declining eGFR and rising albuminuria. Despite high cardiovascular mortality among patients with CKD, these patients may be less likely to undergo coronary revascularization procedures, possibly because of the increased risk for contrast-induced nephropathy (see Special Considerations, Imaging Contrast Agents).

In patients with CKD, serum biomarkers for myocardial ischemia such as cardiac troponins may be chronically elevated due to decreased renal clearance. Serial troponin measurements and other markers such as creatine kinase-MB can help distinguish acute ischemia from stable elevations.

KEY POINTS

- Both the Kidney Disease: Improving Global Outcomes group and the 2017 high blood pressure guideline from the American College of Cardiology (ACC), the American Heart Association (AHA), and nine other organizations recommend a target blood pressure of <130/80 mm Hg in patients with hypertension and chronic kidney disease.

- Treatment of hypertension in patients with chronic kidney disease includes an ACE inhibitor or angiotensin receptor blocker, dietary sodium restriction to <2000 mg/d, and addition of a diuretic as needed to control vascular volume. *(Continued)*

KEY POINTS *(continued)*

- The Kidney Disease: Improving Global Outcomes guidelines recommend treatment with a statin in all patients with non-dialysis–dependent chronic kidney disease (CKD) who are over 50 years of age and in adults 18 to 49 years of age with non-dialysis–dependent CKD and any one of the following: coronary disease, diabetes mellitus, prior ischemic stroke, or a >10% estimated risk of coronary death or nonfatal myocardial infarction.

Chronic Kidney Disease-Mineral and Bone Disorder

As kidney function declines, the normal homeostasis of calcium and phosphorus levels by the kidney becomes compromised, resulting in alterations in bone mineralization. The term *chronic kidney disease-mineral and bone disorder* (CKD-MBD) encompasses these changes. The KDIGO guidelines for CKD-MBD are available at kdigo.org.

Calcium and Phosphorus Homeostasis

Three hormones are largely responsible for regulating calcium and phosphorus homeostasis: parathyroid hormone (PTH), vitamin D, and fibroblast growth factor 23 (FGF-23). PTH is the most important regulator of calcium and phosphorus concentrations. PTH has three separate mechanisms to increase serum calcium: It stimulates osteoclasts to resorb bone, stimulates hydroxylation of 25-hydroxyvitamin D in the kidneys, and stimulates tubular reabsorption of calcium (**Figure 20**). Concurrently, PTH induces renal phosphorus excretion.

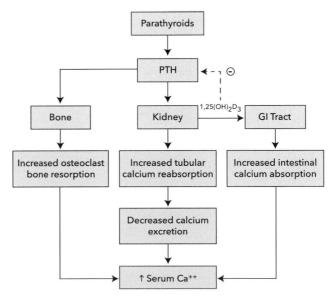

FIGURE 20. Overview of the metabolic systems that maintain calcium homeostasis. Parathyroid hormone (PTH) stimulates increased 1,25-dihydroxyvitamin D_3 [1,25(OH)$_2$D$_3$] synthesis by the kidneys, and 1,25(OH)$_2$D$_3$ causes feedback suppression of PTH production. Ca^{++} = ionized calcium; GI = gastrointestinal; 1,25(OH)$_2$D$_3$ = 1,25-dihydroxyvitamin D$_3$; PTH = parathyroid hormone; ↑ = increased.

FGF-23 is a peptide secreted by osteocytes and osteoclasts. It acts on the kidney to induce phosphaturia and downregulates 1α-hydroxylase to inhibit synthesis of 1,25 dihydroxyvitamin D. FGF-23 rises in stage G3a CKD, preceding PTH elevation. As GFR falls and PTH rises, PTH directly stimulates further FGF-23 production by osteocytes, resulting in a massive increase of FGF-23 blood levels, upwards of 100-fold from normal. Initially, the high FGF-23 serves to increase renal phosphorus excretion and helps maintain normal phosphorus levels as GFR declines.

As CKD progresses, increased FGF-23 and decreased nephron mass reduce the conversion of 25-hydroxyvitamin D to 1,25-dihydroxyvitamin D by renal tubular cells. Reduction in 1,25-dihydroxyvitamin D levels results in lower intestinal absorption of calcium and phosphorus in the gut, mitigating phosphorus retention but also contributing to hypocalcemia, especially late in CKD. Reduced 1,25-dihydroxyvitamin D levels also increase PTH production by the parathyroid glands, and hypocalcemia is a potent stimulus for further increases in PTH levels.

Increased plasma PTH as a result of CKD is referred to as *secondary hyperparathyroidism*. Increased PTH levels result in reduced calcium excretion, increased calcium absorption from the gut, increased phosphorus excretion by the kidneys, and activation of osteoclast bone resorption. Early in CKD, the PTH-induced increase in renal phosphorus excretion enables normal phosphorus levels despite reduced renal excretory capacity. However, as CKD progresses, the kidney is unable to compensate for the increased release of phosphorus from bone, and phosphorus levels rise. This results in a vicious cycle as hyperphosphatemia stimulates PTH production.

If secondary hyperparathyroidism cannot be adequately controlled, tertiary hyperparathyroidism can ensue. Tertiary hyperparathyroidism is the result of the prolonged PTH stimulation needed to maintain eucalcemia. This prolonged stimulation results in increased calcium levels and severe hyperparathyroid hyperplasia with elevated PTH levels that are no longer responsive to the plasma calcium concentration.

Laboratory Abnormalities

Serum calcium and phosphorus levels typically remain in the normal range until the eGFR drops below 20 to 30 mL/min/1.73 m² (stages G4-G5), at which point the ability of elevated FGF-23 and PTH levels to promote phosphorus excretion becomes overwhelmed, and hyperphosphatemia develops. Progressive decline in 1,25-dihydroxyvitamin D levels results in reduced intestinal calcium absorption, and hyperphosphatemia promotes precipitation of calcium and phosphorus in extraskeletal tissues, leading to hypocalcemia.

In addition to reduced conversion of 25-hydroxyvitamin D to 1,25-dihydroxyvitamin D, patients with CKD also have a higher prevalence of 25-hydroxyvitamin D deficiency. KDIGO guidelines recommend that patients with an eGFR <60 mL/min/1.73 m² (stage G3-G5) be evaluated for 25-hydroxyvitamin D deficiency and supplemented as per guidelines for the general population.

PTH levels are often elevated in patients with an eGFR <60 mL/min/1.73 m² (stage G3-G5) and progressively increase with worsening CKD. KDIGO guidelines recommend measuring intact PTH levels in these patients to aid in the detection and management of secondary hyperparathyroidism and its complications.

Vascular Calcification

An increased prevalence of arterial calcification, including the coronary arteries, has been noted in patients with CKD; the burden of calcification is highest in patients with ESKD. Arterial calcification reduces vascular compliance and likely contributes to the increased prevalence of left ventricular hypertrophy observed in patients with CKD. Arterial calcification is also strongly associated with cardiovascular and all-cause mortality; KDIGO guidelines therefore suggest treating patients with CKD and arterial calcification as is appropriate for patients in the highest category of cardiovascular risk, although treatments specifically targeted at reducing vascular calcification have not been shown to improve clinical outcomes.

Renal Osteodystrophy

Renal osteodystrophy refers to alteration of bone morphology in patients with CKD, which occurs as part of the systemic disorder of CKD-MBD. Four main types of histologic changes in bone can occur as part of renal osteodystrophy and are discussed in this section. KDIGO guidelines recommend a bone biopsy if knowledge of the type of renal osteodystrophy will affect treatment decisions in patients with CKD stages G3a to G5. This recommendation is based on the growing experience with osteoporosis medications in patients with CKD, low bone mineral density, and a high risk of fracture. The lack of ability to perform a bone biopsy may not justify withholding antiresorptive therapy from patients at high risk of fracture.

Osteitis Fibrosa Cystica

Osteitis fibrosa cystica is due to abnormally high bone turnover that can occur after prolonged exposure of bone to sustained high levels of PTH in secondary hyperparathyroidism. It is associated with an increased number and activity of osteoblasts and osteoclasts and expansion of osteoid surfaces, resulting in an increased risk for fracture. Patients can be asymptomatic or have bone pain. Classic skeletal changes on radiograph include subperiosteal resorption of bone, most prominently at the phalanges of the hands, and radiolucent bone cysts of the long bones.

Adynamic Bone Disease

Adynamic bone disease occurs when there is a lack of bone cell activity and a markedly reduced rate of bone turnover. Histopathologic abnormalities include decreased osteoclast activity with an increase in osteoid, resulting in an increased risk for fracture. Patients have suppressed PTH levels (due to chronic illness or aggressive treatment with vitamin D

CONT.

analogues) or skeletal resistance to PTH from down-regulation of the bone PTH receptor due to high circulating PTH levels. Patients may be asymptomatic or have bone pain. Adynamic bone disease should be excluded prior to bisphosphonate therapy because these drugs can cause and/or worsen the disease by inhibiting osteoclast activity.

Osteomalacia

Osteomalacia is characterized by decreased mineralization of osteoid at sites of bone turnover, with increased risk of fracture. The most common symptoms include bone pain and tenderness. Although patients with CKD are at increased risk for osteomalacia, CKD does not cause osteomalacia per se; vitamin D deficiency caused by coexisting factors such as intestinal malabsorption due to gastrointestinal disorders or restricted access to sunlight is often present.

Osteoporosis

Patients with CKD have many causes of reduced bone density. Current KDIGO guidelines indicate that in patients with CKD stages G3a to G5 with evidence of CKD-MBD and/or risk factors for osteoporosis, bone mineral density testing is suggested to assess fracture risk if results will affect treatment decisions.

Management

In patients with CKD stages G3a to G5, treatment of CKD-MBD is based on serial assessments of phosphorus, calcium, and PTH levels. Current KDIGO guidelines recommend that in patients with CKD stages G3a to G5, elevated phosphorus levels should be lowered *toward* the normal range, not into the normal range, because there is an absence of data showing that efforts to maintain phosphorus in the normal range are of benefit and safety concerns. Thus, treatment should be aimed at overt hyperphosphatemia, and decisions to start phosphate-lowering treatment should be based solely on progressively or persistently elevated serum phosphorus levels.

KDIGO guidelines recommend avoiding hypercalcemia. Mild and asymptomatic hypocalcemia (for example, in the context of calcimimetic treatment) can be tolerated to avoid inappropriate calcium loading. KDIGO guidelines also now recommend restricting the dose of calcium-based phosphate binders (calcium carbonate and calcium acetate) in CKD stages G3a to G5, rather than restriction only in those with hypercalcemia. This change was based on published trials suggesting that exposure to exogenous calcium is harmful in terms of vascular calcification in all stages of CKD, along with data suggestive of lower mortality risk with non–calcium-containing phosphate binders (sevelamer and lanthanum) versus calcium-containing binders.

For patients with CKD stages G3a to G5 who are not on dialysis, optimal PTH levels are not known. Previously, patients with PTH levels above the upper normal limit were targeted for management. The 2016 KDIGO update suggests that patients with levels of intact PTH "*progressively rising or persistently above the upper normal limit* for the assay be evaluated for modifiable factors, including hyperphosphatemia, hypocalcemia, high phosphate intake, and vitamin D deficiency." KDIGO guidelines recommend against routine use of calcitriol and vitamin D analogues to lower PTH levels in patients with CKD stages G3a to G5 not on dialysis, because trials of these agents failed to demonstrate improvements in clinically relevant outcomes. Instead, these agents should be reserved for patients with CKD stages G4 to G5 with severe and progressive hyperparathyroidism.

In patients on dialysis, KDIGO guidelines recommend use of calcimimetics, calcitriol, or vitamin D analogues, or a combination of calcimimetics and calcitriol or vitamin D analogues, to lower PTH levels. This recommendation was largely due to the EVOLVE (EValuation Of Cinacalcet Hydrochloride Therapy to Lower CardioVascular Events) trial and several secondary analyses of data from this trial. The EVOLVE trial evaluated the effect of cinacalcet versus placebo in hemodialysis patients by using a composite end point of all-cause mortality, nonfatal myocardial infarction, hospitalization for unstable angina, heart failure, and peripheral vascular events. Although the primary analysis demonstrated a nonsignificant reduction in the primary composite end point with cinacalcet, multiple sensitivity analyses demonstrated statistically significant reductions in the composite end point, including in those aged ≥65 years. Given these mostly positive but mixed findings, the KDIGO Work Group listed calcimimetic therapy among the acceptable treatment options while still recognizing the utility and efficacy of active vitamin D compounds.

Tertiary hyperparathyroidism does not respond to phosphate binders or calcitriol therapy, and patients often require parathyroidectomy for definitive treatment.

KEY POINTS

- Chronic kidney disease-mineral and bone disorder is defined by the changes to the normal homeostasis of calcium and phosphorus levels as kidney function declines, resulting in alterations in bone mineralization.
- According to current Kidney Disease: Improving Global Outcomes (KDIGO) guidelines, management of chronic kidney disease-mineral and bone disorder focuses upon normalizing serum phosphorus, avoiding hypercalcemia, and addressing modifiable factors.

Anemia

Anemia in the setting of CKD is common, and its prevalence increases as CKD progresses into stages G4 and G5. Most often normocytic, anemia in CKD largely results from lack of erythropoietin production due to the decline in functional renal mass. Other contributors include erythropoietin resistance, neocytolysis (decreased survival time of erythrocytes), and iron deficiency.

Although modest declines in hemoglobin are well tolerated, concern for inducing or contributing to the development

CONT.

of left ventricular hypertrophy has been the key driver in the belief that higher hemoglobin values are beneficial. Moreover, observational data suggest that higher hemoglobin values are associated with better outcomes in patients with CKD and ESKD. However, several large randomized controlled trials conducted in the past 15 to 20 years demonstrated no benefit or increased harm regarding some cardiovascular events in groups randomly assigned to higher hemoglobin targets via erythropoiesis-stimulating agents (ESAs). Moreover, these trials revealed only modest improvements in fatigue and no benefit in physical functioning with higher hemoglobin targets. The mechanisms underlying the lack of benefit or harm for the higher hemoglobin groups are not well understood but may include off-target effects of ESAs on extrarenal organs. Thus, current KDIGO recommendations are to consider ESAs for patients with CKD who have hemoglobin concentrations <10 g/dL (100 g/L). Black box warnings for use of ESAs include the risk for increased mortality and/or tumor progression in patients with active malignancy, increased risk for thromboembolic events in postsurgical patients not receiving anticoagulant therapy, and increased risk for serious cardiovascular events when ESAs are administered to patients with hemoglobin values >11 g/dL (110 g/L) or with a history of stroke.

All patients with CKD and anemia should have iron profiles assessed, including total iron-binding capacity and ferritin levels. KDIGO recommendations suggest maintaining transferrin saturation levels of >30% and serum ferritin levels of >500 ng/mL (500 µg/L) using either oral or intravenous iron supplementation. Inadequate iron stores will contribute to ESA hyporesponsiveness. Blood transfusions can be used in patients with severe anemia or modest anemia with symptoms; however, the goal is to minimize the number of erythrocyte transfusions in patients with CKD and ESKD due to concerns for iron overload and sensitization to HLA antigens, which may lead to allosensitization and increased waiting times for kidney transplantation.

KDIGO guidelines for the diagnosis and management of CKD-related anemia can be found at kdigo.org.

Metabolic Acidosis

Metabolic acidosis frequently occurs in patients with CKD due to defective acid excretion (resulting in reduced bicarbonate generation), most commonly due to impaired ammoniagenesis. Untreated metabolic acidosis can lead to muscle loss (due to increased muscle proteolysis) and bone loss (due to increased bone resorption and impaired bone formation). In early CKD, metabolic acidosis is typically a normal anion gap hyperchloremic metabolic acidosis. As eGFR declines, organic and inorganic anions are retained, and an increased anion gap metabolic acidosis develops.

Large observational studies have shown a strong association between lower serum bicarbonate levels and both increased progression of CKD and mortality. Alkali therapy, most commonly sodium bicarbonate or sodium citrate, can

delay the progression of CKD. Therefore, KDIGO guidelines recommend starting alkali therapy when the serum bicarbonate is chronically <22 mEq/L (22 mmol/L). The alkali salt therapy dose should be titrated to achieve a serum bicarbonate level within the normal range; excessive alkali therapy in the setting of a reduced eGFR may induce a metabolic alkalosis, which is associated with increased mortality. Despite the administration of excess sodium, alkali salts are not associated with volume expansion, even among patients with chronic heart failure or overt edema, most likely because the accompanying anion is not chloride. ⬛

Nephrotoxins

Two major issues exist regarding drug administration in patients with CKD: 1) Renally excreted drugs require dose adjustment to avoid accumulation and potential side effects; and 2) Reduced functional nephron mass increases the probability that a potentially nephrotoxic drug will cause nephrotoxicity.

Conceptually, it is useful to compartmentalize nephrotoxic medications by their main site of action. For example, several medications, including NSAIDs, calcineurin inhibitors, and ACE inhibitors/angiotensin receptor blockers, can have effects on glomerular blood flow. Patients with AKI who are on NSAIDs should have the medications immediately discontinued. For patients with CKD, the American Society of Nephrology recommends the avoidance of NSAIDs, including cyclooxygenase-2 inhibitors, due to the risk of worsening kidney function. ACE inhibitors or angiotensin receptor blockers are the cornerstone of treatment for patients with CKD; however, during episodes of acute illness and/or volume depletion, these drugs increase the risk for AKI due to their effects on intraglomerular pressure. Drugs that cause glomerular injury, tubular injury, or tubulointerstitial nephritis are reviewed in Acute Kidney Injury.

Emerging literature suggests that proton pump inhibitors, in addition to their classic association with acute interstitial nephritis/AKI, may contribute to the development and progression of CKD. The association is robust and has been confirmed in three independent cohorts. These studies used careful comparators, including the use of H_2 blockers, and adjusted for numerous potential confounding variables, including chronic NSAID use.

Proteinuria

The severity of proteinuria is strongly associated with adverse clinical outcomes, including progression of CKD to ESKD, cardiovascular morbidity, and mortality. It is unclear whether proteinuria is simply a marker of the underlying severity of kidney damage and disease, or if proteinuria itself activates inflammatory pathways and contributes to tubulointerstitial fibrosis. Although dual renin-angiotensin system blockade via combinations of ACE inhibitors, angiotensin receptor blockers, or direct renin inhibitors have been shown to decrease proteinuria, several clinical trials have revealed that use of combination renin-angiotensin system antagonism results in more adverse events (hyperkalemia, hypotension, AKI) without additional cardiovascular or renal benefits.

Protein Restriction

In animal models, protein-restricted diets have been shown to slow the progression of kidney disease by reducing glomerular filtration pressure, thereby preventing progressive injury and fibrosis. However, in the Modification of Diet in Renal Disease study, no definitive benefit was seen in renal outcomes in patients randomly assigned to the low protein (0.6 g/kg/d) group. Although there is insufficient evidence to recommend routine use of low protein diets to slow progression of CKD, high protein diets may precipitate or exacerbate symptoms of uremia in patients with stage G5 CKD. Small studies suggest that low protein diets might delay the onset of symptomatic uremia and the need for renal replacement therapy in patients with stage G5 CKD not yet on dialysis.

KEY POINTS

- Erythropoiesis-stimulating agents are associated with an increased risk for serious cardiovascular events when administered to patients with hemoglobin values >11 g/dL (110 g/L) or a history of stroke.

- Kidney Disease: Improving Global Outcomes (KDIGO) guidelines recommend treatment of metabolic acidosis with alkali therapy in patients with chronic kidney disease when the serum bicarbonate is chronically <22 mEq/L (22 mmol/L).

- ACE inhibitors and angiotensin receptor blockers decrease proteinuria and slow progression of proteinuric kidney diseases, but use of both drug classes in combination results in more adverse events without additional cardiovascular or renal benefits.

Special Considerations

Imaging Contrast Agents

Intravenous iodinated contrast can cause contrast-induced nephropathy (CIN), and risk for CIN increases with increasing severity of CKD. Patients with CKD should receive intravenous hydration with isotonic saline or bicarbonate-containing solutions before and after receiving contrast unless there is evidence of frank pulmonary edema. See Acute Kidney Injury for more information on CIN.

Gadolinium contrast used in MRI is associated with risk for nephrogenic systemic fibrosis (NSF) and must be avoided in patients with an eGFR <30 mL/min/1.73 m². In life-threatening situations in which benefit outweighs the risk for NSF, MRI is performed with low doses of stable gadolinium agents. Prior nephrology consult should be obtained to assess risks of gadolinium administration and guide the use

of dialysis in advanced CKD and ESKD. In those with severe CKD who require gadolinium, daily dialysis for 3 days appears to be effective at clearing the gadolinium and reducing the risk for NSF. See MKSAP 18 Dermatology for more information on NSF.

Vaccination

Patients with CKD are at increased risk for infections that can be prevented by vaccination; however, these patients also have impaired immune responses to vaccines. The Centers for Disease Control and Prevention guidelines state that vaccinations in patients with CKD may be more effective when performed before the need for chronic dialysis or kidney transplantation. Patients with CKD should otherwise receive vaccinations according to guidelines, with a few exceptions:

- Patients with advanced CKD near dialysis dependence or those with ESKD on hemodialysis should be vaccinated against hepatitis B virus.

- Patients with CKD (stage not specified) or the nephrotic syndrome should receive the 23- and 13-valent pneumococcal vaccines, with revaccination with the 23-valent vaccine after a minimum of 5 years.

- Influenza vaccine should be administered annually to patients with CKD, but patients with ESKD should only receive the inactivated influenza vaccine due to risks associated with the live vaccines in immunocompromised patients.

Vascular Access

Patients with advanced CKD may ultimately require renal replacement therapy; for those who choose hemodialysis, timely vascular access creation is essential. Referral to an experienced surgeon many months before dialysis is critical because arteriovenous fistula placement can be technically challenging and may require several months for full maturation. Arteriovenous fistulas have superior clinical outcomes compared with arteriovenous grafts and tunneled catheters.

Protecting the nondominant arm veins is paramount and involves limiting phlebotomy and intravenous catheters in that arm. Peripherally inserted central venous catheters should be avoided in patients with an eGFR <60 mL/min/1.73 m². A recent study demonstrated that peripherally inserted central catheters placed before or after hemodialysis initiation were independently associated with approximately 15% to 20% lower likelihoods of transition to any working fistula or graft. Avoidance of subclavian venous catheters helps to limit subclavian stenosis, which could impair the proper functioning of an arteriovenous fistula or arteriovenous graft used for dialysis.

Older Patients

CKD stages G1 through G3a in elderly patients without albuminuria is of minimal clinical importance; some may refer to this mild decrement in eGFR as normal aging. For elderly persons with progressing or severe CKD necessitating discussions about renal replacement therapy and/or referral for evaluation for kidney transplantation, a patient-centered approach is preferred. Comorbid medical conditions, functional status, expected outcomes, and patient preferences regarding goals of care should be considered. For patients aged ≥80 years at the start of hemodialysis treatment, data demonstrate better survival among those who received pre-hemodialysis nephrology care that followed a planned management pathway, those who had a good nutritional status, and those with an arteriovenous fistula as vascular access for hemodialysis at the time of hemodialysis initiation.

> **KEY POINTS**
>
> - Gadolinium contrast used in MRI is associated with the risk for nephrogenic systemic fibrosis and must be avoided in patients with an estimated glomerular filtration rate <30 mL/min/1.73 m².
>
> - In patients with chronic kidney disease, peripherally inserted central venous catheters and subclavian venous catheters should be avoided in the nondominant arm veins for possible future dialysis vascular access.

End-Stage Kidney Disease

CKD stage G5 is defined as an eGFR <15 mL/min/1.73 m², and ESKD is defined as CKD stage G5 treated with chronic dialysis or kidney transplantation. About 10% of patients with CKD stage G3 progress to ESKD, but most die from cardiovascular disease or infection before they progress to advanced CKD.

Patients with an eGFR <30 mL/min/1.73 m² should be educated about renal replacement therapy (RRT) treatment options, including hemodialysis, peritoneal dialysis, and kidney transplantation. Patients with advanced age or multiple comorbidities may not want any of these life-sustaining options. There has been increasing support of "kidney supportive care," which involves services aimed at improving the quality of life for patients with advanced CKD. It includes aligning treatment with a patient's goals through culturally sensitive shared decision-making and advance care planning, along with treating symptoms resulting from uremia, hypervolemia, hyperkalemia, and/or acidosis. For patients amenable to RRT, studies demonstrate no benefit in starting RRT in asymptomatic patients or at a specific eGFR cutoff compared with watchful waiting and initiating RRT for symptoms or metabolic abnormalities that are refractory to medical treatment. For the elderly and frail patients, physicians need to balance the management of symptoms with optimal care, with less emphasis being placed on maximizing long-term health outcomes, such as survival. Care should align with patient preferences and maximize the patient's quality of life. **Table 30** compares goals of care for patients with ESKD treated with standard dialysis versus kidney supportive care.

Dialysis

Patients who choose hemodialysis should be referred for arteriovenous fistula creation in a timely manner to allow for arteriovenous fistula maturation. Arteriovenous grafts for hemodialysis and peritoneal dialysis catheters for peritoneal dialysis can be placed weeks before starting RRT but ideally should be planned months in advance. Tunneled dialysis catheters can be placed within days or the same day prior to starting hemodialysis but are associated with increased risk for bloodstream infections and death. Therefore, arteriovenous fistula or arteriovenous graft is preferred.

Hemodialysis

Hemodialysis achieves clearance of blood solutes by convection and diffusion against a concentration gradient provided

TABLE 30.	Goals of Care for Patients with End-Stage Kidney Disease Treated with Dialysis Versus Kidney Supportive Care	
Issue	**Current Disease-Focused Metrics for Conventional Delivery of Dialysis Care**	**Kidney Supportive Care**
Vascular access	Creation and maintenance of an AVF; avoid central venous catheters as much as possible	Central venous catheter acceptable if patient chooses hemodialysis
Dialysis adequacy	Target small solute clearance based on current standards, intensifying the dialysis prescription as needed to achieve targets	Lower clearance acceptable if changes in dialysis prescription increase demands inconsistent with patient preference; may involve fewer hemodialysis sessions or more frequent but shorter sessions
Cardiovascular disease	Treat cardiovascular risk factors, potentially targeting BP and dyslipidemia	Tolerate hypertension to avoid symptoms; no indication for dyslipidemia treatment
Mineral and bone disorder	Dietary counseling; binders to control hyperphosphatemia; vitamin D analogues with or without calcimimetics for secondary hyperparathyroidism	Limited restrictions; more permissive hyperphosphatemia and hyperparathyroidism
Nutrition	Encourage dietary protein intake while limiting potassium, sodium, and phosphorus intake	Reduce dietary restrictions
Laboratory monitoring	Routine monthly laboratory tests	Minimal necessary

AVF = arteriovenous fistula; BP = blood pressure.

CONT.

by dialysate flowing opposite to blood flow and separated by a semipermeable dialyzer membrane. Hemodialysis is commonly performed three times per week for 3- to 4-hour treatment sessions at an outpatient dialysis unit. Frequent and/or longer treatments provide better control of volume status and serum electrolytes. Some patients perform hemodialysis at home four to five times per week but with shorter treatment sessions.

Peritoneal Dialysis

Peritoneal dialysis utilizes an indwelling catheter to perform exchanges of dialysate with a specified solute concentration and osmolality into the peritoneum, which serves as a semipermeable membrane and allows for diffusion of solutes and osmosis of water. Dialysate needs to be exchanged about three to five times per day to maintain a high concentration gradient and maintain adequate solute clearance. Patients can perform these exchanges during the day, or a cycler can be used to exchange the fluid overnight while the patient sleeps; these options provide greater autonomy because the patient can work or perform activities during the day, rather than the need to be present at a hemodialysis unit three times per week. Clinical outcomes are similar for patients on peritoneal dialysis compared with hemodialysis, although patients starting RRT who have residual renal function may have better outcomes with peritoneal dialysis. Furthermore, residual renal function is preserved longer in peritoneal dialysis compared with hemodialysis and, although small, helps maintain adequate solute clearance and euvolemia.

Peritonitis is an important complication because repeated infections can cause peritoneal fibrosis and reduce the efficacy of the dialysis treatments. Dialysis-associated peritoneal peritonitis is infrequent, with an average of one episode every 2 to 3 years. It is usually caused by gram-positive skin flora and less commonly by gram-negative intestinal flora. Proper skin hygiene and sterile technique when handling the peritoneal dialysis catheter are critical in preventing peritonitis.

Non-dialytic Palliative Therapy

Some patients with CKD stage G5/ESKD may choose not to initiate RRT, or patients already on RRT may decide to discontinue treatment. Palliative care and hospice services play an important role in caring for these patients. Non-dialytic therapy is a reasonable treatment option for elderly patients with ESKD and multiple comorbidities. Treatment focuses on symptom management and results in less hospitalization with similar or better quality of life compared with patients on RRT. For patients who withdraw from RRT, death usually occurs within 2 weeks. Recent studies have shown that the withdrawal rate from dialysis is approximately 3 per 100 person-years of dialysis, and this rate is increasing over time. **H**

KEY POINTS

- Clinical outcomes are similar for patients on peritoneal dialysis compared with hemodialysis, although patients starting renal replacement therapy who have residual renal function may have better outcomes with peritoneal dialysis.
- Non-dialytic palliative therapy is a reasonable option for elderly patients with end-stage kidney disease and multiple comorbidities, with treatment focusing on symptom management and quality of life.

HVC

Kidney Transplantation

Kidney transplantation is the preferred treatment for ESKD. It improves life expectancy and quality of life, and provides a significant cost savings to the health care system compared with dialysis. However, demand far exceeds supply, and waiting lists for deceased-donor kidneys are several years long in most regions of the United States.

Referral

Patients should be referred to a kidney transplant center for evaluation when the eGFR is <20 mL/min/1.73 m². Early referral is important because preemptive kidney transplants (transplants before needing dialysis) are associated with improved clinical outcomes compared with receiving a transplant after starting dialysis. Early referral also allows adequate time to identify suitable living donors; if no living donor is available, early listing is essential to begin the waiting process for a deceased-donor kidney.

Patients and donors undergo extensive health screening to identify issues that may affect the safety and/or outcome of the transplant. In the potential recipient, these include active malignancy, coronary ischemia, or active infections. An adequate social support system and financial resources are also important to ensure medication adherence and long-term survival of the transplanted allograft. Donors are screened for intrinsic kidney disease, hypertension, and diabetes to ensure there is minimal risk related to reduced renal mass resulting from donation nephrectomy.

Patients are generally managed by a transplant nephrologist for at least the first 6 months posttransplant and are then comanaged with a general nephrologist and/or internist, especially for comorbidities.

Immunosuppressive Therapy

Immunosuppressive medications are required to prevent allograft rejection. Induction therapy is started perioperatively with polyclonal anti–T-cell antibodies (thymoglobulin) or monoclonal anti–interleukin-2 receptor antibody (basiliximab). Calcineurin inhibitors with pulse glucocorticoids are started at this time as well.

Long-term maintenance therapy for most patients includes a combination of calcineurin inhibitors (tacrolimus or cyclosporine), antimetabolites (mycophenolate mofetil or azathioprine), and glucocorticoids. However, some patients with well-matched allografts can discontinue glucocorticoids. Doses of these medications are highest immediately posttransplant and are gradually decreased over the next several months to minimize side effects (**Table 31**), including long-term nephrotoxicity, while maintaining adequate immunosuppression.

Risks of Transplantation

Immediately posttransplant, patients need to be monitored for acute rejection and postoperative complications. Thereafter, minimizing risk for infection and medication side effects becomes the focus while maintaining adequate immunosuppression to prevent acute and chronic rejection.

Infection

Immunosuppression significantly increases the risk for infection. Within the first month after surgery, the most common infectious complications are similar to other surgical patients and include urinary tract infections and wound infections. Afterward, opportunistic infections become more prevalent.

Cytomegalovirus (CMV) is an important pathogen, and the risk for infection depends on the serologic status of the donor and recipient at the time of transplant. The highest risk occurs when a seropositive donor kidney is transplanted into a seronegative recipient. Most patients receive prophylaxis against CMV with valganciclovir during the first 6 to 12 months; however, CMV infections can occur after the medication is discontinued. Signs and symptoms include fever, pneumonitis, hepatitis, and gastroenteritis/colitis.

TABLE 31. Common Side Effects of Medications Used for Chronic Maintenance Immunosuppression After Kidney Transplantation

Class	Medication	Common Side Effects
Calcineurin inhibitor	Cyclosporine	Hypertension; decreased GFR; dyslipidemia; hirsutism; gingival hyperplasia
	Tacrolimus	New-onset diabetes mellitus; decreased GFR; hypertension; gastrointestinal symptoms
Antimetabolite	Mycophenolate mofetil	Diarrhea; nausea/vomiting; leukopenia; anemia
	Azathioprine	Leukopenia; hepatitis; pancreatitis
mTOR inhibitor	Sirolimus; everolimus	Proteinuria; dyslipidemia; new-onset diabetes mellitus; anemia; leukopenia
Glucocorticoid	Prednisone	Osteopenia, osteoporosis, osteonecrosis; hypertension; edema; new-onset diabetes mellitus; glaucoma; cataracts

GFR = glomerular filtration rate; mTOR = mammalian target of rapamycin.

Prophylaxis against *Pneumocystis jirovecii* pneumonia with trimethoprim-sulfamethoxazole is most commonly used, but atovaquone can be used for sulfa-allergic or hyperkalemic patients.

Polyoma BK virus uniquely affects kidney transplant patients, only rarely occurring with other organ transplants or in other immunosuppressed states. The most common clinical manifestation is an acute or indolent rise in serum creatinine due to tubulointerstitial nephritis or ureteral stenosis. Treatment requires reduction in the immunosuppression dose, but this must be balanced against the risk of allograft rejection.

Cancer

Because kidney transplant recipients are at higher risk for developing cancer, it is important to screen recipients for the presence of active malignancy prior to transplant.

Immunosuppressive medications increase the risk for several forms of malignancy, with non-melanoma skin cancers being the most common. Transplant patients therefore should be screened regularly for skin cancer and other age- and sex-appropriate cancer.

Posttransplant lymphoproliferative disorders can occur with long-term immunosuppression. These malignancies are caused by uncontrolled B-lymphocyte proliferation associated with Epstein-Barr virus infection and impaired T-cell surveillance. Treatment involves reduction in immunosuppression and administration of the anti–B-cell monoclonal antibody rituximab. Additionally, calcineurin inhibitors may be switched to the mammalian target of rapamycin inhibitor sirolimus because of its antiproliferative effects.

Kaposi sarcoma is also common and is associated with human herpesvirus-8 infection. Treatment involves reduction in immunosuppression dosing and switching to a sirolimus-based regimen.

Special Considerations in Transplant Recipients

Acute Kidney Injury

AKI is a common posttransplant complication and can occur immediately posttransplant or any time in the future. Acute rejection should always be part of the differential diagnosis, because early recognition and treatment are associated with better long-term outcomes. Posttransplant AKI may also be due to renal vasoconstriction from calcineurin inhibitor toxicity, calcineurin inhibitor–induced thrombotic microangiopathy, BK nephropathy, acute tubular necrosis, acute interstitial nephritis, or volume depletion/prerenal causes.

Disease Recurrence

Glomerular diseases can recur in the transplant allograft. Focal segmental glomerulosclerosis is one of the most common forms of glomerular disease to recur posttransplant and can occur within a few days to weeks after transplantation. Focal segmental glomerulosclerosis and thrombotic microangiopathy should be treated aggressively if disease recurrence is seen in the transplanted kidney, because these conditions are associated with high rates of graft failure. Patients with lupus or ANCA vasculitis should have quiescent disease for several months preceding transplantation to reduce risk for disease recurrence posttransplant. Diabetic nephropathy and IgA nephropathy can affect allograft function after transplant but are unlikely to cause graft failure.

Cardiovascular Disease

Cardiovascular disease is the leading cause of death in kidney transplant recipients (about 50% of deaths). Kidney transplantation, despite restoration of kidney function, should be treated as a cardiovascular disease equivalent for purposes of risk factor modification.

Calcineurin inhibitors induce hypertension by activating the sodium chloride cotransporter in the distal convoluted tubule of the kidney. Therefore, thiazide diuretics may be efficacious in these patients. Dyslipidemia is a common side effect of calcineurin inhibitors, sirolimus, and glucocorticoids. Treatment with a statin improves cardiac outcomes; however, statins have drug-drug interactions with calcineurin inhibitors and can increase toxicities of both drugs.

Bone Disease

Secondary and tertiary hyperparathyroidism, common in patients with ESKD, can persist for several months posttransplant; continuation of vitamin D analogues or calcimimetics may be warranted if the patient is hypercalcemic. Additionally, hypophosphatemia secondary to hyperparathyroidism is common posttransplant due to renal phosphorus wasting. Long-term glucocorticoids can cause osteopenia, osteoporosis, and osteonecrosis. Calcineurin inhibitors induce magnesium wasting. See Chronic Kidney Disease-Mineral and Bone Disorder for more information.

Vaccination

Most transplant centers do not recommend immunization within the first 3 to 6 months posttransplant due to increased immunosuppression and therefore decreased likelihood of developing long-term immunity from the vaccine. Influenza vaccine, however, may be administered within 1 month of transplant in the setting of an influenza outbreak. Live attenuated vaccines are generally contraindicated in transplant recipients.

KEY POINTS

- Patients should be referred to a kidney transplant center for evaluation when the estimated glomerular filtration rate is <20 mL/min/1.73 m^2.

- Preemptive kidney transplants are associated with improved clinical outcomes compared with transplantation after dialysis.

- Within the first month following kidney transplantation, the most common infectious complications are similar to other surgical patients and include urinary tract infections and wound infections; afterward, opportunistic infections (such as cytomegalovirus, *Pneumocystis jirovecii*, and polyoma BK virus) become more prevalent.

(Continued)

KEY POINTS *(continued)*

- Immunosuppression of kidney transplant recipients increases the risk for several malignancies, including non-melanoma skin cancers, Kaposi sarcoma, and posttransplant lymphoproliferative disorders; regular screening for skin cancer and other age- and sex-appropriate cancer is recommended.

Complications of End-Stage Kidney Disease

Cardiovascular Disease

Sudden cardiac death is the leading cause of death in ESKD. This population is at increased risk due to rapid shifts of serum electrolytes during dialysis and chronic volume overload that contribute to left ventricular hypertrophy and cardiac fibrosis. Uremic toxins also contribute to left ventricular hypertrophy and cardiac fibrosis and may play a role in arrhythmogenesis. Avoiding rapid changes in serum potassium during dialysis may help limit arrhythmias, and adherence to dietary salt and fluid restriction may help limit volume overload. However, intradialytic hypotension induced by rapid volume removal during dialysis may cause cardiovascular and central nervous system injury due to organ hypoperfusion. Vascular calcification is accelerated by uremic toxins, chronic inflammation, and calcium-based medications/vitamin D analogues. Limiting medications that raise serum calcium and achieving adequate clearance during dialysis may help delay the progression of atherosclerosis. KDGIO guidelines recommend continuing a statin if a patient with CKD progresses to ESKD, but statins should not be newly started if progression to ESKD has already occurred.

Infection

Infection is the second leading cause of death in ESKD. Patients are at increased risk due to a relatively immunosuppressed state from chronic inflammation and frequent exposure to the health care environment. Tunneled dialysis catheters increase the risk for bacteremia, and empiric antibiotics should be administered while waiting for blood culture results in patients with suspected bacteremia. Tunneled catheters should be removed immediately for severe sepsis, evidence of metastatic infection, evidence of an exit-site or tunnel infection, persistent fever, or bacteremia despite antibiotics. Exchange of the catheter over a guidewire may be an option for clinically stable patients without a tunnel infection or for patients who clear the bacteremia within 48 hours of antibiotic administration. Antibiotic lock therapy consists of the instillation of a highly concentrated antibiotic solution into an intravascular catheter lumen to treat catheter-related bloodstream infections. Antibiotic lock therapy with vancomycin and/or ceftazidime is an alternative option for stable patients with less virulent organisms such as *Staphylococcus epidermitis*, but catheter salvage should not be attempted for *Staphylococcus aureus* infections and some gram-negative organisms.

Acquired Cystic Kidney Disease

Acquired cystic kidney disease is common among patients with severe CKD and ESKD. Cysts are usually detected during routine kidney ultrasonography or incidentally found on abdominal CT or MRI. These cysts are at increased risk for transformation into renal cell carcinoma, but routine screening is not recommended for most patients. A high index of suspicion is warranted for patients with new gross hematuria or unexplained flank pain. For cysts that are highly suspicious for malignancy, partial nephrectomy and nephron-sparing approaches are indicated for less severe stages of CKD. For patients with advanced CKD or ESKD, radical nephrectomy is the most prudent option.

KEY POINT

- Complications of end-stage kidney disease include cardiovascular disease, infection, and acquired cystic kidney disease.

Bibliography

Clinical Evaluation of Kidney Function

Corapi KM, Chen JL, Balk EM, Gordon CE. Bleeding complications of native kidney biopsy: a systematic review and meta-analysis. Am J Kidney Dis. 2012;60:62-73. [PMID: 22537423]

Davis R, Jones JS, Barocas DA, Castle EP, Lang EK, Leveille RJ, et al; American Urological Association. Diagnosis, evaluation and follow-up of asymptomatic microhematuria (AMH) in adults: AUA guideline. J Urol. 2012;188:2473-81. [PMID: 23098784]

Fähling M, Seeliger E, Patzak A, Persson PB. Understanding and preventing contrast-induced acute kidney injury. Nat Rev Nephrol. 2017;13:169-180. [PMID: 28138128]

Inker LA, Schmid CH, Tighiouart H, Eckfeldt JH, Feldman HI, Greene T, et al; CKD-EPI Investigators. Estimating glomerular filtration rate from serum creatinine and cystatin C. N Engl J Med. 2012;367:20-9. [PMID: 22762315]

Ix JH, Wassel CL, Stevens LA, Beck GJ, Froissart M, Navis G, et al. Equations to estimate creatinine excretion rate: the CKD epidemiology collaboration. Clin J Am Soc Nephrol. 2011;6:184-91. [PMID: 20966119]

Levey AS, Fan L, Eckfeldt JH, Inker LA. Cystatin C for glomerular filtration rate estimation: coming of age [Editorial]. Clin Chem. 2014;60:916-9. [PMID: 24871681]

Margulis V, Sagalowsky AI. Assessment of hematuria. Med Clin North Am. 2011;95:153-9. [PMID: 21095418]

Moyer VA; U.S. Preventive Services Task Force. Screening for bladder cancer: U.S. Preventive Services Task Force recommendation statement. Ann Intern Med. 2011;155:246-51. [PMID: 21844550]

Nielsen M, Qaseem A; High Value Care Task Force of the American College of Physicians. Hematuria as a marker of occult urinary tract cancer: advice for high-value care from the American College of Physicians. Ann Intern Med. 2016;164:488-97. [PMID: 26810935]

Subramaniam RM, Suarez-Cuervo C, Wilson RF, Turban S, Zhang A, Sherrod C, et al. Effectiveness of prevention strategies for contrast-induced nephropathy: a systematic review and meta-analysis. Ann Intern Med. 2016;164:406-16. [PMID: 26830221]

Fluids and Electrolytes

Adrogué HJ, Madias NE. Hypernatremia. N Engl J Med. 2000;342:1493-9. [PMID: 10816188]

Agus ZS. Hypomagnesemia. J Am Soc Nephrol. 1999;10:1616-22. [PMID: 10405219]

Ahamed S, Anpalahan M, Savvas S, Gibson S, Torres J, Janus E. Hyponatraemia in older medical patients: implications for falls and adverse outcomes of hospitalisation. Intern Med J. 2014;44:991-7. [PMID: 25039672]

Almond CS, Shin AY, Fortescue EB, Mannix RC, Wypij D, Binstadt BA, et al. Hyponatremia among runners in the Boston Marathon. N Engl J Med. 2005;352:1550-6. [PMID: 15829535]

Felsenfeld AJ, Levine BS. Approach to treatment of hypophosphatemia. Am J Kidney Dis. 2012;60:655-61. [PMID: 22863286]

Greenlee M, Wingo CS, McDonough AA, Youn JH, Kone BC. Narrative review: evolving concepts in potassium homeostasis and hypokalemia. Ann Intern Med. 2009;150:619-25. [PMID: 19414841]

Hoorn EJ, Betjes MG, Weigel J, Zietse R. Hypernatraemia in critically ill patients: too little water and too much salt. Nephrol Dial Transplant. 2008;23:1562-8. [PMID: 18065827]

Huang CL, Kuo E. Mechanism of hypokalemia in magnesium deficiency. J Am Soc Nephrol. 2007;18:2649-52. [PMID: 17804670]

Jain G, Ong S, Warnock DG. Genetic disorders of potassium homeostasis. Semin Nephrol. 2013;33:300-9. [PMID: 23953807]

Mohmand HK, Issa D, Ahmad Z, Cappuccio JD, Kouides RW, Sterns RH. Hypertonic saline for hyponatremia: risk of inadvertent overcorrection. Clin J Am Soc Nephrol. 2007;2:1110-7. [PMID: 17913972]

Moritz ML, Kalantar-Zadeh K, Ayus JC. Ecstasy-associated hyponatremia: why are women at risk? Nephrol Dial Transplant. 2013;28:2206-9. [PMID: 23804804]

Palmer BF. Regulation of potassium homeostasis. Clin J Am Soc Nephrol. 2015;10:1050-60. [PMID: 24721891]

Regolisti G, Cabassi A, Parenti E, Maggiore U, Fiaccadori E. Severe hypomagnesemia during long-term treatment with a proton pump inhibitor. Am J Kidney Dis. 2010;56:168-74. [PMID: 20493607]

Sterns RH, Silver SM. Complications and management of hyponatremia. Curr Opin Nephrol Hypertens. 2016;25:114-9. [PMID: 26735146]

Acid-Base Disorders

Gennari FJ. Pathophysiology of metabolic alkalosis: a new classification based on the centrality of stimulated collecting duct ion transport. Am J Kidney Dis. 2011;58:626-36. [PMID: 21849227]

Kraut JA, Kurtz I. Toxic alcohol ingestions: clinical features, diagnosis, and management. Clin J Am Soc Nephrol. 2008;3:208-25. [PMID: 18045860]

Kraut JA, Madias NE. Metabolic acidosis of CKD: an update. Am J Kidney Dis. 2016;67:307-17. [PMID: 26477665] doi:10.1053/j.ajkd.2015.08.028

Kraut JA, Nagami GT. The serum anion gap in the evaluation of acid-base disorders: what are its limitations and can its effectiveness be improved? Clin J Am Soc Nephrol. 2013;8:2018-24. [PMID: 23833313]

Madias NE. Renal acidification responses to respiratory acid-base disorders. J Nephrol. 2010;23 Suppl 16:S85-91. [PMID: 21170892]

Melcescu E, Phillips J, Moll G, Subauste JS, Koch CA. 11Beta-hydroxylase deficiency and other syndromes of mineralocorticoid excess as a rare cause of endocrine hypertension. Horm Metab Res. 2012;44:867-78. [PMID: 22932914]

Raimondi GA, Gonzalez S, Zaltsman J, Menga G, Adrogué HJ. Acid-base patterns in acute severe asthma. J Asthma. 2013;50:1062-8. [PMID: 23947392]

Rastegar M, Nagami GT. Non-anion gap metabolic acidosis: a clinical approach to evaluation. Am J Kidney Dis. 2017;69:296-301. [PMID: 28029394]

Treger R, Pirouz S, Kamangar N, Corry D. Agreement between central venous and arterial blood gas measurements in the intensive care unit. Clin J Am Soc Nephrol. 2010;5:390-4. [PMID: 20019117]

Vichot AA, Rastegar A. Use of anion gap in the evaluation of a patient with metabolic acidosis. Am J Kidney Dis. 2014;64:653-7. [PMID: 25132207]

Hypertension

ALLHAT Officers and Coordinators for the ALLHAT Collaborative Research Group. The Antihypertensive and Lipid-Lowering Treatment to Prevent Heart Attack Trial. Major outcomes in high-risk hypertensive patients randomized to angiotensin-converting enzyme inhibitor or calcium channel blocker vs diuretic: The Antihypertensive and Lipid-Lowering Treatment to Prevent Heart Attack Trial (ALLHAT). JAMA. 2002;288:2981-97. [PMID: 12479763]

Appel LJ, Wright JT Jr, Greene T, Agodoa LY, Astor BC, Bakris GL, et al; AASK Collaborative Research Group. Intensive blood-pressure control in hypertensive chronic kidney disease. N Engl J Med. 2010;363:918-29. [PMID: 20818902]

Braam B, Taler SJ, Rahman M, Fillaus JA, Greco BA, Forman JP, et al. Recognition and management of resistant hypertension. Clin J Am Soc Nephrol. 2017;12:524-535. [PMID: 27895136]

Brook RD, Appel LJ, Rubenfire M, Ogedegbe G, Bisognano JD, Elliott WJ, et al; American Heart Association Professional Education Committee of the Council for High Blood Pressure Research, Council on Cardiovascular and Stroke Nursing, Council on Epidemiology and Prevention, and Council on Nutrition, Physical Activity. Beyond medications and diet: alternative approaches to lowering blood pressure: a scientific statement from the american heart association. Hypertension. 2013;61:1360-83. [PMID: 23608661]

Eckel RH, Jakicic JM, Ard JD, de Jesus JM, Houston Miller N, Hubbard VS, et al; American College of Cardiology/American Heart Association Task Force on Practice Guidelines. 2013 AHA/ACC guideline on lifestyle management to reduce cardiovascular risk: a report of the American College of Cardiology/American Heart Association Task Force on Practice Guidelines. J Am Coll Cardiol. 2014;63:2960-84. [PMID: 24239922]

Fried LF, Emanuele N, Zhang JH, Brophy M, Conner TA, Duckworth W, et al; VA NEPHRON-D Investigators. Combined angiotensin inhibition for the treatment of diabetic nephropathy. N Engl J Med. 2013;369:1892-903. [PMID: 24206457]

Pierdomenico SD, Cuccurullo F. Prognostic value of white-coat and masked hypertension diagnosed by ambulatory monitoring in initially untreated subjects: an updated meta analysis. Am J Hypertens. 2011;24:52-8. [PMID: 20847724]

Qaseem A, Wilt TJ, Rich R, Humphrey LL, Frost J, Forciea MA; Clinical Guidelines Committee of the American College of Physicians and the Commission on Health of the Public and Science of the American Academy of Family Physicians. Pharmacologic treatment of hypertension in adults aged 60 years or older to higher versus lower blood pressure targets: a clinical practice guideline from the American College of Physicians and the American Academy of Family Physicians. Ann Intern Med. 2017;166:430-437. [PMID: 28135725]

Siu AL; U.S. Preventive Services Task Force. Screening for high blood pressure in adults: U.S. Preventive Services Task Force recommendation statement. Ann Intern Med. 2015;163:778-86. [PMID: 26458123]

Stergiou GS, Asayama K, Thijs L, Kollias A, Niiranen TJ, Hozawa A, et al; International Database on HOme blood pressure in relation to Cardiovascular Outcome (IDHOCO) Investigators. Prognosis of white-coat and masked hypertension: International Database of HOme blood pressure in relation to Cardiovascular Outcome. Hypertension. 2014;63:675-82. [PMID: 24420553]

Whelton PK, Carey RM, Aronow WS, Casey DE Jr, Collins KJ, Dennison Himmelfarb C, et al. 2017 ACC/AHA/AAPA/ABC/ACPM/AGS/APhA/ASH/ASPC/NMA/PCNA guideline for the prevention, detection, evaluation, and management of high blood pressure in adults: a report of the American College of Cardiology/American Heart Association Task Force on Clinical Practice Guidelines. J Am Coll Cardiol. 2017. [PMID: 29146535]

Yusuf S, Teo KK, Pogue J, Dyal L, Copland I, Schumacher H, et al; ONTARGET Investigators. Telmisartan, ramipril, or both in patients at high risk for vascular events. N Engl J Med. 2008;358:1547-59. [PMID: 18378520]

Chronic Tubulointerstitial Nephritis

François H, Mariette X. Renal involvement in primary Sjögren syndrome. Nat Rev Nephrol. 2016;12:82-93. [PMID: 26568188]

Hutchison CA, Batuman V, Behrens J, Bridoux F, Sirac C, Dispenzieri A, et al; International Kidney and Monoclonal Gammopathy Research Group. The pathogenesis and diagnosis of acute kidney injury in multiple myeloma. Nat Rev Nephrol. 2011;8:43-51. [PMID: 22045243]

Lazarus B, Chen Y, Wilson FP, Sang Y, Chang AR, Coresh J, et al. Proton pump inhibitor use and the risk of chronic kidney disease. JAMA Intern Med. 2016;176:238-46. [PMID: 26752337]

Saeki T, Kawano M. IgG4-related kidney disease. Kidney Int. 2014;85:251-7. [PMID: 24107849]

Shah S, Carter-Monroe N, Atta MG. Granulomatous interstitial nephritis. Clin Kidney J. 2015;8:516-23. [PMID: 26413275]

Shirali AC, Perazella MA. Tubulointerstitial injury associated with chemotherapeutic agents. Adv Chronic Kidney Dis. 2014;21:56-63. [PMID: 24359987]

Stefanovic V, Toncheva D, Polenakovic M. Balkan nephropathy. Clin Nephrol. 2015;83:64-9. [PMID: 25725245]

Glomerular Diseases

Almaani S, Meara A, Rovin BH. Update on lupus nephritis. Clin J Am Soc Nephrol. 2017;12:825-835. [PMID: 27821390]

Fogo AB, Lusco MA, Najafian B, Alpers CE. AJKD Atlas of Renal Pathology: membranoproliferative glomerulonephritis. Am J Kidney Dis. 2015;66:e19-20. [PMID: 26300204]

Geetha D, Specks U, Stone JH, Merkel PA, Seo P, Spiera R, et al; Rituximab for ANCA-Associated Vasculitis Immune Tolerance Network Research Group. Rituximab versus cyclophosphamide for ANCA-associated vasculitis with renal involvement. J Am Soc Nephrol. 2015;26:976-85. [PMID: 25381429]

Glassock RJ. Antiphospholipase A2 receptor autoantibody guided diagnosis and treatment of membranous nephropathy: a new personalized medical approach [Editorial]. Clin J Am Soc Nephrol. 2014;9:1341-3. [PMID: 25035274]

Glassock RJ, Alvarado A, Prosek J, Hebert C, Parikh S, Satoskar A, et al. Staphylococcus-related glomerulonephritis and poststreptococcal glomerulonephritis: why defining "post" is important in understanding and treating infection-related glomerulonephritis. Am J Kidney Dis. 2015;65:826-32. [PMID: 25890425]

Hogan JJ, Markowitz GS, Radhakrishnan J. Drug-induced glomerular disease: immune-mediated injury. Clin J Am Soc Nephrol. 2015;10:1300-10. [PMID: 26092827]

Maas RJ, Deegens JK, Smeets B, Moeller MJ, Wetzels JF. Minimal change disease and idiopathic FSGS: manifestations of the same disease. Nat Rev Nephrol. 2016;12:768-776. [PMID: 27748392]

Magistroni R, D'Agati VD, Appel GB, Kiryluk K. New developments in the genetics, pathogenesis, and therapy of IgA nephropathy. Kidney Int. 2015;88:974-89. [PMID: 26376134]

Markowitz GS, Bomback AS, Perazella MA. Drug-induced glomerular disease: direct cellular injury. Clin J Am Soc Nephrol. 2015;10:1291-9. [PMID: 25862776]

Sethi S, Haas M, Markowitz GS, D'Agati VD, Rennke HG, Jennette JC, et al. Mayo Clinic/Renal Pathology Society Consensus Report on pathologic classification, diagnosis, and reporting of GN. J Am Soc Nephrol. 2016;27:1278-87. [PMID: 26567243]

Kidney Manifestations of Deposition Diseases

Alpers CE, Kowalewska J. Fibrillary glomerulonephritis and immunotactoid glomerulopathy. J Am Soc Nephrol. 2008;19:34-7. [PMID: 18045849]

Bridoux F, Leung N, Hutchison CA, Touchard G, Sethi S, Fermand JP, et al; International Kidney and Monoclonal Gammopathy Research Group. Diagnosis of monoclonal gammopathy of renal significance. Kidney Int. 2015;87:698-711. [PMID: 25607108]

Heher EC, Rennke HG, Laubach JP, Richardson PG. Kidney disease and multiple myeloma. Clin J Am Soc Nephrol. 2013;8:2007-17. [PMID: 23868898]

Rosner MH, Edeani A, Yanagita M, Glezerman IG, Leung N; American Society of Nephrology Onco-Nephrology Forum. Paraprotein-related kidney disease: diagnosing and treating monoclonal gammopathy of renal significance. Clin J Am Soc Nephrol. 2016;11:2280-2287. [PMID: 27526705]

Genetic Disorders and Kidney Disease

Chapman AB, Devuyst O, Eckardt KU, Gansevoort RT, Harris T, Horie S, et al; Conference Participants. Autosomal-dominant polycystic kidney disease (ADPKD): executive summary from a Kidney Disease: Improving Global Outcomes (KDIGO) Controversies Conference. Kidney Int. 2015;88:17-27. [PMID: 25786098]

Eckardt KU, Alper SL, Antignac C, Bleyer AJ, Chauveau D, Dahan K, et al; Kidney Disease: Improving Global Outcomes. Autosomal dominant tubulointerstitial kidney disease: diagnosis, classification, and management-a KDIGO consensus report. Kidney Int. 2015;88:676-83. [PMID: 25738250]

El Dib R, Gomaa H, Carvalho RP, Camargo SE, Bazan R, Barretti P, et al. Enzyme replacement therapy for Anderson-Fabry disease. Cochrane Database Syst Rev. 2016;7:CD006663. [PMID: 27454104]

Friedman DJ, Pollak MR. Apolipoprotein L1 and kidney disease in African Americans. Trends Endocrinol Metab. 2016;27:204-215. [PMID: 26947522]

Hall G, Gbadegesin RA. Translating genetic findings in hereditary nephrotic syndrome: the missing loops. Am J Physiol Renal Physiol. 2015;309:F24-8. [PMID: 25810439]

Savige J, Storey H, Il Cheong H, Gyung Kang H, Park E, Hilbert P, et al. X-Linked and autosomal recessive alport syndrome: pathogenic variant features and further genotype-phenotype correlations. PLoS One. 2016;11:e0161802. [PMID: 27627812]

Acute Kidney Injury

Durand F, Graupera I, Ginès P, Olson JC, Nadim MK. Pathogenesis of hepatorenal syndrome: implications for therapy. Am J Kidney Dis. 2016;67:318-28. [PMID: 26500178]

Grodin JL, Stevens SR, de Las Fuentes L, Kiernan M, Birati EY, Gupta D, et al. Intensification of medication therapy for cardiorenal syndrome in acute decompensated heart failure. J Card Fail. 2016;22:26-32. [PMID: 26209004]

Kidney Disease: Improving Global Outcomes (KDIGO) Acute Kidney Injury Work Group. KDIGO Clinical Practice Guideline for Acute Kidney Injury. Kidney inter., Suppl. 2012;2: 1-138.

Mehta RL, Cerdá J, Burdmann EA, Tonelli M, García-García G, Jha V, et al. International Society of Nephrology's 0by25 initiative for acute kidney injury (zero preventable deaths by 2025): a human rights case for nephrology. Lancet. 2015;385:2616-43. [PMID: 25777661]

Patel DM, Connor MJ Jr. Intra-abdominal hypertension and abdominal compartment syndrome: an underappreciated cause of acute kidney injury. Adv Chronic Kidney Dis. 2016;23:160-6. [PMID: 27113692]

Pendergraft WF 3rd, Herlitz LC, Thornley-Brown D, Rosner M, Niles JL. Nephrotoxic effects of common and emerging drugs of abuse. Clin J Am Soc Nephrol. 2014;9:1996-2005. [PMID: 25035273]

Raghavan R, Eknoyan G. Acute interstitial nephritis - a reappraisal and update. Clin Nephrol. 2014;82:149-62. [PMID: 25079860]

Wichmann JL, Katzberg RW, Litwin SE, Zwerner PL, De Cecco CN, Vogl TJ, et al. Contrast-induced nephropathy. Circulation. 2015;132:1931-6. [PMID: 26572669]

Wilson FP, Berns JS. Tumor lysis syndrome: new challenges and recent advances. Adv Chronic Kidney Dis. 2014;21:18-26. [PMID: 24359983]

Kidney Stones

Eisner BH, Goldfarb DS, Pareek G. Pharmacologic treatment of kidney stone disease. Urol Clin North Am. 2013;40:21-30. [PMID: 23177632]

Fink HA, Wilt TJ, Eidman KE, Garimella PS, MacDonald R, Rutks IR, et al. Medical management to prevent recurrent nephrolithiasis in adults: a systematic review for an American College of Physicians Clinical Guideline. Ann Intern Med. 2013;158:535-43. [PMID: 23546565]

Shoag J, Tasian GE, Goldfarb DS, Eisner BH. The new epidemiology of nephrolithiasis. Adv Chronic Kidney Dis. 2015;22:273-8. [PMID: 26088071]

Tan JA, Lerma EV. Nephrolithiasis for the primary care physician. Dis Mon. 2015;61:434-41. [PMID: 26362879]

The Kidney in Pregnancy

American College of Obstetricians and Gynecologists. Hypertension in Pregnancy. Report of the American College of Obstetricians and Gynecologists Task Force on Hypertension in Pregnancy. Obstet Gynecol. 2013;122:1122-31. [PMID: 24150027]

Cheung KL, Lafayette RA. Renal physiology of pregnancy. Adv Chronic Kidney Dis. 2013;20:209-14. [PMID: 23928384]

Coscia LA, Constantinescu S, Davison JM, Moritz MJ, Armenti VT. Immunosuppressive drugs and fetal outcome. Best Pract Res Clin Obstet Gynaecol. 2014;28:1174-87. [PMID: 25175414]

Hladunewich MA, Hou S, Odutayo A, Cornelis T, Pierratos A, Goldstein M, et al. Intensive hemodialysis associates with improved pregnancy outcomes: a Canadian and United States cohort comparison. J Am Soc Nephrol. 2014;25:1103-9. [PMID: 24525032]

Kattah AG, Garovic VD. The management of hypertension in pregnancy. Adv Chronic Kidney Dis. 2013;20:229-39. [PMID: 23928387]

Nadeau-Fredette AC, Hladunewich M, Hui D, Keunen J, Chan CT. End-stage renal disease and pregnancy. Adv Chronic Kidney Dis. 2013;20:246-52. [PMID: 23928389]

Vellanki K. Pregnancy in chronic kidney disease. Adv Chronic Kidney Dis. 2013;20:223-8. [PMID: 23928386]

Zhang JJ, Ma XX, Hao L, Liu LJ, Lv JC, Zhang H. A systematic review and meta-analysis of outcomes of pregnancy in CKD and CKD outcomes in pregnancy. Clin J Am Soc Nephrol. 2015;10:1964-78. [PMID: 26487769]

Chronic Kidney Disease

Coresh J, Turin TC, Matsushita K, Sang Y, Ballew SH, Appel LJ, et al. Decline in estimated glomerular filtration rate and subsequent risk of end-stage renal disease and mortality. JAMA. 2014;311:2518-2531. [PMID: 24892770]

Dierickx D, Habermann TM. Post-transplantation lymphoproliferative disorders in adults. N Engl J Med. 2018;378:549-562. [PMID: 29414277]

Grubbs V, Moss AH, Cohen LM, Fischer MJ, Germain MJ, Jassal SV, et al; Dialysis Advisory Group of the American Society of Nephrology. A palliative approach to dialysis care: a patient-centered transition to the end of life. Clin J Am Soc Nephrol. 2014;9:2203-9. [PMID: 25104274]

Kidney Disease: Improving Global Outcomes (KDIGO) Anemia Work Group. KDIGO Clinical Practice Guideline for Anemia in Chronic Kidney Disease. Kidney Int Suppl. 2012;2:279-335. Available at www.kdigo.org.

Kidney Disease: Improving Global Outcomes (KDIGO) CKD Work Group. KDIGO 2012 clinical practice guideline for the evaluation and management of chronic kidney disease. Kidney Int Suppl. 2013;3:1-150. Available at www.kdigo.org.

Kidney Disease: Improving Global Outcomes (KDIGO) CKD-MBD Update Work Group. KDIGO 2017 clinical practice guideline update for the diagnosis, evaluation, prevention, and treatment of chronic kidney disease-mineral and bone disorder (CKD-MBD). Kidney Int Suppl. 2017;7:1-59. Available at www.kdigo.org.

Kidney Disease: Improving Global Outcomes (KDIGO) Transplant Work Group. KDIGO clinical practice guideline for the care of kidney transplant recipients. Am J Transplant. 2009;9 Suppl 3:S1-155. [PMID: 19845597]

McMahon EJ, Campbell KL, Bauer JD, Mudge DW. Altered dietary salt intake for people with chronic kidney disease. Cochrane Database Syst Rev. 2015:CD010070. [PMID: 25691262]

Mills KT, Chen J, Yang W, Appel LJ, Kusek JW, Alper A, et al; Chronic Renal Insufficiency Cohort (CRIC) Study Investigators. Sodium excretion and the risk of cardiovascular disease in patients with chronic kidney disease. JAMA. 2016;315:2200-10. [PMID: 27218629]

Murphy D, McCulloch CE, Lin F, Banerjee T, Bragg-Gresham JL, Eberhardt MS, et al; Centers for Disease Control and Prevention Chronic Kidney Disease Surveillance Team. Trends in prevalence of chronic kidney disease in the United States. Ann Intern Med. 2016;165:473-481. [PMID: 27479614]

Saunders MR, Cifu A, Vela M. Screening for chronic kidney disease. JAMA. 2015;314:615-6. [PMID: 26262800]

Tangri N, Grams ME, Levey AS, Coresh J, Appel LJ, Astor BC, et al; CKD Prognosis Consortium. Multinational assessment of accuracy of equations for predicting risk of kidney failure: a meta-analysis. JAMA. 2016;315:164-74. [PMID: 26757465]

Whelton PK, Carey RM, Aronow WS, Casey DE Jr, Collins KJ, Dennison Himmelfarb C, et al. 2017 ACC/AHA/AAPA/ABC/ACPM/AGS/APhA/ASH/ASPC/NMA/PCNA guideline for the prevention, detection, evaluation, and management of high blood pressure in adults: a report of the American College of Cardiology/American Heart Association task force on clinical practice guidelines. J Am Coll Cardiol. 2017. [PMID: 29146535]

Xie Y, Bowe B, Li T, Xian H, Balasubramanian S, Al-Aly Z. Proton pump inhibitors and risk of incident CKD and progression to ESRD. J Am Soc Nephrol. 2016;27:3153-3163. [PMID: 27080976]

Nephrology Self-Assessment Test

This self-assessment test contains one-best-answer multiple-choice questions. Please read these directions carefully before answering the questions. Answers, critiques, and bibliographies immediately follow these multiple-choice questions. The American College of Physicians (ACP) is accredited by the Accreditation Council for Continuing Medical Education (ACCME) to provide continuing medical education for physicians.

The American College of Physicians designates MKSAP 18 Nephrology for a maximum of 25 *AMA PRA Category 1 Credits*™. Physicians should claim only the credit commensurate with the extent of their participation in the activity.

Successful completion of the CME activity, which includes participation in the evaluation component, enables the participant to earn up to 25 medical knowledge MOC points in the American Board of Internal Medicine's Maintenance of Certification (MOC) program. It is the CME activity provider's responsibility to submit participant completion information to ACCME for the purpose of granting MOC credit.

Earn Instantaneous CME Credits or MOC Points Online

Print subscribers can enter their answers online to earn instantaneous CME credits or MOC points. You can submit your answers using online answer sheets that are provided at mksap.acponline.org, where a record of your MKSAP 18 credits will be available. To earn CME credits or to apply for MOC points, you need to answer all of the questions in a test and earn a score of at least 50% correct (number of correct answers divided by the total number of questions). Please note that if you are applying for MOC points, you must also enter your birth date and ABIM candidate number. Take either of the following approaches:

- Use the printed answer sheet at the back of this book to record your answers. Go to mksap.acponline.org, access the appropriate online answer sheet, transcribe your answers, and submit your test for instantaneous CME credits or MOC points. There is no additional fee for this service.

- Go to mksap.acponline.org, access the appropriate online answer sheet, directly enter your answers, and submit your test for instantaneous CME credits or MOC points. There is no additional fee for this service.

Earn CME Credits or MOC Points by Mail or Fax

Pay a $20 processing fee per answer sheet and submit the printed answer sheet at the back of this book by mail or fax, as instructed on the answer sheet. Make sure you calculate your score and enter your birth date and ABIM candidate number, and fax the answer sheet to 215-351-2799 or mail the answer sheet to Member and Customer Service, American College of Physicians, 190 N. Independence Mall West, Philadelphia, PA 19106-1572, using the courtesy envelope provided in your MKSAP 18 slipcase. You will need your 10-digit order number and 8-digit ACP ID number, which are printed on your packing slip. Please allow 4 to 6 weeks for your score report to be emailed back to you. Be sure to include your email address for a response.

If you do not have a 10-digit order number and 8-digit ACP ID number, or if you need help creating a username and password to access the MKSAP 18 online answer sheets, go to mksap.acponline.org or email custserv@acponline.org.

CME credits and MOC points are available from the publication date of December 31, 2018, until December 31, 2021. You may submit your answer sheet or enter your answers online at any time during this period.

Directions

Each of the numbered items is followed by lettered answers. Select the ONE lettered answer that is BEST in each case.

Item 1

A 72-year-old man is evaluated for near-syncope and a recent fall. History is significant for hypertension, hyperlipidemia, and coronary artery disease. Medications are hydrochlorothiazide, amlodipine, carvedilol, pravastatin, and aspirin. The hydrochlorothiazide dose was increased from 25 mg to 50 mg 1 month ago.

On physical examination, blood pressure is 164/88 mm Hg sitting and 140/76 mm Hg standing after 3 minutes, and pulse rate is 64/min sitting and 66/min standing; other vital signs are normal. Ecchymosis is noted over the left elbow. The remainder of the examination, including the neurologic examination, is unremarkable.

Laboratory studies:

Creatinine	1.4 mg/dL (123.8 µmol/L); 1 month ago: 1.0 mg/dL (88.4 µmol/L)
Bicarbonate	30 mEq/L (30 mmol/L); 1 month ago: 26 mEq/L (26 mmol/L)
Potassium	3.0 mEq/L (3.0 mmol/L); 1 month ago: 3.8 mEq/L (3.8 mmol/L)
Sodium	132 mEq/L (132 mmol/L); 1 month ago: 136 mEq/L (136 mmol/L)

A 12-lead electrocardiogram shows no changes from previous tracings.

Which of the following is the most appropriate management?

(A) Decrease hydrochlorothiazide dose and obtain ambulatory blood pressure monitoring
(B) Order telemetry and cardiac enzyme testing
(C) Schedule bilateral carotid ultrasonography
(D) Schedule head CT

Item 2

An 81-year-old man is hospitalized for an acute onset of edema in his legs and abdomen. History is significant for chronic back pain, for which he takes daily ibuprofen. He has no other symptoms.

On physical examination, vital signs are normal. There is no rash. Cardiac examination is without extra sounds or murmurs, and the estimated central venous pressure is normal. The lungs are clear on examination. Ascites is noted. There is 3-mm pitting edema of the extremities to the mid thigh.

Laboratory studies:

Albumin	2.1 g/dL (21 g/L)
Creatinine	2.9 mg/dL (256.4 µmol/L)
Electrolytes	Normal
Urinalysis	No blood; 4+ protein
Urine protein-creatinine ratio	7200 mg/g
24-Hour urine output	1.5 L

Doppler ultrasound of the kidneys is unremarkable.

Which of the following is the most appropriate next step in management?

(A) Initiate dialysis
(B) Schedule a kidney biopsy

(C) Start heparin
(D) Start intravenous glucocorticoids

Item 3

A 56-year-old man is seen during a routine evaluation for stage G4 chronic kidney disease (CKD). History is also significant for hypertension. Medications are losartan, labetalol, furosemide, and amlodipine. He has no symptoms and remains physically active.

On physical examination, blood pressure is 129/76 mm Hg, and pulse rate is 68/min; other vital signs are normal. The physical examination is otherwise unremarkable.

Laboratory studies:

Hemoglobin	11 g/dL (110 g/L)
Bicarbonate	19 mEq/L (19 mmol/L)
Creatinine	3.1 mg/dL (274 µmol/L)
Phosphorus	5.7 mg/dL (1.8 mmol/L)
Potassium	5.1 mEq/L (5.1 mmol/L)

The addition of which of the following will most likely slow progression of this patient's CKD?

(A) ACE inhibitor
(B) Erythropoiesis-stimulating agent
(C) Phosphate binder
(D) Sodium bicarbonate

Item 4

A 69-year-old woman is evaluated in the emergency department for new-onset dependent edema that began 3 weeks ago. She says it is difficult to walk, and she has gained 4.5 kg (10 lb) of fluid weight. History is significant for obesity and hypertension. Her only medication is lisinopril.

On physical examination, vital signs are normal. BMI is 32. There is no rash. There is 3-mm bilateral dependent edema stopping just below the abdomen; it is equal on both sides. The remainder of the examination is unremarkable.

Laboratory studies:

Albumin	2.1 g/dL (21 g/L)
Creatinine	1.3 mg/dL (114.9 µmol/L)
Urine protein-creatinine ratio	8700 mg/g

Kidney biopsy findings are consistent with a diagnosis of minimal change glomerulopathy with superimposed acute tubular necrosis.

In addition to initiating diuretic therapy, which of the following is the most appropriate treatment?

(A) Cyclosporine
(B) High-dose oral prednisone
(C) Rituximab
(D) No additional treatment

Item 5

A 67-year-old man is seen for an increase in serum creatinine level and an abnormal urinalysis found during the evaluation of monoclonal gammopathy of undetermined significance. His evaluation revealed an M-protein spike of 1.5 g/dL, <10% clonal plasma cells on bone marrow biopsy, and no evidence of anemia, hypercalcemia, or lytic bone lesions on skeletal survey. Immunofixation revealed IgG as the monoclonal type. He has no constitutional symptoms, no other medical problems, and takes no medications.

On physical examination, vital signs are normal. Trace lower extremity edema is noted. The remainder of the examination is unremarkable.

Laboratory studies:

Albumin	3.6 g/dL (36 g/L)
Creatinine	1.6 mg/dL (141.4 μmol/L)
Urinalysis	pH 5.5; 2+ blood; 3+ protein; 5-8 erythrocytes/hpf
Urine albumin-creatinine ratio	400 mg/g

Which of the following is the most appropriate next diagnostic test?

(A) ANCA testing

(B) β_2-Microglobulin levels

(C) Kidney biopsy

(D) Serum free light chains

Item 6

A 31-year-old man is evaluated during a follow-up visit for IgA nephropathy found on kidney biopsy 3 months ago, at which time lisinopril was initiated. He is asymptomatic.

Physical examination and vital signs are unremarkable.

Laboratory studies:

	Current	3 Months Ago
Creatinine	1.1 mg/dL (97. 2 μmol/L)	1.0 mg/dL (88.4 μmol/L)
Potassium	4.8 mEq/L (4.8 mmol/L)	4.4 mEq/L (4.4 mmol/L)
Urinalysis	3+ blood; 2+ protein	3+ blood; 3+ protein
Urine protein-creatinine ratio	700 mg/g	1200 mg/g

Which of the following is the most appropriate next step in management?

(A) Add losartan

(B) Add oral glucocorticoid therapy

(C) Start alternating courses of intravenous and oral glucocorticoid therapy

(D) Make no changes to the current medication regimen

Item 7

A 48-year-old woman is evaluated in the emergency department for a 1-day history of hearing voices. History is significant for bipolar disorder. Medications are lithium carbonate and quetiapine.

On physical examination, the patient is disheveled and looks chronically ill. She is alert and oriented but appears anxious. Blood pressure is 138/78 mm Hg, and pulse rate is 80/min without orthostatic changes. There is no edema. The remainder of the examination is normal.

Laboratory studies:

Blood urea nitrogen	6 mg/dL (2.1 mmol/L)
Creatinine	0.9 mg/dL (79.6 μmol/L)
Electrolytes:	
Sodium	126 mEq/L (126 mmol/L)
Potassium	3.5 mEq/L (3.5 mmol/L)
Chloride	94 mEq/L (94 mmol/L)
Bicarbonate	26 mEq/L (26 mmol/L)
Glucose	156 mg/dL (8.7 mmol/L)
Urine sodium	12 mEq/L (12 mmol/L)
Urine osmolality	96 mOsm/kg H_2O

Which of the following is the most likely cause of this patient's hyponatremia?

(A) Hyperglycemia

(B) Nephrogenic diabetes insipidus

(C) Polydipsia

(D) Syndrome of inappropriate antidiuretic hormone secretion

(E) Volume depletion

Item 8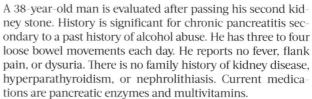

A 38-year-old man is evaluated after passing his second kidney stone. History is significant for chronic pancreatitis secondary to a past history of alcohol abuse. He has three to four loose bowel movements each day. He reports no fever, flank pain, or dysuria. There is no family history of kidney disease, hyperparathyroidism, or nephrolithiasis. Current medications are pancreatic enzymes and multivitamins.

Physical examination reveals a thin man. Vital signs and the remainder of the examination are unremarkable.

Laboratory studies:

Calcium	8.5 mg/dL (2.1 mmol/L)
Creatinine	0.7 mg/dL (61.9 μmol/L)
Electrolytes:	
Sodium	137 mEq/L (137 mmol/L)
Potassium	3.5 mEq/L (3.5 mmol/L)
Chloride	104 mEq/L (104 mmol/L)
Bicarbonate	21 mEq/L (21 mmol/L)
Urinalysis	Specific gravity; pH 5.0; negative dipstick; positive for calcium oxalate crystals

In addition to increasing fluid intake, which of the following is the most appropriate management?

(A) Add allopurinol

(B) Add potassium citrate

(C) Add vitamin C

(D) Decrease calcium intake

(E) Increase protein intake

Item 9

A 33-year-old man is hospitalized for headache, hypertension, and an elevated serum creatinine level. He has a 10-year

CONT.

history of poorly controlled type 2 diabetes mellitus and hypertension. Medications are insulin glargine, insulin lispro, atorvastatin, amlodipine, and low-dose aspirin.

On physical examination, blood pressure is 145/94 mm Hg; other vital signs are normal. Funduscopic examination reveals nonproliferative diabetic retinopathy. There is 1-mm pitting edema of the lower extremities to the ankles, equal on both sides. Dorsalis pedis and posterior tibial pulses are decreased bilaterally, and the feet are insensate.

Laboratory studies:

Complete blood count	Normal
Albumin	3.3 g/dL (33 g/L)
Creatinine	1.8 mg/dL (159.1 µmol/L)
Hemoglobin A_{1c}	8.1%
Antinuclear antibodies	Negative
Hepatitis B virus antibodies	Negative
Hepatitis C virus antibodies	Negative
HIV antibodies	Negative
Urinalysis	No blood; 3+ protein
Urine protein-creatinine ratio	6700 mg/g

Kidney ultrasound reveals mildly increased echogenicity bilaterally, and both kidneys are enlarged at 12 cm.

In addition to improved glycemic control, which of the following is the most appropriate management?

(A) Add an ACE inhibitor
(B) Obtain ANCA titers
(C) Obtain serum and urine protein electrophoresis
(D) Schedule a kidney biopsy

Item 10

A 32-year-old woman is brought to the emergency department by her boyfriend after she was found unresponsive and lying on the ground. She was last seen more than 24 hours ago. History is significant for substance use disorder. She has no other medical problems and takes no prescription drugs.

On physical examination, the patient is intubated and on mechanical ventilation. She is minimally responsive. Blood pressure is 120/75 mm Hg, and pulse rate is 110/min. The remainder of the vital signs and the cardiac, pulmonary, and abdominal examinations are unremarkable. The neurologic examination is nonfocal. Urine output has been <20 mL/h for the past 2 hours.

Laboratory studies:

Calcium	6.9 mg/dL (1.7 mmol/L)
Creatine kinase	40,000 U/L
Creatinine	2.8 mg/dL (247.5 µmol/L)
Electrolytes:	
Sodium	150 mEq/L (150 mmol/L)
Potassium	5.5 mEq/L (5.5 mmol/L)
Chloride	110 mEq/L (110 mmol/L)
Bicarbonate	16 mEq/L (16 mmol/L)
Phosphorous	5.9 mg/dL (1.9 mmol/L)
Fractional excretion of sodium	<1%
Urine myoglobin	300 mg/mL
Urinalysis	Reddish brown urine; pH 5.2; 4+ blood; 2+ protein; granular casts
Toxicology screen	Positive for cocaine and opiates

Which of the following is the most appropriate treatment?

(A) Hemodialysis
(B) Intravenous 0.9% saline
(C) Intravenous 5% dextrose
(D) Intravenous calcium gluconate infusion
(E) Intravenous isotonic sodium bicarbonate in 5% dextrose

Item 11

A 68-year-old woman is hospitalized for a non–ST-elevation myocardial infarction. History is significant for hypertension, hyperlipidemia, type 2 diabetes mellitus, and stage G3b chronic kidney disease. Medications on admission are furosemide, irbesartan, atorvastatin, basal and prandial insulin, and low-dose aspirin.

Vital signs and the physical examination are normal.

Transthoracic echocardiogram shows anterolateral hypokinesis with an estimated left ventricular ejection fraction of 35% to 40%.

Coronary angiography is scheduled.

In addition to stopping furosemide, which of the following is the most appropriate measure to prevent acute kidney injury?

(A) Begin intravenous 0.9% saline
(B) Begin oral N-acetylcysteine
(C) Discontinue atorvastatin
(D) Discontinue irbesartan

Item 12

A 75-year-old woman is hospitalized for a 1-week history of dizziness, nausea, vomiting, increased urination, and decreased appetite. History is significant for hypertension treated with hydrochlorothiazide. She also takes calcium carbonate for bone health.

On physical examination, blood pressure is 150/85 mm Hg supine and 122/70 mm Hg standing, pulse rate is 78/min supine and 100/min standing, and respiration rate is 18/min. There is no neck vein distention. Cardiac, pulmonary, and abdominal examinations are unremarkable. There is no lower extremity edema.

Laboratory studies:

Hematocrit	30%
Leukocyte count	3000/µL (3.0×10^9/L)
Platelet count	82,000/µL (82×10^9/L)
Calcium	12.8 mg/dL (3.2 mmol/L)
Creatinine	3.7 mg/dL (327.1 µmol/L)
Electrolytes:	
Sodium	132 mEq/L (132 mmol/L)
Potassium	4.9 mEq/L (4.9 mmol/L)
Chloride	115 mEq/L (115 mmol/L)
Bicarbonate	17 mEq/L (17 mmol/L)
Phosphorus	6.2 mg/dL (2.0 mmol/L)
Urine sodium	15 mEq/L (15 mmol/L)
Urinalysis	Specific gravity 1.018; trace protein; few erythrocytes/hpf; occasional leukocytes/hpf; few granular casts; numerous hyaline casts

CONT.

Which of the following is the most likely cause of this patient's hypercalcemia and acute kidney injury?

(A) Hydrochlorothiazide therapy
(B) Milk alkali syndrome
(C) Multiple myeloma
(D) Primary hyperparathyroidism

Item 13

A 57-year-old man is evaluated during a routine visit. History is significant for hypertension. Medications are hydrochlorothiazide, 25 mg/d, and amlodipine, 5 mg/d.

On physical examination, blood pressure is 135/86 mm Hg, and pulse rate is 70/min; other vital signs are normal. There is 1+ bilateral ankle edema. The remainder of the examination is normal.

Laboratory studies show a serum creatinine level of 1.0 mg/dL (88.4 µmol/L), a serum potassium level of 3.6 mEq/L (3.6 mmol/L), and an estimated glomerular filtration rate >60 mL/min/1.73 m².

Which of the following is the most appropriate treatment?

(A) Add hydralazine
(B) Add losartan
(C) Double the amlodipine dose
(D) Double the hydrochlorothiazide dose

Item 14

A 25-year-old woman is evaluated in the emergency department after a suicide attempt. History is significant for major depression. She takes no medication.

On physical examination, temperature is normal, blood pressure is 142/92 mm Hg, pulse rate is 110/min, and respiration rate is 22/min. The patient is obtunded. The remainder of the examination is normal.

Laboratory studies:

Blood urea nitrogen	28 mg/dL (10 mmol/L)
Creatinine	2.2 mg/dL (194.5 µmol/L)
Electrolytes:	
Sodium	136 mEq/L (136 mmol/L)
Potassium	4.0 mEq/L (4.0 mmol/L)
Chloride	100 mEq/L (100 mmol/L)
Bicarbonate	12 mEq/L (12 mmol/L)
Ethanol	Undetected
Glucose	90 mg/dL (5.0 mmol/L)
Osmolality	314 mOsm/kg H$_2$O
Arterial blood gases:	
pH	7.25
P$_{CO_2}$	28 mm Hg (3.7 kPa)

Which of the following is the most appropriate management?

(A) Activated charcoal gastric decontamination
(B) Intravenous ethanol
(C) Intravenous hydration, fomepizole, and hemodialysis
(D) Intravenous sodium bicarbonate

Item 15

A 68-year-old woman is evaluated during a follow-up visit for a 3-week history of the nephrotic syndrome. She otherwise has been well and reports no additional symptoms. She has a 50-pack-year history of cigarette smoking with ongoing tobacco use.

On physical examination, vital signs are normal. Pitting edema to the ankles is present. The remainder of the examination is unremarkable.

Laboratory studies:

Albumin	2.9 g/dL (29 g/L)
C3	Normal
C4	Normal
Creatinine	Normal
Rapid plasma reagin	Normal
Antinuclear antibodies	Negative
Hepatitis B antibodies	Negative
Hepatitis C antibodies	Negative
24-Hour urine protein excretion	10,000 mg/24 h

Kidney ultrasound shows normal-appearing kidneys with no evidence of thrombus in the renal veins. Lower extremity Doppler ultrasound shows no evidence of deep venous thrombosis.

Kidney biopsy shows membranous glomerulopathy with negative staining for the phospholipase A2 receptor (PLA2R) on immunofluorescence.

Which of the following is the most appropriate management?

(A) Age- and sex-appropriate cancer screening
(B) Immunosuppression therapy
(C) Prophylactic anticoagulation
(D) Serologic testing for anti-PLA2R antibodies

Item 16

A 42-year-old man is evaluated for a 2-month history of painless gross hematuria. He was diagnosed with chronic kidney disease 4 years ago. His only medication is occasional ibuprofen. He is a recent immigrant from Bosnia.

On physical examination, blood pressure is 150/86 mm Hg. The remainder of the examination is unremarkable.

Laboratory studies:

Hemoglobin	10.5 g/dL (105 g/L)
Creatinine	4.0 mg/dL (353.6 µmol/L)
Urinalysis	1+ protein; numerous nondysmorphic erythrocytes; 5-8 leukocytes/hpf; occasional granular casts
Urine protein-creatinine ratio	900 mg/g

Kidney ultrasound shows echogenic kidneys measuring 8.0 cm and 8.5 cm in length; an irregular bladder wall is noted.

Which of the following is the most appropriate diagnostic test to perform next?

(A) CT urography
(B) Endoscopic urologic evaluation

(C) Kidney biopsy

(D) Urine cultures

Item 17

A 46-year-old man is evaluated for increased urination and thirst of 3 days' duration. History is significant for pulmonary sarcoidosis diagnosed 4 months ago; prednisone, 40 mg/d, was initiated and subsequently tapered to 10 mg/d. Initial symptoms were cough and dyspnea on exertion, which had improved with treatment. He is taking no other medications.

Physical examination and vital signs are normal.

Laboratory studies:

Blood urea nitrogen	16 mg/dL (5.7 mmol/L)
Calcium	9.9 mg/dL (2.5 mmol/L)
Creatinine	1.1 mg/dL (97.2 μmol/L)
Electrolytes:	
Sodium	146 mEq/L (146 mmol/L)
Chloride	110 mEq/L (110 mmol/L)
Potassium	3.8 mEq/L (3.8 mmol/L)
Bicarbonate	26 mEq/L (26 mmol/L)
Urine sodium	20 mEq/L (20 mmol/L)
Urine osmolality	115 mOsm/kg H_2O

In addition to increasing the prednisone, which of the following is the most appropriate treatment?

(A) Desmopressin acetate

(B) Hydrochlorothiazide

(C) Intravenous 5% dextrose

(D) Tolvaptan

Item 18

A 52-year-old woman was hospitalized 3 days ago for laparoscopic resection of the sigmoid colon secondary to recurrent diverticulitis. Diet has been advanced to a full diet. She has a 20-year history of hypertension, stage G3 chronic kidney disease, and migraine headaches. Medications are amlodipine, heparin, topiramate, and as-needed intravenous morphine.

On physical examination, vital signs are normal. Mild incisional tenderness is present. The remainder of the physical examination is unremarkable.

Laboratory studies:

	On Admission	Today
Creatinine	1.6 mg/dL (141.4 μmol/L)	1.9 mg/dL (168 μmol/L)
Electrolytes:		
Sodium	140 mEq/L (140 mmol/L)	138 mEq/L (138 mmol/L)
Potassium	4.9 mEq/L (4.9 mmol/L)	5.6 mEq/L (5.6 mmol/L)
Chloride	102 mEq/L (102 mmol/L)	110 mEq/L (110 mmol/L)
Bicarbonate	25 mEq/L (25 mmol/L)	20 mEq/L (20 mmol/L)
Glucose	116 mg/dL (6.4 mmol/L)	128 mg/dL (7.1 mmol/L)

Urine output during the past 24 hours is 1400 mL.

Which of the following is the most likely cause of this patient's elevated serum potassium?

(A) Acute kidney injury

(B) Heparin

(C) Hyperglycemia

(D) Metabolic acidosis

(E) Topiramate

Item 19

A 40-year-old man is evaluated for a 2-month history of fatigue, nausea, and poor appetite. History is significant for stage G5 chronic kidney disease and hypertension. He has no history of abdominal surgery. Medications are iron, sodium bicarbonate, sevelamer, furosemide, losartan, and amlodipine. He works full time as an on-site supervisor of a team of software engineers. He is on the kidney transplant waiting list.

On physical examination, vital signs are normal. BMI is 25. Conjunctival pallor is noted. There is no pericardial friction rub, jugular venous distention, lung crackles, or asterixis.

Laboratory studies are notable for a hemoglobin level of 8.7 g/dL (87 g/L) and an estimated glomerular filtration rate of 8 mL/min/1.73 m².

Which of the following considerations might favor the choice of peritoneal dialysis as the preferred pretransplant renal replacement therapy for this patient?

(A) Greater autonomy

(B) Improvement in anemia

(C) Improvement in mortality

(D) Lack of infectious complications

Item 20

A 44-year-old man is evaluated during a follow-up visit for treatment of persistently elevated blood pressure. He takes no medications.

Physical examination reveals a well-developed muscular man in no apparent distress. Blood pressure is 165/98 mm Hg, and pulse rate is 70/min; other vital signs are normal. BMI is 26. Jugular venous pressure is normal. Cardiac examination is unremarkable.

Laboratory studies:

Bicarbonate	27 mEq/L (27 mmol/L)
Creatinine	1.3 mg/dL (114.9 μmol/L)
Potassium	4.5 mEq/L (4.5 mmol/L)
Estimated glomerular filtration rate	>60 mL/min/1.73 m²
Urine toxicology screen	Negative

Electrocardiogram reveals normal sinus rhythm; voltage criteria for left ventricular hypertrophy are present.

Which of the following is the most appropriate treatment?

(A) Amlodipine/benazepril combination once daily

(B) Doxazosin and metoprolol, each once daily

(C) Hydralazine three times daily

(D) Telmisartan and ramipril, each once daily

Item 21

An 83-year-old man is evaluated for a 1-week history of poor appetite, myalgia, fatigue, arthralgia, and low-grade fever. He was previously healthy and active. His only medication is acetaminophen as needed.

On physical examination, the patient is afebrile. Blood pressure is 155/95 mm Hg, and pulse rate is 80/min; there are no orthostatic changes. There is trace lower extremity edema. A faint red-blue reticular rash is present over the lower extremities.

Laboratory studies:

Hemoglobin	12 g/dL (120 g/L)
Calcium	9.8 mg/dL (2.5 mmol/L)
Creatinine	Current: 3.1 mg/dL (274 µmol/L)
	Baseline 2 months ago: 0.9 mg/dL
	(79.6 µmol/L)
Urinalysis	3+ blood; 2+ protein; 20-30 dysmorphic
	erythrocytes/hpf; 5-10 leukocytes/hpf

Chest radiograph shows no acute infiltrates. Kidney ultrasound shows no masses or obstruction.

Which of the following is the most likely diagnosis?

(A) ANCA-associated glomerulonephritis
(B) Anti–glomerular basement membrane antibody disease
(C) Minimal change glomerulopathy
(D) Myeloma cast nephropathy
(E) Proliferative lupus nephritis

H Item 22

A 79-year-old woman is evaluated in the emergency department for worsening confusion over the past 5 days. She also reports lower back pain for the past 3 months. History is significant for hypertension and coronary artery disease with stenting of the left anterior descending artery 2 years ago. Daily medications are metoprolol, hydrochlorothiazide, atorvastatin, low-dose aspirin, and acetaminophen. Her husband confirms that the patient takes all medications as directed.

On physical examination, temperature is normal, blood pressure is 128/76 mm Hg, pulse rate is 72/min, respiration rate is 20/min, and oxygen saturation is 95% on ambient air. BMI is 19. There is no abdominal pain. The patient is weak, confused to time and place, and sleepy but easily arousable. The remainder of the neurologic examination is normal.

Laboratory studies:

Blood urea nitrogen	35 mg/dL (12.5 mmol/L)
Creatinine	1.4 mg/dL (123.8 µmol/L)
Electrolytes:	
Sodium	138 mEq/L (138 mmol/L)
Potassium	4.8 mEq/L (4.8 mmol/L)
Chloride	102 mEq/L (102 mmol/L)
Bicarbonate	14 mEq/L (14 mmol/L)
Lactate	0.7 mEq/L (0.7 mmol/L)
Arterial blood gases:	
pH	7.31
P_{CO_2}	29 mm Hg (3.9 kPa)
Urinalysis	Specific gravity 1.025; no protein,
	ketones, cells, or crystals

Which of the following is the most likely diagnosis?

(A) D-Lactic acidosis
(B) Propylene glycol toxicity
(C) Pyroglutamic acidosis
(D) Salicylate toxicity

Item 23

An 18-year-old man is evaluated in the ICU for oliguric acute kidney injury. Eighteen hours ago he underwent hepatectomy for a giant fibrolamellar hepatic carcinoma. During the procedure he developed coagulopathy and hepatic bleeding and required resuscitation with eight units of packed red blood cells, multiple units of fresh frozen plasma, and several liters of crystalloid fluids. He is receiving cefepime, gentamicin, propofol, and fentanyl. Urine output has decreased to 10 mL/h since ICU admission 14 hours ago.

On physical examination, the patient is mechanically ventilated. Blood pressure is 120/70 mm Hg, pulse rate is 115/min, and respiration rate is 12/min. Breath sounds are decreased bilaterally. The abdomen is distended and tense with intact midline incision and wall edema. The remainder of the examination is noncontributory.

Laboratory studies:

Hemoglobin	10 g/dL (100 g/L)
Creatine kinase	1250 U/L
Creatinine	1.7 mg/dL (150.3 µmol/L); on admission:
	0.9 mg/dL (79.6 µmol/L)
Potassium	5.2 mEq/L (5.2 mmol/L)
Urine sodium	<20 mEq/L (20 mmol/L)
Urinalysis	Specific gravity 1.030; pH 5.5; 4+ blood;
	trace protein; too numerous to count
	erythrocytes; few hyaline casts

Kidney ultrasound reveals normal-sized kidneys and no hydronephrosis; a large volume of ascites is noted.

Which of the following is the most appropriate diagnostic test to perform next?

(A) Fractional excretion of sodium
(B) Intra-abdominal pressure measurement
(C) Urine myoglobin levels
(D) Urine stain for eosinophils

Item 24

A 45-year-old man is evaluated for one episode of macroscopic hematuria. He currently does not see blood in his urine. He reports no flank pain and no associated trauma or exertion. He is a nonsmoker and takes no medications.

Physical examination and vital signs are normal.

Laboratory studies show a normal serum creatinine level; urinalysis shows 1+ blood, no protein, 10-15 isomorphic erythrocytes/hpf, 0-2 leukocytes/hpf, no nitrites, and no leukocyte esterase.

Contrast-enhanced CT urogram shows no kidney stones, masses, or cysts.

Which of the following is the most appropriate diagnostic test to perform next?

(A) Cystoscopy
(B) Kidney biopsy
(C) Kidney and renal vein Doppler ultrasonography
(D) Urine cytology

Item 25

A 27-year-old woman is evaluated for a 6-month history of fatigue, arthralgia, and myalgia. She has a history of urinary tract infections. Medications are an oral contraceptive pill and as-needed naproxen for pain.

On physical examination, temperature is 38.2 °C (100.8 °F), blood pressure is 142/90 mm Hg, and pulse rate is 90/min. Cardiac, lung, and abdominal examinations are normal.

Laboratory studies show a serum creatinine level of 1.4 mg/dL (123.8 µmol/L); urinalysis shows 2+ blood, 3+ protein, positive leukocyte esterase, no nitrites, 10-15 erythrocytes/hpf, 5-10 leukocytes/hpf, and no crystals.

Urine microscopy is shown.

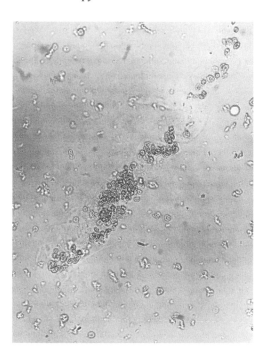

Which of the following is the most likely diagnosis?

(A) Bladder cancer
(B) Glomerulonephritis
(C) Tubulointerstitial nephritis
(D) Urinary tract infection

Item 26

A 61-year-old woman is evaluated in the ICU for acute kidney injury. She was discharged from the hospital 10 days ago following elective cholecystectomy. Seven days ago she was readmitted to the hospital with sepsis. A CT scan of the abdomen with intravenous contrast did not show any abdominal pathology but confirmed pneumonia.

She was treated with intravenous fluids, norepinephrine infusion, vancomycin, and cefepime. The norepinephrine was stopped yesterday. History is significant for hypertension and stage G3a chronic kidney disease. Her baseline serum creatinine is 1.4 mg/dL (123.8 µmol/L). On admission the serum creatinine was 1.9 mg/dL (168 µmol/L) and returned to baseline by hospital day 2; it is 3.1 mg/dL (274 µmol/L) today. Outpatient medications are lisinopril and chlorthalidone.

On physical examination, temperature is 37.6 °C (99.7 °F), blood pressure is 140/82 mm Hg, pulse rate is 103/min, and respiration rate is 20/min. Examination of the lungs reveals bilateral crackles. There is 1+ pedal edema of the extremities. The remainder of the physical examination is noncontributory.

Current laboratory studies:

Serum creatinine	3.1 mg/dL (274 µmol/L)
Vancomycin trough	25 mg/L
Fractional excretion of sodium	2.5%
Urinalysis	Specific gravity 1.012; pH 5.5; no blood; 1+ protein; trace leukocyte esterase; no nitrites; no glucose; 2-4 leukocytes/hpf; 5-10 renal tubular epithelial cells/hpf; 5-10 coarse granular casts/hpf

Kidney ultrasound reveals normal-sized kidneys and no hydronephrosis.

Which of the following is the most likely cause of this patient's acute kidney injury?

(A) Cefepime
(B) Intravenous contrast
(C) Omeprazole
(D) Vancomycin

Item 27

An 18-year-old woman is brought to the emergency department by friends. She is confused and febrile. Her friends state that she took 3,4-methylenedioxymethamphetamine (ecstasy) at a party and was previously well. There is no other medical history.

On physical examination, the patient is confused and oriented to her name only. Temperature is 38.9 °C (102.0 °F), blood pressure is 148/94 mm Hg, pulse rate is 108/min, respiration rate is 20/min, and oxygen saturation is 96% breathing 2 L/min oxygen by nasal cannula. The remainder of the examination is unremarkable.

Laboratory studies:

Blood urea nitrogen	11 mg/dL (3.9 mmol/L)
Creatinine	0.8 mg/dL (70.7 µmol/L)
Electrolytes:	
Sodium	118 mEq/L (118 mmol/L)
Potassium	3.5 mEq/L (3.5 mmol/L)
Chloride	88 mEq/L (88 mmol/L)
Bicarbonate	21 mEq/L (21 mmol/L)
Glucose	88 mg/dL (4.9 mmol/L)
Urine osmolality	405 mOsm/kg H$_2$O

Self-Assessment Test

H
CONT.

Which of the following is the most appropriate initial treatment?

(A) 0.9% sodium chloride, 100 mL/h
(B) 100-mL bolus of 3% saline
(C) Fluid restriction
(D) Oral urea
(E) Tolvaptan

H **Item 28**

A 26-year-old woman is evaluated during a follow-up visit for hypertension diagnosed 1 month ago. She is a marathon runner with previously normal blood pressure. Family history is significant for her mother who died of a ruptured cerebral aneurysm at the age of 50 years. Medications are lisinopril and an oral contraceptive.

On physical examination, blood pressure is 146/92 mm Hg, and pulse rate is 59/min. A systolic-diastolic abdominal bruit that lateralizes to the left side is heard. There is no lower extremity edema. The remainder of the examination is unremarkable.

Laboratory studies show a serum creatinine level of 1.4 mg/dL (123.8 µmol/L) (1 month ago: 0.8 mg/dL [70.7 µmol/L]). Urinalysis is normal with no blood, protein, or leukocyte esterase. A pregnancy test is negative.

A 12-lead electrocardiogram is normal.

Which of the following is the most appropriate diagnostic test to perform next?

(A) Plasma aldosterone concentration/plasma renin activity ratio
(B) Plasma fractionated metanephrines
(C) Renal artery imaging
(D) Transthoracic echocardiography

H **Item 29**

A 75-year-old man is evaluated in the hospital for an acute anterior ST-elevation myocardial infarction. He was hospitalized for chest pain and shortness of breath 45 minutes ago. History is significant for stage G4 chronic kidney disease (estimated glomerular filtration rate, 24 mL/min/1.73 m²), hypertension, and peripheral vascular disease. Medications are lisinopril, metoprolol, furosemide, sevelamer, sodium bicarbonate, aspirin, clopidogrel, and unfractionated heparin.

On physical examination, blood pressure is 145/88 mm Hg, pulse rate is 94/min, and respiration rate is 18/min. Cardiopulmonary examination reveals jugular venous distension, a grade 2/6 mitral regurgitation murmur, an S_4 gallop, and end-expiratory bilateral basilar crackles.

Which of the following is the most appropriate immediate management?

(A) Cardiac catheterization
(B) Cardiac magnetic resonance imaging
(C) Emergent dialysis followed by coronary catheterization
(D) Medical management

H **Item 30**

A 36-year-old man is evaluated in the emergency department for renal colic. He is in otherwise good health and takes no medications.

Physical examination reveals left costovertebral angle tenderness. The remainder of the examination is normal.

Noncontrast helical CT scan shows an 11-mm stone at the left ureteral pelvic junction and mild left caliectasis.

Analgesics are initiated.

Which of the following is the most appropriate next step in management?

(A) Extracorporeal shock wave lithotripsy
(B) Forced diuresis with intravenous normal saline
(C) Nifedipine
(D) Tamsulosin

Item 31

A 41-year-old woman is evaluated for a 3-month history of increasing nonproductive cough, fatigue, anorexia, and malaise. History is significant for hypertension. Medications are hydrochlorothiazide, lisinopril, and self-prescribed vitamin D and calcium for bone health.

On physical examination, vital signs are normal. Bilateral crackles are heard on pulmonary auscultation. Trace pedal edema is present. The remainder of the examination is unremarkable.

Laboratory studies:

Calcium	11.3 mg/dL (2.8 mmol/L)
Creatinine	1.6 mg/dL (141.4 µmol/L); 1 year ago: 1.0 mg/dL (88.4 µmol/L)
Phosphorus	3.4 mg/dL (1.1 mmol/L)
Parathyroid hormone	12 pg/mL (12 ng/L)
25-Hydroxyvitamin D	43 ng/mL (107.3 nmol/L)
Urinalysis	Specific gravity 1.010; 1+ protein; 5-20 leukocytes/hpf; occasional granular casts
Urine protein-creatinine ratio	400 mg/g
24-Hour urine calcium	Elevated

Chest radiograph shows diffuse reticular opacities. Kidney ultrasound demonstrates nephrocalcinosis.

Which of the following is the most likely cause of this patient's findings?

(A) Hydrochlorothiazide
(B) Primary hyperparathyroidism
(C) Sarcoidosis
(D) Vitamin D intoxication

Item 32

A 25-year-old woman is evaluated in the emergency department for chest pain after a belted motor vehicle accident. She is pregnant at approximately 23 weeks' gestation. She reports no additional symptoms and is otherwise well. Her only medication is a prenatal vitamin.

On physical examination, the patient is afebrile, blood pressure is 102/62 mm Hg, and pulse rate is 80/min. Pain and bruising over the left chest wall are noted. Abdominal examination findings are consistent with changes of pregnancy.

Laboratory studies are significant for a serum sodium level of 132 mEq/L (132 mmol/L).

Which of the following is the most likely cause of this patient's low serum sodium level?

(A) Excessive water intake

(B) Hypotension-induced antidiuretic hormone release

(C) Normal physiologic change in pregnancy

(D) Syndrome of inappropriate antidiuretic hormone secretion

Item 33

A 51-year-old man is evaluated during a routine follow-up visit for stage G4 chronic kidney disease and hypertension. He is asymptomatic. Medications are valsartan, amlodipine, and furosemide.

On physical examination, blood pressure is 140/70 mm Hg, and pulse rate is 70/min. BMI is 32. The remainder of the physical examination is noncontributory.

Laboratory studies:

HDL cholesterol	32 mg/dL (0.83 mmol/L)
LDL cholesterol	119 mg/dL (3.08 mmol/L)
Total cholesterol	208 mg/dL (5.39 mmol/L)
Triglycerides	289 mg/dL (3.27 mmol/L)

Which of the following is the most appropriate management for this patient's dyslipidemia?

(A) Gemfibrozil

(B) Niacin

(C) Omega-3 fish oil

(D) Rosuvastatin

Item 34

A 28-year-old man is evaluated in the emergency department for acute right-sided flank pain and blood in the urine. He reports no prior episodes of hematuria or flank pain. He takes no medications.

On physical examination, vital signs are normal. Costovertebral angle tenderness is noted. The abdomen is soft and nontender.

Urinalysis shows 3+ blood, trace protein, and too numerous to count erythrocytes.

A kidney ultrasound shows normal-appearing kidneys, no hydronephrosis, and no nephrolithiasis.

Which of the following is the most appropriate test to perform next?

(A) Contrast MRI

(B) Contrast-enhanced helical abdominal CT

(C) Kidney, ureter, and bladder plain radiography

(D) Noncontrast helical abdominal CT

Item 35

A 26-year-old man is evaluated during a follow-up visit after presenting to an urgent care clinic for back pain 1 week ago. Laboratory studies at that time were significant for a serum creatinine level of 1.4 mg/dL (123.8 µmol/L); other laboratory studies, including urinalysis, were normal. A urine albumin-creatinine ratio obtained in preparation for this visit is 10 mg/g. He is a personal trainer, and his daily exercise regimen includes weightlifting. He states that his back pain has resolved. He occasionally takes ibuprofen; the last use was 1 week ago. He takes no over-the-counter supplements.

On physical examination today, vital signs are normal. BMI is 29. The patient is muscular, without signs of obesity. There is no muscle tenderness.

Which of the following is the most appropriate management?

(A) Avoid all NSAID medications

(B) Measure the serum creatine kinase level

(C) Measure the serum cystatin C level

(D) Schedule a kidney biopsy

Item 36

A 42-year-old man is evaluated during a follow-up visit for kidney stones. He had his first stone 4 years ago. Despite increasing his water intake, he has had two additional episodes. Stone analysis has revealed only calcium oxalate. He is in otherwise good health. He has no history of urinary tract infections. There is no family history of kidney disease, hyperparathyroidism, or nephrolithiasis.

The physical examination and vital signs are unremarkable. The patient weighs 80 kg (176 lb).

Laboratory studies:

Calcium	9.6 mg/dL (2.4 mmol/L)
Creatinine	0.9 mg/dL (79.6 µmol/L)
Electrolytes:	
Sodium	138 mEq/L (138 mmol/L)
Potassium	4.1 mEq/L (4.1 mmol/L)
Chloride	105 mEq/L (105 mmol/L)
Bicarbonate	25 mEq/L (25 mmol/L)
Urinalysis	Specific gravity 1.008; pH 5.5; no blood, protein, leukocyte esterase, or nitrites
24-Hour Urine Studies:	
Volume	2945 mL
pH	5.2
Calcium	320 mg/24 h (normal range, <320 mg/24 h)
Citrate	790 mg/24 h (normal range, 300-1100 mg/24 h)
Oxalate	32 mg/24 h (normal range, <40 mg/24 h)
Sodium	140 mEq/24 h (normal range, 40-220 mEq/24 h)
Uric acid	640 mg/24 h (normal range, <800 mg/24 h)

Noncontrast helical CT scan shows a 4-mm stone in the lower pole of the left kidney and a 3-mm stone in the mid pole of the right kidney.

CONT.

Which of the following is the most appropriate next step to decrease this patient's stone recurrence?

(A) Add allopurinol
(B) Add hydrochlorothiazide
(C) Add potassium citrate
(D) Increase urine volume
(E) Recommend a low calcium diet

Item 37

A 25-year-old man is evaluated during a physical examination for a new job. He is adopted, with no knowledge of his biological parents' medical history. He takes no medications.

On physical examination, blood pressure is 100/60 mm Hg; other vital signs are normal. The remainder of the examination, including cardiac examination, is unremarkable.

Urinalysis shows 2+ blood and no protein.

Kidney ultrasound shows a 15-cm right kidney, a 16-cm left kidney, and multiple cysts bilaterally.

Screening for *PKD* mutations is performed, and the *PKD1* variant associated with autosomal dominant polycystic kidney disease is detected.

Which of the following is the most appropriate next step in management?

(A) Obtain echocardiography
(B) Obtain MR angiography of the brain
(C) Start amlodipine
(D) Start tolvaptan

Item 38

A 44-year-old man is evaluated during a follow-up visit for membranous glomerulopathy, which was diagnosed last week on kidney biopsy. He has no other pertinent personal or family history. His only medication is furosemide.

On physical examination, vital signs are normal. There is trace bilateral lower extremity edema to the ankles. The remainder of the examination is unremarkable.

Laboratory studies performed before kidney biopsy:

Albumin	3.0 g/dL (30 g/L)
Total cholesterol	310 mg/dL (8.0 mmol/L)
Creatinine	0.8 mg/dL (70.7 µmol/L)
Antinuclear antibodies	Negative
Anti–phospholipase A2 receptor antibodies	Titer: 1:80
Hepatitis B surface Ag and Ab antibodies	Negative
Hepatitis C Ab antibodies	Negative
HIV antibodies	Negative
24-Hour urine protein excretion	6500 mg/24 h

Ultrasound of the kidneys shows normal appearance with no evidence of thrombus in the renal veins.

An ACE inhibitor and a statin are initiated.

Which of the following is the most appropriate additional management?

(A) Alternating course of glucocorticoids and alkylating agents
(B) Anti–double-stranded DNA antibody measurement
(C) Cyclosporine
(D) Hepatitis B and hepatitis C viral polymerase chain reaction testing
(E) No additional management at this time

Item 39

A 65-year-old man is seen in the hospital for preoperative evaluation prior to an umbilical hernia repair. Medical history is significant for hypertension, hyperlipidemia, and chronic kidney disease. Medications are metoprolol, amlodipine, furosemide, hydralazine, simvastatin, and aspirin.

On physical examination, average blood pressure is 150/96 mm Hg, and pulse rate is 54/min; other vital signs are normal. BMI is 26. Cardiac examination reveals no murmurs, gallops, or rubs. The lungs are clear. The abdomen is nontender, with a bruit heard over the umbilical region. Lower extremity pulses are diminished. The remainder of the examination is unremarkable.

Laboratory studies:

Creatinine	1.7 mg/dL (150.3 µmol/L); 3 months ago: 1.8 mg/dL (159.1 µmol/L)
HDL cholesterol	46 mg/dL (1.2 mmol/L)
LDL cholesterol	100 mg/dL (2.6 mmol/L)
Total cholesterol	180 mg/dL (4.7 mmol/L)
Urine albumin-creatinine ratio	300 mg/g

Abdominal ultrasound with Doppler reveals 75% ostial right renal artery stenosis; there is no aortic aneurysm.

Which of the following is the most appropriate next step in management?

(A) Begin lisinopril
(B) Obtain renal intra-arterial angiography
(C) Perform percutaneous transluminal renal artery angioplasty and stenting
(D) Perform renal artery surgical revascularization

Item 40

A 68-year-old woman is hospitalized for chest pain. History is significant for stage G3 chronic kidney disease, hypertension, coronary artery disease, and type 2 diabetes mellitus. Medications are aspirin, losartan, basal and prandial insulin, metoprolol, nitroglycerin paste, and unfractionated heparin.

On physical examination, blood pressure is 130/80 mm Hg; other vital signs are normal. S_1 and S_2 are normal. There is no S_3, lung crackles, or leg edema.

Laboratory studies show a serum creatinine level of 1.8 mg/dL (159.1 µmol/L) and an elevated serum troponin level.

CONT.

Electrocardiogram shows a 2-mm ST-segment depression in leads I, aVL, and V_4 through V_6.
Cardiac catheterization is planned.

Which of the following is the most appropriate peri-procedure management?

(A) Administer furosemide before cardiac catheterization

(B) Administer intravenous isotonic fluids before and after cardiac catheterization

(C) Administer oral sodium bicarbonate before catheterization

(D) Initiate hemodialysis following cardiac catheterization

Item 41

A 40-year-old woman is evaluated for arthralgia, dry eyes, and dry mouth of several weeks' duration. She has been taking naproxen and acetaminophen daily for about 1 week. She has no pertinent personal or family history.

On physical examination, vital signs are normal. Mucous membranes and conjunctivae are dry. Bilateral parotid gland enlargement is present.

Laboratory studies:

Creatinine	0.9 mg/dL (79.6 µmol/L)
Electrolytes:	
Sodium	138 mEq/L (138 mmol/L)
Potassium	3.1 mEq/L (3.1 mmol/L)
Chloride	118 mEq/L (118 mmol/L)
Bicarbonate	12 mEq/L (12 mmol/L)
Glucose	74 mg/dL (4.1 mmol/L)
Urinalysis	pH 7.0; no blood, protein, glucose, erythrocytes, or leukocytes

Kidney ultrasound shows echogenic normal-sized kidneys.

Which of the following is the most likely cause of the patient's laboratory findings?

(A) Naproxen

(B) Type 1 (hypokalemic distal) renal tubular acidosis

(C) Type 2 (proximal) renal tubular acidosis

(D) Type 4 (hyperkalemic distal) renal tubular acidosis

Item 42

A 49-year-old man is evaluated in the emergency department for abdominal pain, vomiting, and nausea after binge drinking. History is significant for alcohol abuse, with numerous hospitalizations for intoxications and withdrawal.

On physical examination, temperature is normal, blood pressure is 122/72 mm Hg sitting and 100/62 mm Hg standing, pulse rate is 100/min sitting and 118/min standing, respiration rate is 22/min, and oxygen saturation is 97% breathing ambient air. BMI is 18. Abdominal examination reveals diffuse abdominal tenderness to palpation; there is no rebound tenderness, ascites, or evidence of trauma. Neurologic examination is normal. There is no edema.

Laboratory studies:

Electrolytes:	
Sodium	137 mEq/L (137 mmol/L)
Potassium	3.7 mEq/L (3.7 mmol/L)
Chloride	96 mEq/L (96 mmol/L)
Bicarbonate	10 mEq/L (10 mmol/L)
Ethanol	10 mg/dL (2.2 mmol/L)
Glucose	94 mg/dL (5.2 mmol/L)
Lactate	0.8 mEq/L (0.8 mmol/L)
Arterial blood gases:	
pH	7.26
P_{CO_2}	23 mm Hg (3.1 kPa)
Urinalysis	Specific gravity 1.020; pH 5.5; positive ketones; no blood or cells

Thiamine and B-complex vitamin are administered.

Which of the following is the most appropriate treatment?

(A) 0.9% saline

(B) 5% dextrose in 0.9% saline

(C) 5% dextrose in water with 150 mEq (150 mmol) of sodium bicarbonate

(D) Insulin and 5% dextrose in 0.9% saline

Item 43

A 45-year-old man is evaluated during a follow-up visit for membranous glomerulopathy diagnosed 3 weeks ago. He reports persistent lower extremity edema and no weight loss despite adhering to a low-salt diet and taking maximal-dose furosemide. He does not have shortness of breath or abdominal discomfort. Other medications are enalapril and simvastatin.

On physical examination, vital signs are normal. The patient weighs 80 kg (176.4 lb), with a baseline weight of 75 kg (165.3 lb). There is no rash. Cardiac examination is normal, and there is no evidence of jugular venous distention. The lungs are clear on examination. There is pitting edema in the legs bilaterally to just below the patellae.

Laboratory studies:

Albumin	2.9 g/dL (29 g/L)
Blood urea nitrogen	Normal
Creatinine	1.0 mg/dL (88.4 µmol/L)
Electrolytes	Normal
Urinalysis	No blood; 4+ protein
Urine protein-creatinine ratio	6100 mg/g

Doppler ultrasound of the lower extremities performed 3 weeks ago showed no evidence of deep venous thrombosis.

Which of the following is the most appropriate management?

(A) Add metolazone

(B) Change furosemide to bumetanide

(C) Hospitalize for intravenous diuresis

(D) Repeat lower extremity Doppler ultrasonography

Item 44

A 27-year-old woman is evaluated for proteinuria identified on urinalysis performed for a life insurance examination. She reports no symptoms. History is significant for premature birth, a 2-year history of hypertriglyceridemia and prediabetes, and a 5-year history of obesity. The remainder of her medical history is unremarkable. Her only medication is gemfibrozil.

On physical examination, vital signs are normal. BMI is 37. The remainder of the examination is unremarkable.

Laboratory studies:

Albumin	3.8 g/dL (38 g/L)
Creatinine	1.0 mg/dL (88.4 µmol/L)
Hemoglobin A$_{1c}$	6.4%
Urinalysis	No blood; 3+ protein
Urine protein-creatinine ratio	2100 mg/g

Kidney ultrasound shows normal-appearing kidneys with no masses or hydronephrosis.

Which of the following is the most likely diagnosis?

(A) Diabetic nephropathy
(B) Lipoprotein glomerulopathy
(C) Minimal change glomerulopathy
(D) Secondary focal segmental glomerulosclerosis

Item 45

A 38-year-old woman is evaluated during a follow-up visit for primary membranous glomerulopathy. Diagnosis was made by kidney biopsy 4 months ago, and she was found to be positive for anti–phospholipase A2 receptor (PLA2R) antibodies. Medications are furosemide, losartan, and simvastatin. Recent age- and sex-appropriate cancer screening tests were normal.

On physical examination, vital signs are normal. There is pitting lower extremity edema to the mid shins bilaterally.

Laboratory studies:

Albumin	2.1 g/dL (21 g/L)
Total cholesterol	288 mg/dL (7.5 mmol/L)
Creatinine	1.1 mg/dL (97.2 µmol/L)
Urine protein-creatinine ratio	9135 mg/g

Which of the following complications is this patient at greatest risk for developing?

(A) Gout
(B) Malignancy
(C) Renal cell carcinoma
(D) Venous thromboembolism

Item 46

A 50-year-old man is evaluated for elevated blood pressure measurements despite an increase in his hydrochlorothiazide dose 1 month ago. History is significant for hypertension and hyperlipidemia. Medications are hydrochlorothiazide and atorvastatin.

On physical examination, blood pressure is 150/92 mm Hg, and pulse rate is 69/min. BMI is 30. The remainder of the examination is normal.

Laboratory studies show a serum creatinine level of 1.0 mg/dL (88.4 µmol/L), a serum potassium level of 3.4 mEq/L (3.4 mmol/L), and a urine albumin-creatinine ratio of 550 mg/g.

In addition to weight loss, which of the following is the most appropriate management?

(A) Add amlodipine
(B) Add losartan
(C) Add spironolactone
(D) Schedule a follow-up visit for 3 months

Item 47

A 37-year-old woman is evaluated for a headache lasting 1 day. She is in the third trimester of her first pregnancy. Until now, the pregnancy has been unremarkable, including blood pressure and urine protein measurements. Her only medication is a prenatal vitamin.

On physical examination, blood pressure is 166/115 mm Hg; other vital signs are normal. There is no papilledema. Cardiac examination is normal. On abdominal examination, the patient has a gravid uterus consistent with her stage of pregnancy, and there is no abdominal tenderness.

Laboratory studies:

Hemoglobin	12.3 g/dL (123 g/L)
Platelet count	70,000/µL (70 × 10^9/L)
Alanine aminotransferase	72 U/L
Aspartate aminotransferase	80 U/L
Bilirubin	Normal
Creatinine	1.4 mg/dL (123.8 µmol/L)
Electrolytes	Normal
Peripheral blood smear	Normal
Urinalysis	2+ protein

Which of the following is the most likely diagnosis?

(A) Chronic hypertension
(B) Eclampsia
(C) Gestational hypertension
(D) HELLP syndrome
(E) Preeclampsia

Item 48

A 29-year-old man is evaluated in the emergency department for a 3-week history of headaches. He reports a painful burning sensation in his toes and feet for the past few years, particularly after he exercises at the gym, and states that he does not sweat as much after exercise compared with his peers. He takes no medications. Family history is notable for the following: His maternal grandfather and maternal granduncle had similar burning sensations in their feet for years and died from strokes in their early 40s; and his mother has occasional burning sensations in her feet as well as corneal dystrophy.

On physical examination, blood pressure is 160/95 mm Hg; other vital signs are normal. Numerous angiokeratomas over the sternal area are present. Reduced pain and temperature sensation in the lower extremities bilaterally is noted.

Laboratory studies show a blood urea nitrogen level of 60 mg/dL (21.4 mmol/L) and a serum creatinine level of 4.1 mg/dL (362.4 µmol/L); urinalysis shows 2+ blood and 3+ protein.

Kidney ultrasound shows increased echogenicity in bilateral kidneys.

Which of the following is the most likely diagnosis?

(A) Fabry disease
(B) Hereditary nephritis
(C) Medullary cystic kidney disease
(D) Tuberous sclerosis complex

Item 49

A 58-year-old woman is evaluated in the emergency department for fever and dysuria of 24 hours' duration. History is significant for frequent urinary tract infections. The patient takes no medications.

On physical examination, the patient appears ill. Temperature is 38.3 °C (101.0 °F), blood pressure is 148/84 mm Hg, pulse rate is 98/min, and respiration rate is 18/min. Abdominal examination reveals right costovertebral angle tenderness. The remainder of the examination is unremarkable.

Laboratory studies:
Creatinine   1.1 mg/dL (97.2 µmol/L)
Urinalysis   Specific gravity 1.010; pH 8.0; trace blood; trace protein; 2+ leukocyte esterase; 2+ nitrites; 3-4 erythrocytes/hpf; 10-12 leukocytes/hpf; positive for bacteria

Abdominal radiograph shows a staghorn calculus in the right kidney.

Empiric antibiotic therapy is initiated.

Which of the following is the most appropriate next step in management?

(A) Chronic antibiotic suppression
(B) Potassium citrate administration
(C) Stone removal
(D) Urease inhibitor administration
(E) Urinary acidification

Item 50

A 78-year-old woman is evaluated in the emergency department for severe pain in the left hip after a fall. History is significant for end-stage kidney disease as of 18 months ago, hypertension, and peripheral vascular disease. Medications are lisinopril, amlodipine, sevelamer, and epoetin alfa. She is also receiving morphine for the hip pain.

On physical examination, blood pressure is 132/70 mm Hg, and pulse rate is 72/min; other vital signs are normal. The left lower extremity is externally rotated at the hip. Peripheral pulses are diminished. The remainder of the physical examination is noncontributory.

Laboratory studies:
Alkaline phosphatase   78 U/L
Calcium   9.7 mg/dL (2.4 mmol/L)
Phosphorus   4.2 mg/dL (1.4 mmol/L)
Parathyroid hormone   62 pg/mL (62 ng/L)
25-Hydroxyvitamin D   32 ng/mL (80 nmol/L)

Radiographs of the hips show a left hip fracture and calcified arteries.

Which of the following is the most likely diagnosis for the underlying bone disease?

(A) Adynamic bone disease
(B) β_2-Microglobulin–associated amyloidosis
(C) Osteitis fibrosis cystica
(D) Osteomalacia

Item 51

A 72-year-old man is hospitalized for a 1-week history of worsening shortness of breath; he also has worsening lower extremity edema despite an increase in his furosemide dose 2 days ago. History is significant for hypertension, stage G3a chronic kidney disease, and heart failure with a preserved ejection fraction. Outpatient medications are amlodipine, lisinopril, furosemide, and low-dose aspirin.

On physical examination, blood pressure is 112/60 mm Hg, and pulse rate is 97/min. BMI is 28. Cardiac examination reveals an elevated jugular venous pressure and an S_4. Breath sounds are diminished at the lung bases. There is 2+ pitting edema of the lower legs.

Laboratory studies:
Blood urea nitrogen   64 mg/dL (22.8 mmol/L); 2 weeks ago, 40 mg/dL (14.3 mmol/L)
Creatinine   2.3 mg/dL (203.3 µmol/L); 2 weeks ago, 1.9 mg/dL (168 µmol/L)
Sodium   130 mEq/L (130 mmol/L); 2 weeks ago, 133 mEq/L (133 mmol/L)
Urinalysis   Specific gravity 1.009; 1+ protein; few hyaline casts

Chest radiograph shows bibasilar effusions and vascular congestion.

Which of the following is the most appropriate treatment?

(A) Add conivaptan
(B) Add dobutamine infusion
(C) Increase furosemide
(D) Start ultrafiltration

Item 52

A 62-year-old woman is evaluated for fatigue and weakness. History is significant for stage G4 chronic kidney disease and hypertension. Her only medication is amlodipine.

On physical examination, blood pressure is 135/85 mm Hg; other vital signs are normal. There is no jaundice. Conjunctival rim pallor is noted, and there is no scleral icterus.

Laboratory studies:
Hemoglobin   8.5 g/dL (85 g/L)
Leukocyte count   Normal
Mean corpuscular volume   80 fL
Platelet count   Normal
Reticulocyte count   1% of erythrocytes
Ferritin   30 ng/mL (30 µg/L)
Transferrin saturation   10%
Estimated glomerular filtration rate   18 mL/min/1.73 m²
Stool testing for occult blood   Negative

Colonoscopy performed at age 60 years was normal.

H
CONT.

Which of the following is the most appropriate treatment?

(A) Blood transfusion

(B) Bone marrow biopsy

(C) Erythropoietin-stimulating agent

(D) Iron supplementation

Which of the following is the most likely diagnosis?

(A) Cushing syndrome

(B) Gitelman syndrome

(C) Primary hyperaldosteronism

(D) Surreptitious vomiting

H Item 53

A 45-year-old woman is evaluated for the recent onset of resistant hypertension. During her last visit, chlorthalidone was added to her medication regimen. She reports no symptoms, and review of the systems is otherwise unremarkable. Current medications are metoprolol, amlodipine, hydralazine, and chlorthalidone.

On physical examination, blood pressure is 160/96 mm Hg, and pulse rate is 65/min; other vital signs are normal. BMI is 24. There is no proptosis. The thyroid gland is not enlarged. The remainder of the examination is unremarkable.

Laboratory studies:

Bicarbonate	34 mEq/L (34 mmol/L)
Creatinine	0.8 mg/dL (70.7 µmol/L)
Potassium	2.9 mEq/L (2.9 mmol/L)
Urine albumin-creatinine ratio	10 mg/g

Which of the following is the most appropriate diagnostic test to perform next?

(A) Kidney ultrasonography with Doppler

(B) Plasma aldosterone concentration/plasma renin activity ratio

(C) Plasma fractionated metanephrines

(D) Polysomnography

H Item 54

A 28-year-old woman is evaluated in the emergency department for muscle cramps and weakness. She notes a weight loss of 15 kg (33 lb) over the past 3 months; baseline weight was 115 kg (254 lb). She reports no abdominal pain or diarrhea. She has a 1-year history of type 2 diabetes mellitus, for which she takes metformin.

On physical examination, temperature is normal, blood pressure is 122/72 mm Hg, pulse rate is 100/min, and respiration rate is 18/min. BMI is 36. Muscle strength of the lower and upper extremities is 4/5. Other than weakness, neurologic examination is normal.

Laboratory studies:

Electrolytes:	
Sodium	138 mEq/L (138 mmol/L)
Potassium	2.4 mEq/L (2.4 mmol/L)
Chloride	92 mEq/L (92 mmol/L)
Bicarbonate	34 mEq/L (34 mmol/L)
Arterial blood gases:	
pH	7.50
P_{CO_2}	45 mm Hg (6.0 kPa)
Urine sodium	40 mEq/L (40 mmol/L)
Urine potassium	60 mEq/L (60 mmol/L)
Urine chloride	5 mEq/L (5 mmol/L)

H Item 55

A 64-year-old man is evaluated for a 2-month history of increasing fatigue and bilateral swelling of the submandibular region. History is significant for autoimmune pancreatitis treated with prednisone 2 years ago, hypertension, and allergic rhinitis. Medications are losartan and fluticasone propionate.

On physical examination, blood pressure is 148/84 mm Hg, and pulse rate is 78/min. There is no rash. Head and neck examination reveals bilateral submandibular gland swelling. Trace edema of the ankles is present. The remainder of the examination is normal.

Laboratory studies:

Hemoglobin	12 g/dL (120 g/L)
Leukocyte count	10,000/µL (10 × 10⁹/L); 33% eosinophils
Platelet count	180,000/µL (180 × 10⁹/L)
C3	65 mg/dL (650 mg/L)
C4	7 mg/dL (70 mg/L)
Creatinine	3.1 mg/dL (274 µmol/L); 6 months ago: 1.8 mg/dL (159.1 µmol/L)
IgG	2600 mg/dL (26 g/L)
IgE	500 U/mL (500 kU/L)
Antinuclear antibodies	1:640
Urinalysis	Specific gravity 1.010; trace protein; 6-10 leukocytes/hpf

Kidney ultrasound demonstrates bilateral markedly enlarged kidneys measuring 15 cm in size with hyperechoic cortex and peripheral cortical nodules.

Which of the following is the most likely diagnosis?

(A) IgG4-related disease

(B) Lupus nephritis

(C) Sarcoidosis

(D) Sjögren syndrome

H Item 56

A 70-year-old man is evaluated for new-onset swelling and fatigue for several weeks' duration, as well as right knee pain occurring during the same time period. History is significant for stage G3a chronic kidney disease and knee osteoarthritis. Medications are lisinopril and over-the-counter naproxen.

On physical examination, blood pressure is 150/80 mm Hg, and pulse rate is 70/min; other vital signs are normal. BMI is 30. There are no lung crackles or jugular venous distension. The bladder is not palpable. There is no abdominal bruit. Examination of the right knee reveals crepitus and

H
CONT.
pain at extremes of flexion and extension. There is 1+ pedal edema.

Laboratory studies:

Bicarbonate	23 mEq/L (23 mmol/L)
Creatinine	2.4 mg/dL (212.2 µmol/L); baseline, 1.8 mg/dL (159.1 µmol/L)
Potassium	5.6 mEq/L (5.6 mmol/L)
Urinalysis	No blood; trace protein

Which of the following is the most appropriate management?

(A) Discontinue naproxen
(B) Obtain CT angiography of the renal arteries
(C) Obtain kidney biopsy
(D) Start furosemide

Item 57

A 40-year-old man is evaluated during a follow-up visit for a kidney transplant he received 2 years ago. History is also significant for hypertension. Medications are tacrolimus, mycophenolate mofetil, prednisone, and nifedipine.

On physical examination, blood pressure is 150/95 mm Hg; other vital signs are normal. BMI is 26. The cardiovascular and pulmonary examinations are normal. The abdomen and renal allograft are nontender to palpation. Trace pedal edema is noted.

Laboratory studies:

Potassium	5.6 mEq/L (5.6 mmol/L)
Sodium	Normal
Estimated glomerular filtration rate	90 mL/min/1.73 m²

Duplex ultrasound of the kidneys shows no evidence of transplant renal artery stenosis.

Which of the following is the most appropriate treatment?

(A) Chlorthalidone
(B) Fludrocortisone
(C) Sodium polystyrene sulfonate
(D) Spironolactone

H Item 58

A 48-year-old woman is evaluated in the emergency department for lower extremity weakness, nausea, and increased somnolence occurring during the past 24 hours. She had constipation for 3 days, for which she drank one bottle of milk of magnesia each night. History is significant for hypertension as well as stage G4 chronic kidney disease secondary to autosomal dominant polycystic kidney disease. Her only medication is lisinopril.

On physical examination, temperature is 36.6 °C (97.9 °F), blood pressure is 94/54 mm Hg, pulse rate is 58/min, respiration rate is 16/min, and oxygen saturation is 92% breathing ambient air. Bilateral flank fullness is present. Deep tendon reflexes are diminished diffusely. Strength in the lower extremities is 3/5.

Laboratory studies:

Calcium	8.0 mg/dL (2 mmol/L)
Creatinine	3.9 mg/dL (344.8 µmol/L)
Electrolytes:	
Sodium	138 mEq/L (138 mmol/L)
Potassium	3.7 mEq/L (3.7 mmol/L)
Chloride	104 mEq/L (104 mmol/L)
Bicarbonate	22 mEq/L (22 mmol/L)
Magnesium	8.1 mg/dL (3.3 mmol/L)
Phosphorous	4.4 mg/dL (1.4 mmol/L)

In addition to administration of 0.9% saline and furosemide, which of the following is the most appropriate treatment?

(A) Hemodialysis
(B) Intravenous calcium
(C) Intravenous potassium
(D) Intravenous sodium bicarbonate
(E) Oral sodium polystyrene sulfonate

Item 59 **H**

A 72-year-old man is evaluated in the hospital after developing acute kidney injury 2 days following coronary artery bypass grafting. He is currently on mechanical ventilation and requires vasopressors for hypotension. He underwent coronary angiography 12 hours prior to surgery. The serum creatinine has increased from 0.8 mg/dL (70.7 µmol/L) at baseline to 2.2 mg/dL (194.5 µmol/L), and urine output has decreased to 350 mL/24 h. History is significant for type 2 diabetes mellitus and coronary artery disease. Current medications are intravenous furosemide, insulin, propofol, fentanyl, and norepinephrine.

On physical examination, the patient is intubated and mechanically ventilated. A urinary catheter is in place. Temperature is 37.9 °C (100.2 °F), blood pressure is 98/60 mm Hg, pulse rate is 105/min, respiration rate is 28/min, and oxygen saturation is 96% on 30% FIO₂. There is no rash. Decreased breath sounds are heard in the lung bases. The remainder of the examination is noncontributory.

Which of the following is the most appropriate test to perform next?

(A) Examination of urine sediment
(B) Fractional excretion of sodium
(C) Kidney ultrasonography
(D) Measurement of central venous pressure

Item 60

A 42-year-old woman is evaluated during a routine visit. She recently had her blood pressure measured at her workplace; two measurements were taken, and both were elevated. The patient feels well, and review of systems is unremarkable. Family history is significant for hypertension in her father, mother, and two siblings; stroke in her father; and heart failure in her mother. She takes no medications.

On physical examination, the average of three blood pressure measurements is 128/78 mm Hg. BMI is 30. The remainder of the examination is normal.

Laboratory studies:

Bicarbonate	24 mEq/L (24 mmol/L)
Creatinine	0.9 mg/dL (79.6 µmol/L)
Potassium	4.0 mEq/L (4.0 mmol/L)
Urine albumin-creatinine ratio	10 mg/g

Electrocardiogram reveals normal sinus rhythm and positive voltage criteria for left ventricular hypertrophy.

Which of the following is the most appropriate test to perform next?

(A) 24-Hour ambulatory blood pressure monitoring

(B) Plasma aldosterone concentration/plasma renin activity ratio

(C) Polysomnography

(D) Thyroid-stimulating hormone measurement

Item 61

A 46-year-old man is evaluated during a follow-up visit for recently diagnosed hypertension. Hydrochlorothiazide, 25 mg/d, was initiated 1 month ago. He tries to adhere to a low sodium, low fat diet. The patient is black.

On physical examination, the average of three blood pressure measurements is 147/97 mm Hg, and pulse rate is 74/min. The remainder of the examination is normal.

Laboratory studies show a serum creatinine level of 1.2 mg/dL (106.1 µmol/L), a serum potassium level of 3.5 mEq/L (3.5 mmol/L), and a urine albumin-creatinine ratio of 15 mg/g.

Which of the following is the most appropriate next step in management?

(A) Add amlodipine

(B) Add lisinopril

(C) Increase hydrochlorothiazide

(D) Reassess blood pressure in 3 months

Item 62

A 28-year-old woman is evaluated during a follow-up visit for elevated blood pressure measurements during pregnancy. She is at 12 weeks' gestation of her first pregnancy. She feels well, and the pregnancy has been otherwise uncomplicated. She did not have routine medical care before her pregnancy. Family history is significant for hypertension in her father and sister. Her only medication is a prenatal vitamin.

On physical examination, blood pressure is 155/95 mm Hg; other vital signs are normal. Funduscopic, neurologic, and cardiac examinations are normal.

Laboratory studies are normal.

Which of the following is the most likely cause of this patient's elevated blood pressure?

(A) Chronic hypertension

(B) Gestational hypertension

(C) Normal physiologic changes in pregnancy

(D) Preeclampsia

Item 63

A 73-year-old woman is hospitalized for an elevated serum creatinine level that has been unresponsive to intravenous fluids. She was evaluated in the emergency department 2 days ago for weakness, myalgia, arthralgia, and cough and admitted to the hospital. She has no other medical history and takes no medications.

On physical examination, the patient is afebrile. Blood pressure is 155/95 mm Hg, pulse rate is 70/min, and oxygen saturation is 98% breathing 2 L of oxygen per minute by nasal cannula. Cardiac examination is normal, without evidence of jugular venous distention. Dullness to percussion and diminished breath sounds are present at the posterior lung bases bilaterally. There is pitting lower extremity edema.

Laboratory studies:

Hemoglobin	9.9 g/dL (99 g/L)
Creatinine	Baseline 6 months ago: 0.7 mg/dL (61.9 µmol/L)
	Emergency department: 4.1 mg/dL (362.4 µmol/L)
	Hospital day 1: 4.3 mg/dL (380.1 µmol/L)
Antinuclear antibodies	Negative
Antimyeloperoxidase antibodies	Positive
Antiproteinase 3 antibodies	Negative
Urinalysis	3+ blood; 2+ protein

Chest radiograph shows diffuse infiltrates at the lung bases bilaterally.

Kidney biopsy shows necrotizing and crescentic glomerulonephritis with linear staining for IgG on immunofluorescence.

Which of the following is the most appropriate diagnostic test to perform in this patient?

(A) Anti–double-stranded DNA antibodies

(B) Anti–glomerular basement membrane antibodies

(C) Anti–phospholipase A2 receptor antibodies

(D) Antihistone antibodies

Item 64

A 24-year-old woman is evaluated during a follow-up visit for elevated blood pressure measurements found on two separate occasions. The measurements were 144/94 mm Hg and 142/92 mm Hg. She states that going to the doctor makes her nervous, so she had her blood pressure measured at the local pharmacy, which was <130/80 mm Hg. Review of systems is otherwise unremarkable. She has no other pertinent personal or family history. She takes no medications.

On physical examination, the average of three blood pressure measurements is 143/93 mm Hg, and pulse rate is 80/min; other vital signs are normal. BMI is 21. The remainder of the examination is normal.

Laboratory studies show a serum creatinine level of 0.8 mg/dL (70.7 µmol/L), and a urine albumin-creatinine ratio is undetectable; pregnancy test results are negative.

Electrocardiogram is normal.

Which of the following is the most appropriate next step in management?

(A) Begin hydrochlorothiazide

(B) Obtain echocardiography

(C) Perform 24-hour ambulatory blood pressure monitoring

(D) Recheck blood pressure in 3 months

Item 65

A 79-year-old woman is evaluated for hyperkalemia. She was admitted to the surgical ICU after having an urgent partial colectomy for a ruptured diverticulum with peritonitis. She was treated with intravenous fluids, antibiotics, and vasopressor therapy. Today, postoperative day 1, she is oliguric with urine output <5 mL/h for the past 4 hours. She is now weaned off the vasopressor therapy. History is significant for hypertension and stage G4 chronic kidney disease. Outpatient medications are amlodipine, irbesartan, and furosemide. Current medications are morphine, propofol, cefotaxime, and metronidazole.

On physical examination, the patient is intubated and mechanically ventilated. A urinary catheter is in place. Temperature is 38.9 °C (102.0 °F), blood pressure is 108/70 mm Hg, and pulse rate is 101/min. There is generalized anasarca. The abdomen is distended and quiet.

Laboratory studies:

Creatinine	3.6 mg/dL (318.2 µmol/L); baseline, 2.0 mg/dL (176.8 µmol/L)
Electrolytes:	
Sodium	142 mEq/L (142 mmol/L)
Potassium	7.1 mEq/L (7.1 mmol/L)
Chloride	102 mEq/L (102 mmol/L)
Total bicarbonate	17 mEq/L (17 mmol/L)
Arterial pH	7.25
Urine sediment	Brown granular casts

Electrocardiogram shows peaked T waves with a QRS of 140 ms.

In addition to intravenous calcium, insulin, and dextrose, which of the following is the most appropriate treatment?

(A) Continuous renal replacement therapy

(B) Hemodialysis

(C) Intravenous furosemide

(D) Sodium bicarbonate

(E) Sodium polystyrene sulfonate enema

Item 66

A 55-year-old man is evaluated for a 4-month history of persistent hyperkalemia. He also has long-standing type 2 diabetes mellitus complicated by retinopathy and nephropathy. Medications are basal and prandial insulin, atorvastatin, and aspirin.

On physical examination, vital signs are normal. Nonproliferative retinopathy is noted on funduscopic examination. The remainder of the physical examination is noncontributory.

Laboratory studies:

Creatinine	1.9 mg/dL (168 µmol/L)
Electrolytes:	
Sodium	138 mEq/L (138 mmol/L)
Potassium	5.1 mEq/L (5.1 mmol/L)
Chloride	112 mEq/L (112 mmol/L)
Bicarbonate	18 mEq/L (18 mmol/L)
Estimated glomerular filtration rate	49 mL/min/1.73 m²
Urinalysis	pH 5.0; no blood, protein, glucose, erythrocytes, or leukocytes
Calculated urine anion gap	Positive

Which of the following is the most likely cause of the patient's acid-base disorder?

(A) Chronic kidney disease

(B) Type 1 (hypokalemic distal) renal tubular acidosis

(C) Type 2 (proximal) renal tubular acidosis

(D) Type 4 (hyperkalemic distal) renal tubular acidosis

Item 67

A 21-year-old woman is evaluated during a follow-up visit for a 1-year history of systemic lupus erythematosus. At the time of diagnosis, she presented with a malar rash and arthritis, along with positive antinuclear and anti–double-stranded DNA antibodies. Medications are hydroxychloroquine, low-dose prednisone, calcium, and vitamin D. She currently feels well and is asymptomatic.

Vital signs are normal, and the physical examination is unremarkable.

Laboratory studies:

C3	40 mg/dL (400 mg/L)
C4	8 mg/dL (80 mg/L)
Anti–double-stranded DNA antibodies	Positive (titer: 1:320)
Urinalysis	2+ blood; 2+ protein; dysmorphic erythrocytes; no casts
Urine protein-creatinine ratio	600 mg/g

Kidney ultrasound shows kidneys of normal size and echogenicity.

Which of the following is the most appropriate next step in management?

(A) Begin pulse glucocorticoids followed by cyclophosphamide

(B) Begin pulse glucocorticoids followed by mycophenolate mofetil

(C) Increase oral prednisone dose and add mycophenolate mofetil

(D) Schedule a kidney biopsy

Item 68

A 45-year-old man is seen for a routine evaluation of his blood pressure. He has gained 1.5 kg (3.3 lb) since his last visit

CONT.

3 weeks ago. History is significant for stage G4 chronic kidney disease, hypertension, type 2 diabetes mellitus, and coronary artery disease. Medications are amlodipine, lisinopril, carvedilol, chlorthalidone, basal and prandial insulin, atorvastatin, and low-dose aspirin.

On physical examination, blood pressure is 165/100 mm Hg, pulse rate is 58/min, and respiration rate is 16/min. There is 1+ bilateral leg edema. The remainder of the physical examination is noncontributory.

Laboratory studies:

Blood urea nitrogen	44 mg/dL (15.7 mmol/L)
Creatinine	2.8 mg/dL (247.5 μmol/L)
Potassium	5.4 mEq/L (5.4 mmol/L)
Estimated glomerular filtration rate	26 mL/min/1.73 m²
Urinalysis	Normal

In addition to maintaining a low sodium diet, which of the following is the most appropriate treatment of this patient's blood pressure?

(A) Add hydralazine
(B) Add losartan
(C) Stop amlodipine; begin spironolactone
(D) Stop chlorthalidone; begin furosemide

 Item 69

A 52-year-old woman is hospitalized for a toe ulcer and foot pain occurring for 1 month. History is significant for stage G4 chronic kidney disease (estimated glomerular filtration rate, 22 mL/min/1.73 m²) and type 2 diabetes mellitus. Medications are lisinopril, sevelamer, sodium bicarbonate, insulin glargine, and insulin aspart.

On physical examination, vital signs are normal. A foul-smelling toe ulcer is present. Probe-to-bone test is positive.

A plain radiograph shows changes compatible with osteomyelitis. The patient undergoes wound débridement and bone biopsy.

Bone cultures are pending, and empiric antibiotic therapy is to be administered.

Which of the following is the most appropriate venous access strategy?

(A) Arteriovenous graft creation followed by peripherally inserted central catheter placement in opposite arm
(B) Peripherally inserted central catheter in the dominant arm
(C) Peripherally inserted central catheter in the nondominant arm
(D) Tunneled internal jugular central venous catheter

Item 70

A 45-year-old woman is evaluated for elevated blood pressure found for the first time at her previous visit 1 month ago. She has a 7-year history of type 2 diabetes mellitus without retinopathy, as well as hyperlipidemia. Medications are metformin and atorvastatin.

On physical examination, blood pressure is 148/94 mm Hg (confirmed by home ambulatory blood pressure monitoring), and pulse rate is 74/min; other vital signs are normal. BMI is 32. The remainder of the physical examination is unremarkable.

Laboratory studies show a serum creatinine level of 0.9 mg/dL (79.6 μmol/L), a serum potassium level of 3.8 mEq/L (3.8 mmol/L), and a urine albumin-creatinine ratio of 50 mg/g.

The patient is instructed in appropriate lifestyle modifications.

Which of the following is the most appropriate treatment?

(A) Begin amlodipine
(B) Begin chlorthalidone
(C) Begin losartan
(D) Remeasure blood pressure in 2 months

Item 71

A 50-year-old man is evaluated during a routine follow-up visit. History is significant for chronic kidney disease, long-standing hypertension, and HIV infection. His antiretroviral regimen was recently adjusted to a once-a-day dosing, with the integrase inhibitor raltegravir discontinued and dolutegravir started 3 weeks ago. In addition to dolutegravir, current medications are abacavir, lamivudine, and lisinopril.

Physical examination and vital signs are normal.

Laboratory studies:

Serum creatinine	1.5 mg/dL (132.6 μmol/L); baseline, 1.3 mg/dL (114.9 μmol/L)
Urinalysis	No blood, protein, or erythrocytes
Urine albumin-creatinine ratio	100 mg/g (unchanged from baseline)

Which of the following is the most appropriate next step in management?

(A) Discontinue lisinopril
(B) Measure a 24-hour urine creatinine clearance
(C) Reassess the serum creatinine level in 1 week
(D) No further assessment

Item 72

A 42-year-old woman is evaluated in the emergency department for right flank pain of 3 hours' duration. History is significant for migraines. There is no family history of kidney stones. Medications are as-needed sumatriptan and daily topiramate.

On physical examination, right costovertebral angle tenderness is present.

Laboratory studies:

Creatinine	0.8 mg/dL (70.7 μmol/L)
Electrolytes:	
Sodium	138 mEq/L (138 mmol/L)
Potassium	3.5 mEq/L (3.5 mmol/L)
Chloride	104 mEq/L (104 mmol/L)
Bicarbonate	21 mEq/L (21 mmol/L)
Urinalysis	Specific gravity 1.005; pH 6.5; 1+ blood; negative leukocyte esterase; negative nitrites; 20-30 erythrocytes/hpf; 1-3 leukocytes/hpf; amorphous crystals

CONT.

Noncontrast helical CT scan shows a 5-mm stone in the right proximal ureter.

Which of the following is the most likely composition of this patient's kidney stone?

(A) Calcium oxalate

(B) Calcium phosphate

(C) Cystine

(D) Struvite

(E) Uric acid

Item 73

A 77-year-old man is evaluated for a 2-month history of worsening fatigue, increasing frequency of urination, nocturia, and anorexia. History is significant for hypertension, hypertriglyceridemia, gastroesophageal reflux disease, and depression. He has been taking low-dose aspirin and valsartan for more than 10 years, omeprazole and St. John's wort for 8 months, and fenofibrate for 2 months.

On physical examination, blood pressure is 150/79 mm Hg, and pulse rate is 82/min. The remainder of the examination is unremarkable.

Laboratory studies:

Creatinine	2.8 mg/dL (247.5 µmol/L); 9 months ago: 1.2 mg/dL (106.1 µmol/L)
Urinalysis	Specific gravity 1.008; trace blood; 2+ protein; 3-5 erythrocytes/hpf; 5-7 leukocytes/hpf

Kidney ultrasound shows 9-cm kidneys without hydronephrosis or calculi bilaterally.

Which of the following is the most likely cause of the patient's kidney findings?

(A) Aspirin

(B) Fenofibrate

(C) Omeprazole

(D) St. John's wort

Item 74

A 54-year-old man is evaluated in the emergency department for a 5-day history of fever, fatigue, and bleeding gums. He was previously feeling well. He takes no medications.

On physical examination, the patient is pale and thin and appears chronically ill. Temperature is 39.0 °C (102.2 °F), blood pressure is 104/62 mm Hg, pulse rate is 108/min, respiration rate is 22/min, and oxygen saturation is 96% breathing ambient air. BMI is 22. Petechiae are present on the conjunctiva, forearms, and distal legs. Cardiac examination reveals tachycardia. There is no hepatosplenomegaly. There is no edema.

Laboratory studies:

Hemoglobin	8.8 g/dL (88 g/L)
Leukocyte count	111,000/µL (111 × 10⁹/L), 98% blasts
Platelet count	28,000/µL (28 × 10⁹/L)
Creatinine	1.2 mg/dL (106.1 µmol/L)

Electrolytes:

Sodium	134 mEq/L (134 mmol/L)
Potassium	6.4 mEq/L (6.4 mmol/L)
Chloride	104 mEq/L (104 mmol/L)
Bicarbonate	21 mEq/L (21 mmol/L)

Electrocardiogram reveals sinus tachycardia but is otherwise normal.

Which of the following is the most appropriate next step in management?

(A) Administer intravenous 0.9% saline

(B) Administer intravenous calcium gluconate

(C) Order a plasma potassium measurement

(D) Start inhaled albuterol

(E) Start sodium bicarbonate

Item 75

A 65-year-old woman is evaluated for a 3-month history of increasing fatigue. History is significant for stage G4 chronic kidney disease and hypertension. Medications are sodium bicarbonate, sevelamer, furosemide, losartan, and amlodipine.

On physical examination, blood pressure is 120/60 mm Hg, and pulse rate is 75/min; other vital signs are normal. Conjunctival rim pallor is noted.

Laboratory studies:

Hemoglobin	8.5 g/dL (85 g/L)
Mean corpuscular volume	90 fL
Ferritin	600 ng/mL (600 µg/L)
Transferrin saturation	40%
Estimated glomerular filtration rate	25 mL/min/1.73 m²

Stool guaiac testing is negative.
Colonoscopy performed within the past 5 years was normal.

Which of the following is the most appropriate treatment?

(A) Discontinue losartan

(B) Schedule packed red blood cell transfusion

(C) Start an erythropoiesis-stimulating agent

(D) Start intravenous iron

Item 76

A 52-year-old woman is evaluated in the emergency department for a 2-day history of lower extremity weakness and nausea. She reports no diarrhea. History is significant for hypertension treated with amlodipine. She has a history of alcohol abuse.

On physical examination, vital signs are normal. On neurologic examination, lower extremity strength is 4/5. The remainder of the examination is unremarkable.

Laboratory studies:

Albumin	3.0 g/dL (30 g/L)
Calcium	8.4 mg/dL (2.1 mmol/L)
Creatinine	0.7 mg/dL (61.9 µmol/L)

CONT.

Electrolytes:
Sodium	136 mEq/L (136 mmol/L)
Potassium	2.1 mEq/L (2.1 mmol/L)
Chloride	104 mEq/L (104 mmol/L)
Bicarbonate	26 mEq/L (26 mmol/L)
Magnesium	1.4 mg/dL (0.58 mmol/L)
Urine potassium	30 mEq/L (30 mmol/L)

Which of the following is the most likely cause of this patient's hypokalemia?

(A) Hypoalbuminemia

(B) Hypocalcemia

(C) Hypomagnesemia

(D) Poor nutrition

Item 77

A 71-year-old man is evaluated in the hospital for an elevated serum creatinine level. He was hospitalized 2 days ago for a 4-day history of progressive right lower leg cellulitis. History is also significant for type 2 diabetes mellitus with prior episodes of cellulitis. Medications are basal and prandial insulin.

On physical examination, temperature is 38.9 °C (102.0 °F), blood pressure is 150/100 mm Hg, pulse rate is 100/min, and respiration rate is 20/min. A well-defined area of tender erythema and edema is present over the right foot and leg to just below the knee. The remainder of the examination is unremarkable.

Laboratory studies:
Leukocyte count	13,500/µL (13.5 × 10⁹/L)
C3	50 mg/dL (500 mg/L)
C4	12 mg/dL (120 mg/L)
Creatinine	On admission: 2.4 mg/dL (212.2 µmol/L); baseline: 1.1 mg/dL (97.2 µmol/L)
Urinalysis	3+ blood; 3+ protein
Urine protein-creatinine ratio	4100 mg/g

Kidney biopsy shows endocapillary proliferation on light microscopy, co-dominant granular staining for C3 and IgA on immunofluorescence microscopy, and subepithelial hump-like deposits on electron microscopy.

Which of the following is the most likely cause of this patient's kidney disease?

(A) *Staphylococcus aureus*

(B) *Streptococcus agalactiae*

(C) *Streptococcus pneumoniae*

(D) *Streptococcus pyogenes*

Item 78

A 72-year-old woman is evaluated during a routine visit. History is significant for hypertension treated with amlodipine and losartan. She has no other medical problems. She remains physically active and routinely plays tennis and golf.

On physical examination, blood pressure is 142/84 mm Hg, and pulse rate is 72/min; other vital signs are normal. BMI is 24. The remainder of the examination is unremarkable.

Laboratory studies show a serum creatinine level of 0.8 mg/dL (70.7 µmol/L) and a serum potassium level of 4.0 mEq/L (4.0 mmol/L).

According to the target blood pressure goals recommended by the American College of Physicians and the American Academy of Family Physicians, which of the following would be an appropriate management?

(A) Add chlorthalidone

(B) Increase the amlodipine dose

(C) Increase the losartan dose

(D) Make no changes to antihypertensive medications

Item 79

A 56-year-old man is evaluated during a follow-up visit for diabetic nephropathy. He has a 15-year history of type 2 diabetes mellitus. Medications are insulin detemir, insulin aspart, lisinopril, furosemide, and atorvastatin.

On physical examination, blood pressure is 129/76 mm Hg; other vital signs are normal. The remainder of the examination is unremarkable.

Laboratory studies:
Calcium	9.5 mg/dL (2.4 mmol/L)
Phosphorus	7.2 mg/dL (2.3 mmol/L)
Intact parathyroid hormone	385 pg/mL (385 ng/L)
25-Hydroxyvitamin D	32 ng/mL (80 nmol/L)
Estimated glomerular filtration rate	25 mL/min/1.73 m²

Which of the following is the most appropriate treatment?

(A) Aluminum hydroxide

(B) Calcitriol

(C) Cinacalcet

(D) Sevelamer

Item 80

A 38-year-old man is evaluated during a follow-up visit for elevated blood pressure found for the first time during his last visit. He reports back pain of several weeks' duration after an episode of heavy lifting at work. History is also notable for seasonal allergies. He currently takes ibuprofen daily for the back pain and loratadine as needed for allergies.

On physical examination, the patient is well developed and muscular, and in no apparent distress. The average of three blood pressure measurements is 139/84 mm Hg, and pulse rate is 52/min; other vital signs are normal. BMI is 26. The remainder of the examination is normal.

Office electrocardiogram is normal.

In addition to follow-up in 1 month, which of the following is the most appropriate management?

(A) Begin amlodipine

(B) Begin hydrochlorothiazide

(C) Discontinue ibuprofen

(D) Discontinue loratadine

Item 81

A 29-year-old man is hospitalized for lower extremity edema and fatigue that has progressed over the past 6 months. Laboratory studies document kidney failure. History is notable for obesity. He has a remote history of intravenous drug use and a 5-year history of multiple sex partners (men and women). He takes no medications.

On physical examination, the patient is afebrile, and blood pressure is 148/94 mm Hg; other vital signs are normal. BMI is 38. There is no rash. There is pitting edema in the lower extremities to the ankles bilaterally. The remainder of the physical examination is unremarkable.

Laboratory studies:

C3	60 mg/dL (600 mg/L)
C4	7.0 mg/dL (70 mg/L)
Creatinine	2.8 mg/dL (247.5 µmol/L)
Urinalysis	3+ blood; 3+protein
Urine protein-creatinine ratio	2900 mg/g

Kidney biopsy shows membranoproliferative glomerulonephritis on light microscopy, with immunofluorescence microscopy showing 3+ staining for IgG, 1+ staining for IgM, 2+ staining for C1q, and 2+ staining for C3.

Results of which of the following tests will most likely explain this patient's findings?

(A) Genetic mutations in alternative complement pathway proteins

(B) Hepatitis B surface antigen and surface antibodies

(C) Hepatitis C antibodies

(D) HIV antibodies

Item 82

A 50-year-old man is evaluated for worsening right toe pain of 3 days' duration. He went to an urgent clinic 6 months ago for similar pain and was diagnosed with gout and hypertension. He has consumed illegally distilled alcohol (moonshine) for years. He is a native of Illinois, and his occupation history includes farming, tractor mechanic, and the postal service. His only medications are losartan and a 7-day course of ibuprofen for his previous gout attack. He reinitiated ibuprofen 2 days ago.

On physical examination, blood pressure is 148/84 mm Hg. The right great toe is red, swollen, warm, and tender to touch. There are no tophi. The remainder of the examination is unremarkable.

Kidney ultrasound shows echogenic but normal-sized kidneys bilaterally and no calculi.

Laboratory studies:

Creatinine	2.0 mg/dL (176.8 µmol/L)
Urate	9.0 mg/dL (0.53 mmol/L)
Urinalysis	Specific gravity 1.009; pH 5.0; 2+ protein; 3-5 leukocytes/hpf; occasional fine granular and waxy casts
Urine protein-creatinine ratio	1200 mg/g

Which of the following is the most likely diagnosis?

(A) Analgesic nephropathy

(B) Balkan nephropathy

(C) Cadmium nephropathy

(D) Lead nephropathy

Item 83

A 24-year-old woman is evaluated for progressive muscle weakness of several months' duration. She provides no pertinent personal or family history and takes no medications.

On physical examination, temperature is normal, blood pressure is 94/58 mm Hg, pulse rate is 98/min, and respiration rate is 16/min. BMI is 19. The remainder of the examination is normal.

Laboratory studies:

Serum electrolytes:	
Sodium	142 mEq/L (142 mmol/L)
Potassium	2.8 mEq/L (2.8 mmol/L)
Chloride	120 mEq/L (120 mmol/L)
Bicarbonate	15 mEq/L (15 mmol/L)
Urine electrolytes:	
Sodium	18 mEq/L (18 mmol/L)
Potassium	8.0 mEq/L (8.0 mmol/L)
Chloride	32 mEq/L (32 mmol/L)
Urinalysis	pH 5.0; no blood or protein

Which of the following is the most likely cause of this patient's metabolic acidosis?

(A) Laxative abuse

(B) Surreptitious vomiting

(C) Type 1 (hypokalemic distal) renal tubular acidosis

(D) Type 4 (hyperkalemic distal) renal tubular acidosis

Item 84

A 51-year-old man is evaluated in the hospital for acute kidney injury. He was admitted 14 days ago with sepsis and community-acquired pneumonia requiring mechanical ventilation. He was treated empirically with ceftriaxone and azithromycin; additional medications included omeprazole, insulin, and subcutaneous heparin. On hospital day 3, blood cultures were positive for *Streptococcus pneumoniae*, and ceftriaxone was continued. Hospital course was complicated by the ICU stay, with mechanical ventilation and pneumothorax requiring thoracostomy tube placement. On admission, his serum creatinine level was 1.0 mg/dL (88.4 µmol/L), increasing to 1.9 mg/dL (168 µmol/L) on hospital day 10; omeprazole and ceftriaxone were discontinued, and he was transferred to the floor. Today, hospital day 14, he is oliguric. History is significant for hypertension and diabetes mellitus. Outpatient medications are losartan and metformin.

On hospital day 14, the patient is on 4-L oxygen by nasal cannula. A right-sided thoracostomy tube is in place. Temperature is 36.1 °C (97.0 °F), blood pressure is 145/78 mm Hg, pulse rate is 92/min, and respiration rate is 12/min. There are coarse rhonchi in the left lower lung field. The remainder of the examination is normal.

Current (hospital day 14) laboratory studies:

Creatinine	2.7 mg/dL (238.7 μmol/L)
Fractional excretion of sodium	3%
Urinalysis	2+ blood; 2+ protein; 5–10 erythrocytes/hpf; 5–10 leukocytes/hpf; 3–5 granular casts/hpf
Urine protein-creatinine ratio	1100 mg/g

Kidney ultrasound is normal and without hydronephrosis.

Which of the following is the most appropriate next step in management?

(A) Empiric glucocorticoids

(B) Kidney biopsy

(C) Normal saline fluid bolus

(D) Urinary catheter placement

Item 85

A 30-year-old woman is evaluated because of her family history of kidney disease. Family history is notable for the following: older brother with end-stage kidney disease due to hereditary nephritis diagnosed by biopsy at age 18 years and now with a transplant at age 32 years; 50-year-old maternal uncle with end-stage kidney disease due to hereditary nephritis at age 31 years; mother and maternal grandmother with microscopic hematuria but normal kidney function; and younger brother and older sister without hematuria or proteinuria. The patient is planning for a pregnancy within the next year.

Physical examination and vital signs are normal.

Laboratory studies show a serum creatinine level of 0.7 mg/dL (61.9 μmol/L), and urinalysis shows 2+ blood and trace protein.

Kidney ultrasound shows bilateral kidneys of normal size and echogenicity with no masses or stones.

Which of the following is the most appropriate to perform next?

(A) Audiometry

(B) Genetic counseling

(C) Kidney biopsy

(D) Skin biopsy

Item 86

A 46-year-old man is evaluated in the emergency department for right flank pain that began 3 hours ago. He describes the pain as sharp and severe with radiation to the right testicle. History is significant for chronic diarrhea from Crohn disease; he has two to three loose bowel movements each day. He reports no nausea, vomiting, or abdominal pain. He has no dysuria.

On physical examination, the patient appears uncomfortable. There is right costovertebral angle tenderness.

Laboratory studies:

Electrolytes:	
Sodium	138 mEq/L (138 mmol/L)
Potassium	3.9 mEq/L (3.9 mmol/L)
Chloride	106 mEq/L (106 mmol/L)
Bicarbonate	21 mEq/L (21 mmol/L)
Urinalysis	Specific gravity 1.025; pH 5.5; moderate blood; no protein, leukocyte esterase, or nitrites

Kidney ultrasound shows a 6-mm stone at the right ureteral pelvic junction.

Which of the following is the most likely composition of this patient's kidney stone?

(A) Calcium oxalate

(B) Calcium phosphate

(C) Cystine

(D) Struvite

(E) Uric acid

Item 87

A 54-year-old woman is evaluated in the emergency department for ataxia, confusion, and slurred speech occurring for several days. History is significant for antiphospholipid antibody syndrome with superior mesenteric artery embolus 1 year ago that required resection of a large segment of the small bowel. Her only medication is warfarin. There is no history of over-the-counter medication use.

On physical examination, blood pressure is 106/65 mm Hg, pulse rate is 95/min, and respiration rate is 20/min. The patient is confused, and her speech is slurred. She also has an unsteady, wide-based gait.

Laboratory studies:

Blood urea nitrogen	14 mg/dL (5.0 mmol/L)
Electrolytes:	
Sodium	141 mEq/L (141 mmol/L)
Potassium	3.8 mEq/L (3.8 mmol/L)
Chloride	105 mEq/L (105 mmol/L)
Bicarbonate	16 mEq/L (16 mmol/L)
Glucose	99 mg/dL (5.5 mmol/L)
Lactate	0.8 mEq/L (0.8 mmol/L)
Osmolality	298 mOsm/kg H_2O
Arterial blood gases:	
pH	7.31
P_{CO_2}	33 mm Hg (4.4 kPa)
Urinalysis	No protein, ketones, cells, or crystals

Noncontrast CT of the head is normal.

Which of the following is the most likely diagnosis?

(A) D-Lactic acidosis

(B) Ethylene glycol toxicity

(C) Methanol toxicity

(D) Pyroglutamic acidosis

Item 88

A 27-year-old woman seeks preconception counseling. She anticipates pregnancy within 3 to 6 months. She has a 10-year history of type 1 diabetes mellitus and a 3-year history of hypertension. Medications are basal and prandial insulin, losartan, and hydrochlorothiazide.

Vital signs include a blood pressure of 110/70 mm Hg and a pulse rate of 70/min. Physical examination findings are normal.

Laboratory studies show a urine albumin-creatinine ratio of 25 mg/g.

Which of the following is the most appropriate next step in management?

(A) Discontinue hydrochlorothiazide
(B) Discontinue losartan
(C) Discontinue losartan; begin lisinopril
(D) No changes until patient is pregnant

Item 89

A 50-year-old man is evaluated during a follow-up visit for hypertension. Losartan was started 3 months ago. He is asymptomatic. Family history is notable for his father who was on chronic hemodialysis and died of a ruptured brain aneurysm at the age of 62 years.

On physical examination, blood pressure is 152/96 mm Hg, and pulse rate is 75/min; other vital signs are normal. BMI is 20. The thyroid gland is not enlarged. Abdominal examination reveals bilateral flank fullness and tenderness on deep palpation; the abdomen is otherwise soft and without bruits. The remainder of the examination is unremarkable.

Laboratory studies:

Bicarbonate	26 mEq/L (26 mmol/L)
Creatinine	1.0 mg/dL (88.4 µmol/L)
Potassium	4.7 mEq/L (4.7 mmol/L)
Urinalysis	Trace protein; 10-20 erythrocytes; 0-5 leukocytes

Which of the following is the most appropriate diagnostic test to perform next?

(A) Kidney ultrasonography
(B) Plasma aldosterone concentration/plasma renin activity ratio
(C) Plasma fractionated metanephrines
(D) Thyroid-stimulating hormone

Item 90

A 31-year-old woman seeks preconception counseling. She has end-stage kidney disease secondary to focal segmental glomerulosclerosis. She received a haploidentical kidney transplant from her brother 2 years ago. She had an acute rejection episode 18 months ago that was successfully treated with glucocorticoids, and kidney function has been stable since that time. She currently feels well and reports no symptoms. Current medications are mycophenolate mofetil, tacrolimus, and prednisone.

On physical examination, vital signs are normal. The allograft is palpable in the right lower quadrant and is nontender.

Laboratory studies show a serum creatinine level of 1.3 mg/dL (114.9 µmol/L).

Which of the following is the most appropriate management?

(A) Advise against pregnancy
(B) Discontinue mycophenolate mofetil; begin azathioprine
(C) Discontinue tacrolimus; begin cyclosporine
(D) Proceed with pregnancy without further intervention

Item 91

A 54-year-old woman is evaluated for a 4-week history of dyspnea on exertion, malaise, fatigue, and anorexia. History is significant for hypertension, gout, and osteoarthritis. Medications are losartan, hydrochlorothiazide, allopurinol, naproxen, and aspirin.

On physical examination, blood pressure is 148/84 mm Hg, and pulse rate is 98/min; other vital signs are normal. Conjunctivae are pale. There is 2+ edema of the ankles.

Laboratory studies:

Hemoglobin	8.0 g/dL (80 g/L)
Albumin	3.0 g/dL (30 g/L)
Calcium	9.8 mg/dL (2.5 mmol/L)
Creatinine	2.2 mg/dL (194.5 µmol/L); 3 weeks ago: 1.2 mg/dL (106.1 µmol/L)
Total protein	8.4 g/dL (84 g/L)
Urate	7.0 g/dL (0.41 mmol/L)
Urinalysis	1+ protein; 2-5 granular casts/hpf; 1-2 erythrocytes/hpf
Urine protein-creatinine ratio	6100 mg/g

Chest radiograph is normal.

Which of the following is the most likely diagnosis?

(A) Light chain cast nephropathy
(B) NSAID-induced acute tubular injury
(C) Renal sarcoidosis
(D) Uric acid nephropathy

Item 92

A 28-year-old woman is evaluated in the emergency department for hematuria of 12 hours' duration. She also reports upper respiratory infection symptoms for the past 2 days. She does not have dysuria or flank pain and is not currently menstruating. She reports a similar incident during college when she had the flu, but the urine cleared up after a few hours; she also had an episode of red urine after completing a half-marathon last year. She takes no medications.

Physical examination and vital signs are unremarkable.

Laboratory studies:

C3	Normal
C4	Normal
Creatinine	Normal
Urinalysis	4+ blood; 1+ protein; no leukocyte esterase; no nitrites
Pregnancy test	Negative

Noncontrast CT scan of the abdomen shows no renal masses, no evidence of nephrolithiasis, and no hydronephrosis.

Which of the following is the most likely diagnosis?

(A) Acute postinfectious glomerulonephritis

(B) IgA nephropathy

(C) IgA vasculitis

(D) Lupus nephritis

Item 93

A 76-year-old man is evaluated in the emergency department for confusion, an unsteady gait, tinnitus, nausea, and vomiting. His family has noticed progressive functional decline over the past 2 weeks. History is significant for osteoarthritis. His only medication is aspirin.

On physical examination, the patient is tachypneic and obtunded. Temperature is normal, blood pressure is 140/68 mm Hg, pulse rate is 96/min, respiration rate is 24/min, and oxygen saturation is 99% breathing ambient air. The neurologic examination is nonfocal.

Laboratory studies:

Electrolytes:

Sodium	142 mEq/L (142 mmol/L)
Potassium	3.2 mEq/L (3.2 mmol/L)
Chloride	100 mEq/L (100 mmol/L)
Bicarbonate	20 mEq/L (20 mmol/L)

Arterial blood gases:

pH	7.56
P_{CO_2}	22 mm Hg (2.9 kPa)

Which of the following is the most likely acid-base diagnosis?

(A) Respiratory alkalosis with chronic compensation

(B) Respiratory alkalosis and increased anion gap metabolic acidosis

(C) Respiratory alkalosis and metabolic alkalosis

(D) Respiratory alkalosis, increased anion gap metabolic acidosis, and metabolic alkalosis

Item 94

A 65-year-old man is evaluated for a 2-month history of low back pain. The pain is worse with movement, but it does not radiate. He reports associated fatigue and a 4.5-kg (10-lb) weight loss. He has osteoarthritis and gastroesophageal reflux disease. He has been taking ibuprofen without any pain relief. His only other medication is omeprazole.

The physical examination, including vital signs and neurologic examination, is normal.

Laboratory studies:

Hemoglobin	9.2 g/dL (92 g/L)
Creatinine	3.0 mg/dL (265.2 µmol/L)
Urinalysis	Trace protein; no blood, erythrocytes, leukocytes, leukocyte esterase, or nitrites
Urine protein-creatinine ratio	2500 mg/g

Ultrasound reveals normal-sized kidneys with slightly increased echogenicity; no hydronephrosis or abnormalities of the collecting system are seen.

In addition to discontinuing ibuprofen, which of the following is the most appropriate next step in management?

(A) Discontinue omeprazole

(B) Obtain a 24-hour urine protein collection

(C) Obtain a noncontrast helical abdominal CT

(D) Obtain a urine protein electrophoresis

Item 95

A 60-year-old woman is evaluated for fatigue and weakness. She reports no nausea or vomiting. History is significant for hypertension, stage G4 chronic kidney disease, and type 2 diabetes mellitus. Medications are labetalol, amlodipine, insulin glargine, insulin lispro, and sodium bicarbonate.

On physical examination, blood pressure is 140/90 mm Hg; other vital signs are normal. A mature radiocephalic arteriovenous fistula (AVF) with a strong thrill and bruit is noted. There are no lung crackles. Trace pedal edema is present.

Laboratory studies show normal serum bicarbonate and potassium levels, a blood urea nitrogen level of 50 mg/dL (17.8 mmol/L), and an estimated glomerular filtration rate of 18 mL/min/1.73 m^2.

Which of the following is the most appropriate management?

(A) Clinical follow-up in 6 months

(B) Fistulography to evaluate patency of AVF

(C) Hemodialysis

(D) Kidney transplant evaluation

Item 96

A 55-year-old woman is evaluated for increasing serum creatinine and oliguria; she has cirrhosis. She was hospitalized 3 days ago for worsening ascites, confusion, and an elevated serum creatinine level of 1.5 mg/dL ([132.6 µmol/L]; baseline, 1.1 mg/dL [97.2 µmol/L]). Her diuretics were held, and lactulose was continued. An abdominal paracentesis was negative for spontaneous bacterial peritonitis. Intravenous albumin was administered at 1 g/kg/d for 2 days, and today her serum creatinine level is 3.0 mg/dL (265.2 µmol/L). Urine output for the previous 24 hours was 300 mL. History is significant for cirrhosis secondary to nonalcoholic steatohepatitis. Outpatient medications are lactulose, spironolactone, furosemide, and propranolol.

On physical examination, the patient is confused. She is afebrile, blood pressure is 100/70 mm Hg (stable since admission), pulse rate is 84/min, and respiration rate is 16/min. Asterixis is noted. The skin and sclera are icteric. The jugular venous pressure is normal. Ascites is present. There is 3+ lower extremity edema. The remainder of the examination is normal.

Current laboratory studies:

Bicarbonate	18 mEq/L (18 mmol/L)
Creatinine	3.0 mg/dL (265.2 µmol/L)
Potassium	5 mEq/L (5 mmol/L)
Sodium	129 mEq/L (129 mmol/L)
Urine sodium	<10 mEq/L (10 mmol/L)
Urinalysis	Specific gravity 1.025; pH 5.0; trace protein; 2-4 erythrocytes/hpf; 1-3 pigmented granular casts/hpf

Abdominal ultrasound demonstrates ascites, and normal-sized kidneys with no hydronephrosis.

Which of the following is the most appropriate treatment?

(A) Hemodialysis

(B) Isotonic crystalloid

(C) Octreotide and oral midodrine

(D) Transjugular intrahepatic portosystemic shunt

Item 97

A 56-year-old woman is evaluated for hypernatremia. She was admitted to the ICU 6 days ago for pyelonephritis and septic shock requiring intubation, administration of fluids, norepinephrine, and cefepime. She developed nonoliguric acute kidney injury. She has been weaned off the norepinephrine, and she has been extubated. Her serum sodium level has increased from 142 mEq/L (142 mmol/L) to 148 mEq/L (148 mmol/L) over the past 72 hours.

Physical examination and vital signs are normal.
Urine output is 2.5 L over the past 24 hours.

Laboratory studies:

Blood urea nitrogen	74 mg/dL (26.4 mmol/L)
Creatinine	2.8 mg/dL (247.5 µmol/L)
Electrolytes:	
Sodium	148 mEq/L (148 mmol/L)
Potassium	3.7 mEq/L (3.7 mmol/L)
Chloride	112 mEq/L (112 mmol/L)
Bicarbonate	26 mEq/L (26 mmol/L)
Glucose	136 mg/dL (7.5 mmol/L)
Urine osmolality	420 mOsm/kg H$_2$O

Which of the following is the most likely cause of this patient's hypernatremia?

(A) Adrenal insufficiency

(B) Central diabetes insipidus

(C) Glycosuria

(D) Osmotic diuresis

Item 98

A 55-year-old man is evaluated for an increase in his serum creatinine level. History is significant for hypertension treated with lisinopril for 3 years. He reports no changes or additions to his medication regimen during the past year.

On physical examination, the patient is afebrile, blood pressure is 145/92 mm Hg, and pulse rate is 84/min. There is no rash, alopecia, or joint abnormalities. The remainder of the examination is unremarkable.

Laboratory studies:

Complete blood count	Normal
Creatinine	First specimen, 1.3 mg/dL (114.9 µmol/L); repeat specimen, 1.5 mg/dL (132.6 µmol/L); baseline 6 months ago, 0.9 mg/dL (79.6 µmol/L)
Estimated glomerular filtration rate (eGFR), using the Chronic Kidney Disease Epidemiology (CKD-EPI) Collaboration creatinine formula	>60 mL/min/1.73 m^2
Urinalysis	Trace protein

Ultrasound reveals normal-sized kidneys with increased echogenicity, and no hydronephrosis or abnormalities of the collecting system are seen.

Which of the following is the most appropriate management?

(A) Discontinue lisinopril

(B) Obtain a 24-hour creatinine clearance

(C) Recalculate the eGFR using the CKD-EPI cystatin C formula

(D) Schedule a kidney biopsy

Item 99

An 82-year-old woman is evaluated during a follow-up visit for stage G5 chronic kidney disease. History is also significant for coronary artery bypass graft surgery 10 years ago, peripheral vascular disease, oxygen-dependent COPD, anemia, mild-moderate vascular dementia, and a transient ischemic attack 2 years ago. She has increasing difficulty with activities of daily living and mobility. She has an 80-pack-year history of smoking, having quit 10 years ago. Medications are albuterol, tiotropium, fluticasone-salmeterol inhalers, metoprolol, atorvastatin, iron, and low-dose aspirin. She currently lives in a nursing home.

On physical examination, the patient appears thin and frail. Vital signs include a blood pressure of 108/62 mm Hg, a respiration rate of 22/min, and an oxygen saturation of 92% on 2-L/min oxygen by nasal cannula. BMI is 19. Diminished breath sounds are present throughout the lungs. There is no edema or asterixis.

Laboratory studies:

Blood urea nitrogen	79 mg/dL (28.2 mmol/L)
Creatinine	4.6 mg/dL (406.6 µmol/L)
Potassium	4.6 mEq/L (4.6 mmol/L)
Estimated glomerular filtration rate	9.7 mL/min/1.73 m^2

Which of the following is the most appropriate care strategy for this patient?

(A) Creation of an arteriovenous fistula for dialysis access

(B) Discussion of non-dialytic options

(C) Placement of a double-lumen catheter for long-term hemodialysis

(D) Placement of a peritoneal dialysis catheter

Item 100

A 62-year-old man is evaluated during a follow-up visit for difficult-to-control hypertension. He also has chronic kidney disease and hyperlipidemia. Medications are atorvastatin and carvedilol, as well as maximum doses of lisinopril, amlodipine, and hydralazine.

On physical examination, the average of three blood pressure measurements is 152/98 mm Hg, and pulse rate is 65/min. There is 1+ pitting pretibial lower extremity edema. The remainder of the examination is normal.

Laboratory studies:

Creatinine	2.5 mg/dL (221 µmol/L)
Potassium	4.8 mEq/L (4.8 mmol/L)
Estimated glomerular filtration rate	28 mL/min/1.73 m²
Urine albumin-creatinine ratio	350 mg/g

Which of the following is the most appropriate additional treatment?

(A) Chlorthalidone
(B) Furosemide
(C) Hydrochlorothiazide
(D) Losartan

⊞ Item 101

A 64-year-old man is evaluated for a 5-day history of increased urination and weakness. He was recently diagnosed with non–small cell lung cancer and started on chemotherapy 10 days ago. Medications are cisplatin, gemcitabine, paclitaxel, bevacizumab, and ondansetron.

Physical examination reveals a chronically ill–appearing man. Blood pressure is 105/72 mm Hg, and pulse rate is 100/min; other vital signs are normal. The remainder of the examination is unremarkable.

Laboratory studies:

Complete blood count	Normal
Calcium	8 mg/dL (2 mmol/L)
Creatinine	2.1 mg/dL (185.6 µmol/L); baseline, 0.9 mg/dL (79.6 µmol/L)
Electrolytes:	
Sodium	132 mEq/L (132 mmol/L)
Potassium	2.8 mEq/L (2.8 mmol/L)
Chloride	105 mEq/L (105 mmol/L)
Bicarbonate	18 mEq/L (18 mmol/L)
Glucose	90 g/dL (5 mmol/L)
Magnesium	1.5 mg/dL (0.62 mmol/L)
Phosphorous	1.9 mg/dL (0.61 mmol/L)
Fractional excretion of sodium	2%
Urinalysis	Specific gravity 1.010; pH 6.0; 1+ protein; 1+ glucose; occasional granular casts

Which of the following is the most likely cause of this patient's acute kidney injury?

(A) Bevacizumab
(B) Cisplatin
(C) Gemcitabine
(D) Paclitaxel

Item 102

A 55-year-old man is evaluated during a routine visit. He was diagnosed with primary focal segmental glomerulosclerosis 2 months ago. History is also significant for hypertension. Medications are furosemide, amlodipine, losartan, and prednisone. He has been instructed on a low-sodium diet.

On physical examination, blood pressure is 136/86 mm Hg, and pulse rate is 70/min; other vital signs are normal. Jugular venous pressure is elevated to 14 cm H₂O. Cardiac examination reveals an S₃ gallop. The lungs are clear to auscultation. There is 1+ pitting pretibial edema bilaterally.

Laboratory studies:

Creatinine	1.6 mg/dL (141.4 µmol/L)
Potassium	4.5 mEq/L (4.5 mmol/L)
Estimated glomerular filtration rate	40 mL/min/1.73 m²
Urine albumin-creatinine ratio	1000 mg/g

Which of the following is the most appropriate treatment?

(A) Increase the amlodipine dose
(B) Increase the furosemide dose
(C) Initiate treatment with lisinopril
(D) No changes to medication regimen

Item 103

A 55-year-old man is evaluated during a follow-up visit for newly diagnosed chronic kidney disease (CKD). He also has a 10-year history of hypertension treated with losartan.

On physical examination, blood pressure is 135/78 mm Hg. BMI is 32. The remainder of the vital signs and examination is unremarkable.

Laboratory studies:

Bicarbonate	22 mEq/L (22 mmol/L)
Blood urea nitrogen	27 mg/dL (9.6 mmol/L)
Creatinine	2.1 mg/dL (185.6 µmol/L)
Potassium	4.9 mEq/L (4.9 mmol/L)
Estimated glomerular filtration rate	34 mL/min/1.73 m²
Urinalysis	No blood; 2+ protein

Which of the following additional measurement could best predict this patient's CKD progression?

(A) Serum albumin
(B) Serum calcium
(C) Serum phosphate
(D) Urine albumin-creatinine ratio

Item 104

A 48-year-old woman is evaluated for edema, dyspnea, and proteinuria. She has a 10-year history of rheumatoid arthritis. She was initially treated with NSAIDs, methotrexate, and prednisone. She stopped taking the NSAIDs 6 months ago because of gastritis. Three months ago she began noticing swelling of her legs, and two weeks ago she began experiencing dyspnea when walking. She has never received penicillamine, gold, or a biologic agent. Current medications are methotrexate, prednisone, and omeprazole.

On physical examination, the patient appears chronically ill. Temperature is 37.2 °C (99.0 °F), blood pressure is 158/90 mm Hg, pulse rate is 96/min, and respiration rate is 20/min. Jugular venous pressure is elevated. Cardiac examination reveals a summation gallop. The lungs are clear. Swelling and tenderness at the metacarpophalangeal joints and wrists are noted. There is 3+ lower extremity edema to the knees.

Laboratory studies:

Albumin	2.8 g/dL (28 g/L)
Creatinine	1.1 mg/dL (97.2 µmol/L)
Serum protein electrophoresis	Polyclonal gammopathy
Urinalysis	Specific gravity 1.0120; pH 5.5; no blood; 4+ protein
Urine protein-creatinine ratio	6000 mg/g

Electrocardiogram reveals low voltage, pronounced in the limb leads, but without acute changes.

Which of the following is the most likely cause of this patient's proteinuria?

(A) AA amyloidosis

(B) Focal segmental glomerulosclerosis

(C) Minimal change glomerulopathy

(D) NSAID-associated interstitial nephritis

(E) Proton pump–associated interstitial nephritis

Item 105

A 46-year-old man is evaluated during a follow-up visit for elevated blood pressure. His average blood pressure with home blood pressure monitoring is 126/77 mm Hg. He has no other pertinent medical history and takes no medications.

On physical examination, blood pressure is 128/78 mm Hg; other vital signs are normal. BMI is 28. The remainder of the examination is unremarkable.

Which of the following is the most appropriate next step in management?

(A) Initiate therapy with an angiotensin receptor blocker

(B) Initiate therapy with a thiazide diuretic

(C) Initiate a trial of lifestyle modification

(D) Remeasure blood pressure in 1 year

Item 106

A 70-year-old man is evaluated for a recent onset of macroscopic hematuria. History is significant for end-stage kidney disease and hypertension. He has been on hemodialysis for 3 years. Urine output is approximately 250 mL/d. Medications are sevelamer, sodium bicarbonate, lisinopril, and amlodipine.

On physical examination, blood pressure is 150/90 mm Hg, and pulse rate is 70/min. Bilateral flank tenderness is noted. There is no abdominal mass.

Laboratory studies show a hemoglobin level of 15 g/dL (150 g/L).

Kidney ultrasound shows several complex cysts and two bilateral solid masses.

Which of the following is the most appropriate management?

(A) Bilateral partial nephrectomy

(B) Bilateral radical nephrectomy

(C) Percutaneous kidney biopsy

(D) Surveillance ultrasonography

Item 107

A 42-year-old man is evaluated for an elevated blood pressure measurement of 136/86 mm Hg found during a routine screening at his workplace. He exercises 5 days a week for 45 minutes and adheres to a low fat, low salt diet. Family history is significant for hypertension in his father and mother; his father died of a stroke at the age of 55 years. He takes no medications. The patient is black.

On physical examination, the patient is well developed and muscular. The average of three blood pressure measurements is 126/75 mm Hg, and pulse rate is 52/min. BMI is 24.5. The remainder of the examination is unremarkable.

Which of the following is the most appropriate management?

(A) Amlodipine

(B) Annual blood pressure screening

(C) Blood pressure screening in 3 months

(D) Hydrochlorothiazide

Item 108

A 62-year-old woman is evaluated during a follow-up visit for stage G5 chronic kidney disease. She is not a transplant candidate. She has opted for hemodialysis for her eventual dialysis modality; an arteriovenous fistula was created 6 months ago. She is active, has a fair appetite, and is sleeping well. She reports no nausea or vomiting. History is also significant for hypertension and secondary hyperparathyroidism. Medications are furosemide, amlodipine, epoetin alfa, sevelamer, calcitriol, and sodium bicarbonate.

On physical examination, blood pressure is 144/85 mm Hg; other vital signs are normal. The left upper extremity arteriovenous fistula appears functioning. There is no asterixis. There is 2+ lower extremity edema.

Laboratory studies:

Bicarbonate	21 mEq/L (21 mmol/L)
Blood urea nitrogen	89 mg/dL (31.7 mmol/L)
Creatinine	4.8 mg/dL (424.3 µmol/L)
Potassium	4.8 mEq/L (4.8 mmol/L)
Estimated glomerular filtration rate	9.7 mL/min/1.73 m²

Which of the following is the most appropriate management for this patient?

(A) Delay dialysis until uremic symptoms occur

(B) Discontinue diuretics

(C) Refer for palliative care

(D) Start dialysis now

Answers and Critiques

Item 1   Answer: A

Educational Objective: Use ambulatory blood pressure monitoring to evaluate antihypertensive treatment.

The most appropriate management is to decrease the hydrochlorothiazide dose and obtain ambulatory blood pressure monitoring (ABPM). The patient presents with orthostatic hypotension that likely resulted in his near-syncope and fall due to a recent increase in the dose of a thiazide diuretic. The maximal daily recommended dose for hydrochlorothiazide is 25 mg for the treatment of hypertension; side effects increase beyond this dose with little further antihypertensive effect. Increasing the daily dose to 50 mg likely resulted in an orthostatic drop in his blood pressure, and his pulse rate did not change because he is on a β-blocker. Additional evidence of overtreatment includes an increase in his serum creatinine level, hyponatremia, hypokalemia, and the development of metabolic alkalosis. The appropriate next step is to lower his hydrochlorothiazide dose and obtain ABPM, which is valuable in providing information supplementary to office blood pressure measurements in clinical situations such as hypotensive symptoms from antihypertensive medication treatment. ABPM may reveal that the patient has an element of white coat hypertension and that his blood pressures at home are well controlled on his previous lower dose of hydrochlorothiazide.

Bilateral carotid ultrasonography is not the appropriate next step for this patient. Although he has evidence of atherosclerotic vascular disease and may have carotid stenosis, it is an unlikely cause of near-syncope and falling. The dizziness and fall were most likely the result of orthostasis.

In a study of 1920 hospitalized patients with syncope, the most commonly ordered tests, in addition to electrocardiography, were telemetry (95%), cardiac enzymes (95%), and CT of the head (63%). These tests, along with echocardiography, carotid ultrasonography, and electroencephalography, aided diagnosis in <2% of patients and altered management decisions in <5% of patients. The most valuable diagnostic and management test was postural blood pressure. The American College of Physicians does not recommend brain imaging, with either CT or MRI, in the evaluation of a patient with simple syncope and a normal neurologic examination.

> **KEY POINT**
> - Ambulatory blood pressure monitoring provides valuable information supplementary to office blood pressure measurements in the evaluation of antihypertensive treatment.

Bibliography

Di Stefano C, Milazzo V, Totaro S, Sobrero G, Ravera A, Milan A, et al. Orthostatic hypotension in a cohort of hypertensive patients referring to a hypertension clinic. J Hum Hypertens. 2015;29:599-603. [PMID: 25631221]

Item 2   Answer: B

Educational Objective: Diagnose glomerulopathy with a kidney biopsy.

A kidney biopsy is the most appropriate next step for this patient who has the nephrotic syndrome most likely caused by minimal change glomerulopathy (MCG). MCG is the cause of the nephrotic syndrome in 10% to 15% of adults, with a significantly higher incidence in elderly patients (≥65 years of age) and very elderly patients (≥80 years of age). Most cases are idiopathic, but secondary causes must be considered in adults, including medications such as NSAIDs. Adults with MCG present with acute kidney injury (AKI) in up to 25% of cases. Factors associated with AKI include older age, male sex, hypertension, low serum albumin levels, and heavier proteinuria. The differential diagnosis for the nephrotic syndrome with AKI is limited to only a few entities: MCG with acute tubular necrosis or allergic interstitial nephritis, membranous glomerulopathy with bilateral renal vein thrombosis, amyloidosis with cast nephropathy, and collapsing focal segmental glomerulosclerosis. A kidney biopsy is therefore required to make the correct diagnosis.

Dialysis is used to control complications of severe AKI. Absolute indications for dialysis include hyperkalemia, metabolic acidosis, and pulmonary edema refractory to medical therapy; uremic symptoms; uremic pericarditis; and certain drug intoxications. This patient has no indication for dialysis.

The pathophysiology of hypercoagulability in the nephrotic syndrome is not well understood, nor has the mechanism underlying the higher propensity for thromboembolism in membranous glomerulopathy been well defined. There are no randomized clinical trials of prophylactic anticoagulation in patients with the nephrotic syndrome to guide clinical decision-making; in the absence of known risk and benefits, many experts recommend against prophylactic anticoagulation. Anticoagulation is typically recommended for patients with documented renal vein thrombosis to prevent further propagation of the thrombus and systemic embolization. The patient's ultrasound does not show evidence of renal vein thrombosis, and anticoagulation should be withheld.

Although this presentation is most suggestive of MCG given the patient's age, empiric glucocorticoids would not be indicated without a biopsy-confirmed diagnosis because glucocorticoids would not be efficacious in the treatment of membranous glomerulopathy or amyloidosis.

> **KEY POINT**
> - A kidney biopsy is required to make the diagnosis of glomerulopathy associated with the nephrotic syndrome in adult patients.

Bibliography

Waldman M, Crew RJ, Valeri A, Busch J, Stokes B, Markowitz G, et al. Adult minimal-change disease: clinical characteristics, treatment, and outcomes. Clin J Am Soc Nephrol. 2007;2:445-53. [PMID: 17699450]

Item 3   Answer: D

Educational Objective: Treat chronic metabolic acidosis in a patient with chronic kidney disease.

Sodium bicarbonate therapy is the most likely treatment to slow progression of this patient's chronic kidney disease (CKD). Metabolic acidosis frequently occurs in patients with CKD due to defective acid excretion (resulting in reduced bicarbonate generation), most commonly due to impaired ammoniagenesis. Untreated metabolic acidosis can lead to muscle loss and bone loss. In early CKD, metabolic acidosis is typically a normal anion gap hyperchloremic metabolic acidosis. As glomerular filtration rate (GFR) declines, organic and inorganic anions are retained, and an anion gap metabolic acidosis develops. Large observational studies have shown a strong association between lower serum bicarbonate levels and both increased progression of CKD and mortality. Alkali therapy, most commonly sodium bicarbonate or sodium citrate, can delay the progression of CKD. Therefore, the Kidney Disease: Improving Global Outcomes (KDIGO) guidelines recommend starting alkali therapy when the serum bicarbonate is chronically <22 mEq/L (22 mmol/L). The alkali salt therapy dose should be titrated to achieve a serum bicarbonate level within the normal range; excessive alkali therapy in the setting of a reduced GFR may induce a metabolic alkalosis, which is associated with increased mortality. Patients with CKD who are treated with alkali should be monitored for symptoms of volume overload.

Blood pressure control, particularly with renin-angiotensin system agents, has been shown to slow progression of proteinuric renal diseases and especially diabetes mellitus. However, this patient is already taking an angiotensin receptor blocker (ARB), and dual therapy with an ACE inhibitor and an ARB may instead be detrimental because studies of dual blockade have shown increased risks of acute kidney disease and hyperkalemia.

As the estimated GFR declines below 30 mL/min/1.73 m^2 (stages G4-G5), anemia can become symptomatic. Erythropoiesis-stimulating agents (ESAs) are highly effective in raising hemoglobin concentrations and alleviating symptoms but have not been shown to slow progression of CKD. These agents are associated with risks and are expensive. Black box warnings for use of ESAs include the risk of increased mortality and/or tumor progression in patients with active malignancy, increased risk of thromboembolic events for postsurgical patients not on anticoagulant therapy, and increased risk of serious cardiovascular events when ESAs are administered to patients with hemoglobin values >11 g/dL (110 g/L).

Although poorly controlled hyperphosphatemia is associated with a greater risk of CKD progression, optimizing mineral metabolism parameters with a phosphate binder has not been shown to slow progression of CKD.

KEY POINT

- The Kidney Disease: Improving Global Outcomes (KDIGO) guidelines recommend treatment of metabolic acidosis with alkali therapy in patients with chronic kidney disease when the serum bicarbonate is chronically <22 mEq/L (22 mmol/L).

Bibliography

Kraut JA, Madias NE. Metabolic acidosis of CKD: an update. Am J Kidney Dis. 2016;67:307-17. [PMID: 26477665]

Item 4   Answer: B

Educational Objective: Treat minimal change glomerulopathy.

Diuretics plus high-dose prednisone is the most appropriate treatment for this patient with minimal change glomerulopathy (MCG; also known as minimal change disease). MCG is the most common cause of the nephrotic syndrome in children and accounts for approximately 10% to 15% of cases in adults. Immunosuppressive therapy is indicated for treatment of primary MCG, which invariably presents with the full nephrotic syndrome. The concomitant acute tubular necrosis makes treatment even more imperative in this case, because primary MCG with acute kidney injury has been shown to be a treatment-responsive lesion if treated in a timely manner. First-line therapy is prednisone at a dose of 1 mg/kg per day or 2 mg/kg every other day for 8 to 12 weeks, followed by a taper. Patients typically respond to glucocorticoids within 8 to 16 weeks. However, relapse is common, and in a substantial percentage of patients, the course of MCG is one of remission followed by relapse. For frequently relapsing or glucocorticoid-dependent disease, treatment options include cyclophosphamide, calcineurin inhibitors (tacrolimus or cyclosporine), mycophenolate mofetil, and rituximab. In addition to immunosuppression, patients should receive standard therapy for the nephrotic syndrome, including an ACE inhibitor or angiotensin receptor blocker (this patient is already taking lisinopril, with well-controlled blood pressure), diuretics for edema management, and cholesterol-lowering medication if total cholesterol >200 mg/dL (5.1 mmol/L). In rare cases of MCG secondary to malignancies (Hodgkin lymphoma, non-Hodgkin lymphoma, thymoma), medications (NSAIDs, lithium), infections (strongyloides, syphilis, mycoplasma, ehrlichiosis), and atopy (pollen, dairy products), treatment of the underlying condition without immunosuppression may be sufficient.

Cyclosporine and rituximab are generally reserved for glucocorticoid-resistant or glucocorticoid-dependent cases of MCG and, except for a clear contraindication to glucocorticoids, should not be used as first-line therapy.

Diuretics alone are not sufficient to manage this patient and prevent progressive kidney disease; immunosuppressive therapy is therefore indicated.

- Glucocorticoids are first-line therapy for primary minimal change glomerulopathy; standard treatment of the nephrotic syndrome (ACE inhibitor or angiotensin receptor blocker, diuretics for edema, and cholesterol-lowering medication if total cholesterol >200 mg/dL [5.1 mmol/L]) is also indicated as needed.

Bibliography

Vivarelli M, Massella L, Ruggiero B, Emma F. Minimal change disease. Clin J Am Soc Nephrol. 2017;12:332-345. [PMID: 27940460]

Item 5   Answer: C

Educational Objective: Diagnose monoclonal gammopathy of renal significance with a kidney biopsy.

The most appropriate next diagnostic test is a kidney biopsy. This patient appears to have monoclonal gammopathy of renal significance (MGRS). This is a recently defined set of kidney disorders found in patients who would otherwise meet the criteria for monoclonal gammopathy of undetermined significance but have an abnormal urinalysis and kidney insufficiency. This patient who otherwise meets the diagnostic criteria for monoclonal gammopathy of undetermined significance has an active urine sediment and an increase in the serum creatinine level and thus has underlying kidney disease. MGRS is an increasingly recognized disorder, and a kidney biopsy is necessary to make the diagnosis by demonstrating the presence of monoclonal immunoglobulin deposition in the kidney. MGRS can affect the kidney in various ways, including amyloidosis, proliferative glomerulonephritis, immunoglobulin deposition disease, C3 glomerulopathy, and proximal tubulopathy. Kidney manifestations of MGRS are usually caused by deposition of monoclonal light chains. Patients can present with both nephrotic and subnephrotic proteinuria, hematuria, and elevated serum creatinine. Despite not meeting the definition of multiple myeloma, MGRS increases morbidity and, in most cases, should be treated with therapy designed to eliminate or suppress the immunoglobulin clone.

Pauci-immune glomerulonephritis is caused by microscopic vessel vasculitis affecting the kidney, resulting in necrotizing lesions in the glomeruli with few or no immune deposits. The renal lesion may occur with or without systemic vasculitis and is the most common cause of rapidly progressive glomerulonephritis. Most patients have circulating ANCA directed against neutrophils. Other than proteinuria, this patient has a bland urinalysis that is not consistent with a pauci-immune glomerulonephritis, and testing for ANCA in lieu of a kidney biopsy will not establish a diagnosis.

β_2-Microglobulin levels can be helpful as prognostic indicators in myeloma but cannot be used to make a diagnosis of a plasma cell disorder.

Serum free light chains can be used to diagnose myeloma and predict the risk of progression in patients with monoclonal gammopathy of undetermined significance; however, a kidney biopsy, not serum free light chain determination, will confirm the cause of this patient's kidney disease.

- Monoclonal gammopathy of renal significance is diagnosed in patients who would otherwise meet the criteria for monoclonal gammopathy of undetermined significance but have an abnormal urinalysis and kidney insufficiency; kidney biopsy confirms the diagnosis.

Bibliography

Rosner MH, Edeani A, Yanagita M, Glezerman IG, Leung N; American Society of Nephrology Onco-Nephrology Forum. Paraprotein-related kidney disease: diagnosing and treating monoclonal gammopathy of renal significance. Clin J Am Soc Nephrol. 2016;11:2280-2287. [PMID: 27526705]

Item 6   Answer: D

Educational Objective: Treat IgA nephropathy with an ACE inhibitor or angiotensin receptor blocker.

No changes need to be made to this patient's current medication regimen. He was diagnosed with IgA nephropathy 3 months ago, at which time the ACE inhibitor lisinopril was initiated. Antiproteinuric therapy using an ACE inhibitor or angiotensin receptor blocker (ARB) is the hallmark for treating IgA nephropathy and remains the most proven therapy in slowing progression of the disease. This patient currently has preserved kidney function and proteinuria <1000 mg/24 h; therefore, continuing conservative therapy with the ACE inhibitor lisinopril is appropriate.

Combined use of any of the three renin-angiotensin system drug classes (ACE inhibitor, ARB, and direct renin inhibitors) is not recommended given the results of several clinical trials that revealed more adverse events with these combinations (hyperkalemia, hypotension, acute kidney injury), without additional cardiovascular or renal benefits. Therefore, adding the ARB losartan to this patient's medication regimen is not recommended.

The risk for disease progression appears to be significantly increased when patients have proteinuria >1000 mg/24 h, particularly in the setting of reduced kidney function. Studies on using immunosuppression (particularly glucocorticoids) have used this 1000 mg/24 h proteinuria threshold for enrollment and have demonstrated conflicting results. Although earlier small studies have shown a clear benefit in adding glucocorticoids (oral or a combination of intravenous and oral) to ACE inhibitors or ARBs when proteinuria is >1000 mg/24 h, more recent larger studies (STOP-IgAN and TESTING studies) have raised concerns about the toxicity of this treatment strategy outweighing any potential benefits. Therefore, the use of immunosuppression in IgA nephropathy remains controversial.

Bibliography

Feehally J. Immunosuppression in IgA nephropathy: guideline medicine versus personalized medicine. Semin Nephrol. 2017;37:464-477. [PMID: 28863793]

Item 7   Answer: C

Educational Objective: Identify polydipsia as the cause of isovolemic hypotonic hyponatremia.

This patient has isovolemic hypotonic hyponatremia secondary to polydipsia. Isovolemia is documented by the presence of normal vital signs and physical examination findings. Hypotonicity is documented by the low calculated serum osmolality of 156 mOsm/kg H_2O, using the following equation:

$$\text{Serum Osmolality (mOsm/kg } H_2O) = (2 \times \text{Serum Sodium [mEq/L]}) + \text{Plasma Glucose (mg/dL)}/18 + \text{Blood Urea Nitrogen (mg/dL)}/2.8$$

Isovolemic hypotonic hyponatremia is secondary either to impaired dilution of urine or to water intake that exceeds the kidney's ability to excrete dilute urine. Urine osmolality distinguishes between these two entities. Urine osmolality <100 mOsm/kg H_2O indicates excessive water intake, as seen with psychogenic polydipsia or poor solute intake. Because the kidney cannot excrete pure water, a minimal solute concentration of 50 mOsm/kg H_2O is required. If solute intake is low while liquid intake remains high (as seen in beer potomania or chronic low food intake), water excretion is limited by available urinary solute.

Hyperglycemia causes the osmotic translocation of water from the intracellular to the extracellular fluid compartment, which results in a decrease in the serum sodium level by approximately 1.6 to 2.0 mEq/L (1.6-2.0 mmol/L) for every 100 mg/dL (5.6 mmol/L) increase in the plasma glucose above 100 mg/dL (5.6 mmol/L). Although the patient has mild hyperglycemia, her glucose is not elevated enough to lower her sodium to 126 mEq/L (126 mmol/L).

Diabetes insipidus, due to either a lack of antidiuretic hormone (ADH) secretion from the posterior pituitary gland or kidney resistance to ADH (nephrogenic diabetes insipidus), will result in low urine osmolality as seen in this patient. In the absence of ADH, excessive water is excreted by the kidneys. Serum sodium is typically normal but may be elevated in patients who do not have access to water. Although lithium can cause nephrogenic diabetes insipidus, the fact that she is hyponatremic rules out this diagnosis.

Hyponatremia most often results from an increase in circulating ADH in response to a true or sensed reduction in effective arterial blood volume with resulting fluid retention. Hyponatremia may also be caused by elevated ADH levels associated with the syndrome of inappropriate antidiuretic hormone secretion. Because she has dilute urine indicating a lack of ADH, neither the syndrome of inappropriate antidiuretic hormone secretion nor volume depletion is the cause of her hyponatremia. Volume depletion is also excluded by the normal blood pressure and pulse measurement and absence of orthostatic changes.

Bibliography

Hoorn EJ, Zietse R. Diagnosis and treatment of hyponatremia: compilation of the guidelines. J Am Soc Nephrol. 2017;28:1340-1349. [PMID: 28174217]

Item 8   Answer: B   H

Educational Objective: Prevent calcium oxalate stones using potassium citrate in a patient who has malabsorption.

In addition to increasing fluid intake, potassium citrate is appropriate to prevent future calcium oxalate stones in this patient. Patients with chronic diarrhea and malabsorption are at increased risk for forming calcium oxalate stones for three reasons. First, because of the diarrhea and concomitant metabolic acidosis, urine citrate, an inhibitor of crystallization, is often reduced. In addition, volume depletion from the diarrhea decreases urine volume and thus increases the concentration of calcium and oxalate in the urine. Finally, in malabsorption, especially fat malabsorption as occurs in chronic pancreatitis, enteric calcium binds to fat as opposed to oxalate, leaving oxalate free to be absorbed and excreted in the urine. Although treatment should be based on the metabolic evaluation in this patient, his low urine pH and low serum bicarbonate level suggest that he has metabolic acidosis. Decreased systemic pH lowers urine citrate excretion. Supplementation with citrate as a base equivalent will help correct the acidosis and increase urine citrate, bind urinary calcium, and decrease the formation of calcium oxalate stones.

If the 24-hour urine metabolic evaluation showed elevated urine uric acid or if stone analysis revealed a uric acid nidus, allopurinol could be considered; however, in the absence of this information, allopurinol should not be prescribed.

Vitamin C increases urine oxalate excretion and would not have the desired effect of decreasing calcium oxalate stone formation.

Restricting dietary calcium intake in patients with hypercalciuria may paradoxically increase the risk of kidney stone formation by causing decreased binding of calcium with oxalate in the gut with increased absorption and urinary excretion of oxalate; therefore, dietary calcium should not be limited.

Increased protein intake increases glomerular filtration, and therefore the excretion of calcium, and would not

CONT.

contribute to decreased kidney stone formation. In addition, high protein diets may exacerbate hypocitraturia.

KEY POINT

- Potassium citrate can be used to help prevent calcium oxalate stones in patients with chronic diarrhea and malabsorption.

Bibliography
Pfau A, Knauf F. Update on nephrolithiasis: core curriculum 2016. Am J Kidney Dis. 2016;68:973-985. [PMID: 27497526]

Item 9   Answer: A

Educational Objective: Treat diabetic nephropathy.

The addition of an ACE inhibitor or angiotensin receptor blocker (ARB) is the most appropriate management for this patient with diabetic nephropathy. The hallmark clinical features include a proteinuric form of chronic kidney disease in a patient with long-standing diabetes mellitus and evidence of other (microvascular and/or macrovascular) complications of disease. Diagnosis can be made clinically for this patient, and he can be treated with the cornerstone of treatment: improved glucose control, and blockade of the renin-angiotensin system (RAS) with an ACE inhibitor or ARB using the maximal tolerated dose. Combined use of any RAS drug class (ACE inhibitors, ARBs, and direct renin inhibitors) is not recommended; several clinical trials have revealed more adverse events with these combinations (hyperkalemia, hypotension, acute kidney injury), without additional cardiovascular or renal benefits.

ANCA-associated glomerulonephritis is associated with the nephritic syndrome. The nephritic syndrome is characterized by hematuria, proteinuria, and leukocytes in the urine sediment. The hallmark is the presence of dysmorphic erythrocytes, with or without erythrocyte casts. Systemic findings may include edema, hypertension, and kidney failure. This patient does not have hematuria, making ANCA testing unnecessary.

Serum and urine protein electrophoresis is used to evaluate for kidney failure secondary to dysproteinemia, which is more common in older patients (>65 years of age). Other potential clues to the presence of dysproteinemia-related kidney disease include anemia, hypercalcemia, and evidence of proximal tubular dysfunction such as hypokalemia, metabolic acidosis, hypophosphatemia, glycosuria (with normoglycemia), or hypouricemia.

The diagnosis of diabetic nephropathy usually does not require a kidney biopsy if the clinical presentation is consistent with its diagnosis. The best predictors of finding diabetic nephropathy are duration of diabetes for more than 8 years followed by presence of the nephrotic syndrome. Therefore, this patient with a 10-year history of poorly controlled diabetes, nephrotic-range proteinuria, and findings of microvascular and macrovascular complications does not require a kidney biopsy or other testing to confirm the diagnosis of diabetic nephropathy.

KEY POINT

- The best predictors for the presence of diabetic nephropathy are duration of diabetes mellitus for more than 8 years followed by the presence of the nephrotic syndrome.

Bibliography
Wylie EC, Satchell SC. Diabetic nephropathy. Clin Med (Lond). 2012;12:480-2; quiz 483-5. [PMID: 23101153]

Item 10   Answer: B

Educational Objective: Treat rhabdomyolysis-induced acute kidney injury.

Intravenous 0.9% saline is the most appropriate treatment for this patient who has severe rhabdomyolysis from cocaine and opiates. Major causes of rhabdomyolysis include trauma, drugs and toxins, seizures, metabolic and electrolyte disorders, endocrinopathies, and exercise. Rhabdomyolysis-induced acute kidney injury (AKI) is associated with elevated serum creatine kinase (usually >5000 U/L) and creatinine levels, hyperkalemia, hypocalcemia, hyperphosphatemia, hyperuricemia, and increased anion gap metabolic acidosis. Patients with rhabdomyolysis tend to be significantly volume depleted due to the sequestration of water in injured muscles. Therefore, initial management is early with aggressive repletion of fluids aimed at maintaining a urine output of 200 to 300 mL/h. Normal saline is the recommended initial fluid of choice, and patients can require 10 liters of fluid per day.

Hemodialysis is reserved for patients with severe AKI who remain oliguric with persistent hyperkalemia, persistent metabolic acidosis, and/or volume overload. This patient does not have an indication for hemodialysis at this time.

Although the patient has hypernatremia, intravenous 5% dextrose is not adequate to expand the extracellular fluid compartment. Due to the osmotic gradient, hypotonic fluids will leave the extracellular fluid compartment for the intracellular compartment.

Hypocalcemia is due to sequestration of calcium in damaged cells. Rebound hypercalcemia occurs during the recovery phase due to release of calcium from damaged muscles and is worsened by exogenous calcium treatment. Calcium should only be given in patients who are symptomatic or in patients at risk for arrhythmia due to severe hyperkalemia with electrocardiogram changes.

Although alkalinization of the urine to a pH >6.5 may prevent intratubular pigment cast formation, decrease the release of free iron from myoglobin, and decrease the risk for tubular precipitation of uric acid, clear benefit is lacking. Intravenous bicarbonate should only be used after diuresis is established with volume repletion. It should not be used if pH is >7.5, serum bicarbonate is >30 mEq/L (30 mmol/L), and/or severe hypocalcemia is present. Intravenous bicarbonate can cause symptomatic hypocalcemia and can promote deposition of calcium phosphate in the renal tubules.

Answers and Critiques

> **KEY POINT**
> - Initial management of rhabdomyolysis-induced acute kidney injury includes aggressive fluid resuscitation with normal saline aimed at maintaining a urine output of 200 to 300 mL/h.

Bibliography

Cervellin G, Comelli I, Benatti M, Sanchis-Gomar F, Bassi A, Lippi G. Nontraumatic rhabdomyolysis: background, laboratory features, and acute clinical management. Clin Biochem. 2017;50:656-662. [PMID: 28235546]

Item 11   Answer: A
Educational Objective: Prevent contrast-induced nephropathy.

The administration of 0.9% saline is an appropriate measure to prevent contrast-induced nephropathy (CIN). CIN is a common cause of reversible acute kidney injury in the hospital. CIN is defined as an increase in serum creatinine within 24 to 48 hours following contrast exposure. Adequate intravenous volume expansion with isotonic crystalloids before the procedure and continued for 6 to 24 hours afterward has been shown to decrease the incidence of CIN in patients at risk. Intravenous hydration induces an increase of urine flow rate, reduces the concentration of contrast in the tubule, and increases the excretion of contrast. Because administration of intravenous crystalloid remains the primary strategy for reducing the risk of CIN, patients with compensated heart failure should still be given intravenous volume. Patients with uncompensated heart failure should undergo hemodynamic monitoring with continuation of diuretics. This patient has compensated heart failure noted on examination and should be given fluids.

A recent large randomized trial among patients at high risk for kidney complications compared three different strategies to prevent CIN: intravenous 1.26% sodium bicarbonate or intravenous 0.9% sodium chloride and 5 days of oral acetylcysteine or oral placebo. For fluid administration, this study used a protocol of 1 to 3 mL/kg/h before angiography, 1 to 1.5 mL/kg/h during angiography, and 1 to 3 mL/kg/h 2 to 12 hours after angiography. There was no benefit of intravenous sodium bicarbonate over intravenous sodium chloride or of oral acetylcysteine over placebo for the prevention of death, need for dialysis, or persistent decline in kidney function at 90 days or for the prevention of CIN.

Some but not all studies suggest that statins may reduce the risk of CIN. A 2016 meta-analysis suggested that statins given with N-acetylcysteine plus intravenous saline reduced the risk of CIN compared with N-acetylcysteine plus intravenous saline alone in relatively low-risk patients. Based on these results, there is no need to discontinue atorvastatin in this patient.

Discontinuation of ACE inhibitors or angiotensin receptor blockers such as irbesartan has not been clearly shown to decrease the risk of CIN.

> **KEY POINT**
> - Intravenous volume expansion with isotonic crystalloids has been shown to decrease the incidence of contrast-induced nephropathy in patients at risk.

Bibliography

Weisbord SD, Gallagher M, Jneid H, Garcia S, Cass A, Thwin SS, et al; PRESERVE Trial Group. Outcomes after angiography with sodium bicarbonate and acetylcysteine. N Engl J Med. 2018;378:603-614. [PMID: 29130810]

Item 12   Answer: C
Educational Objective: Diagnose multiple myeloma–associated hypercalcemia as a cause of acute kidney injury.

This patient's acute kidney injury (AKI) is due to hypercalcemia from multiple myeloma. Classic symptoms of polyuria, polydipsia, and nocturia sometimes occur with elevated serum calcium levels of 11 mg/dL (2.8 mmol/L) or less. Other symptoms such as anorexia, nausea, abdominal pain, constipation, increased serum creatinine levels, and mild mental status changes are more likely to occur with levels >11 mg/dL (2.8 mmol/L). Kidney dysfunction is found in about 30% of patients diagnosed with multiple myeloma, often due to cast nephropathy (also termed myeloma kidney), a condition in which excess monoclonal free light chains precipitate in the distal tubules and incite tubulointerstitial damage. Hypercalcemia and exposure to nephrotoxic agents are other frequent causes of kidney dysfunction. Hypercalcemia can decrease glomerular filtration rate through renal vasoconstriction, the natriuretic effects of high serum calcium levels, and impaired renal concentrating ability. This patient has orthostatic hypotension, a bland urinalysis with hyaline casts, and a fractional excretion of sodium <1%, consistent with a prerenal AKI from hypovolemia. The constellation of hypercalcemia, normal anion gap metabolic acidosis, pancytopenia, and AKI suggests multiple myeloma as the etiology.

Hydrochlorothiazide can cause volume depletion, decreased excretion of calcium and mild hypercalcemia, prerenal AKI, and metabolic alkalosis (due to hypovolemic stimulation of aldosterone release). However, the effect on serum calcium is usually minimal, and the patient has a metabolic acidosis, not metabolic alkalosis as might be seen with thiazide therapy.

Milk alkali syndrome occurs with the ingestion of large amounts of calcium and absorbable alkali (for example, calcium carbonate). It presents as hypercalcemia, metabolic alkalosis, and AKI. This patient has a metabolic acidosis, not a metabolic alkalosis, making this diagnosis unlikely.

Primary hyperparathyroidism is the most common cause of hypercalcemia in otherwise healthy outpatients and is diagnosed with a simultaneously elevated serum calcium level and an inappropriately normal or elevated intact parathyroid hormone level. Serum phosphorus levels are typically low or low-normal in these patients. This patient's phosphorus level is elevated, making the diagnosis of primary hyperparathyroidism unlikely.

- A diagnosis of multiple myeloma is suggested by the constellation of anemia, hypercalcemia, normal anion gap metabolic acidosis, and acute kidney injury.

Bibliography

Rosner MH, Perazella MA. Acute kidney injury in patients with cancer. N Engl J Med. 2017;376:1770-1781. [PMID: 28467867]

Item 13   Answer: B

Educational Objective: Adjust an antihypertensive medication regimen to achieve a target blood pressure goal.

The addition of losartan is the most appropriate treatment. As antihypertensive agents are titrated or added when there is inadequate blood pressure control, it is important to recognize that there is a nonlinear and diminishing blood pressure–lowering effect when titrating from 50% maximal dose to 100% maximal dose of any agent. A general rule of thumb is that 75% of an agent's blood pressure–lowering effect may be achieved with 50% of its maximal dose. If blood pressure control requires an additional >5-mm Hg reduction, it is unlikely to be achieved by increasing the single agent from 50% to 100% maximal dose. The better strategy is to add a second drug or a third drug to a two-drug regimen, as seen in this patient.

Hydralazine is not the best option because it is a thrice-daily medication and may pose problems with adherence, considering that once-daily medication options have not been exhausted in this patient. In addition, hydralazine is a direct vasodilator and is associated with sodium and water retention and reflex tachycardia; use with a diuretic and a β-blocker is recommended. Hydralazine is typically reserved for patients with resistant hypertension or hypertensive urgencies.

Increasing the amlodipine or hydrochlorothiazide dose is not appropriate because there is diminishing return in blood pressure lowering if the dose is titrated up from 50% to 100% of maximum. Also, it is unlikely that increasing the dose from 50% to 100% of maximum will result in an additional >5-mm Hg reduction to bring this patient's blood pressure to a target of <130/80 mm Hg. In addition, titration to maximum doses may result in manifestation of undesirable side effects and decreased adherence. In this case, the patient already has dependent edema, which may increase with uptitration of the amlodipine dose. His serum potassium is borderline at 3.6 mEq/L (3.6 mmol/L), and increasing the dose of hydrochlorothiazide may further decrease his serum potassium and necessitate a potassium supplement, adding yet another medication to his drug regimen.

- Three strategies can be used for antihypertensive dose adjustment in the treatment of hypertension: (1) maximize the medication dose before adding another; (2) add another class of medication before reaching the maximum dose of the first; and (3) start with two medication classes separately or as fixed-dose combinations.

Bibliography

Whelton PK, Carey RM, Aronow WS, Casey DE Jr, Collins KJ, Dennison Himmelfarb C, et al. 2017 ACC/AHA/AAPA/ABC/ACPM/AGS/APhA/ASH/ASPC/NMA/PCNA guideline for the prevention, detection, evaluation, and management of high blood pressure in adults: a report of the American College of Cardiology/American Heart Association Task Force on Clinical Practice Guidelines. Hypertension. 2017. [PMID: 29133356]

Item 14   Answer: C

Educational Objective: Treat ethylene glycol toxicity.

The most appropriate management is intravenous hydration, fomepizole, and hemodialysis. This patient has typical findings of ethylene glycol toxicity, including central nervous system depression, an increased anion gap metabolic acidosis, and an increased osmolal gap. In patients with an increased anion gap acidosis, calculation of the serum osmolal gap is helpful in assessing the presence of unmeasured solutes, such as ingestion of certain toxins (for example, methanol or ethylene glycol). The serum osmolal gap is the difference between the measured and calculated serum osmolality. Serum osmolality can be calculated using the following formula:

$$\text{Serum Osmolality (mOsm/kg } H_2O) = (2 \times \text{Serum Sodium} \\ [\text{mEq/L}]) + \text{Plasma Glucose (mg/dL)}/18 \\ + \text{Blood Urea Nitrogen (mg/dL)}/2.8$$

When the measured osmolality exceeds the calculated osmolality by >10 mOsm/kg H_2O, the osmolal gap is considered elevated. This patient has an osmolal gap of 27 mOsm/kg H_2O. Finally, this patient has kidney failure likely resulting from deposition of calcium oxalate crystals in the renal tubules. Because laboratory confirmation of ethylene glycol intoxication may take days, empiric therapy with fomepizole and aggressive fluid resuscitation with crystalloids (250-500 mL/h intravenous initially) should be instituted in all cases to increase kidney clearance of the toxin and to limit deposition of oxalate in the renal cortex. Hemodialysis to clear the alcohol and toxic metabolites should be instituted in the context of any organ-specific toxicity (central nervous system depression, acute kidney injury, systemic collapse), severe acidemia, or very large ingestions.

Activated charcoal gastric decontamination and nasogastric lavage have no role in toxic alcohol poisoning; both ethylene glycol and methanol are typically absorbed too rapidly for either of these modalities to be useful.

Intravenous ethanol was traditionally used as a competitive inhibitor of alcohol dehydrogenase. However, fomepizole has been found to be superior to alcohol with few side effects. Therefore, fomepizole is the preferred agent, and there is no additional benefit to coadministration of the two.

Adjunct therapy with intravenous sodium bicarbonate therapy in the context of pH <7.30 may reduce penetration of toxic metabolites of ethylene glycol (glycolate, glyoxylate, and oxalate) and methanol (formate) into the tissues and enhance renal excretion of glycolate and formate. However, the initiation of dialysis in this patient is more efficacious.

KEY POINT

- Management of ethylene glycol toxicity in the context of organ-specific toxicity, severe acidemia, or very large ingestions includes aggressive fluid resuscitation, fomepizole, and hemodialysis.

Bibliography

Kruse JA. Methanol and ethylene glycol intoxication. Crit Care Clin. 2012;28:661-711. [PMID: 22998995]

Item 15   Answer: A

Educational Objective: Evaluate for secondary causes of membranous glomerulopathy.

Age- and sex-appropriate cancer screening is the most appropriate management. The initial step in the management of newly diagnosed membranous glomerulopathy is to evaluate for secondary forms of the disease, which account for approximately 25% of cases. Some of this evaluation is often done in the prebiopsy screening laboratory tests (for example, screening for hepatitis B and C viruses, lupus, and syphilis). Secondary forms of membranous glomerulopathy correlate with age. Cancer screening is particularly important in evaluating for secondary forms of membranous glomerulopathy in patients over the age of 65 years. Up to 25% of such patients will have a malignancy discovered within 1 year of diagnosis, essentially accounting for all forms of secondary membranous glomerulopathy in this age group. This 68-year-old woman with newly diagnosed membranous glomerulopathy has a 50-pack-year history of smoking. She should be sent for age- and sex-appropriate cancer screening, which would include cervical cytology and human papillomavirus testing, mammography, colonoscopy, and low-dose chest CT.

Immunosuppression should not be offered in this case until a secondary form has definitively been ruled out and the patient has been carefully monitored for at least 3 to 6 months to allow for the possibility, if this is a primary form of membranous glomerulopathy, for spontaneous remission, which occurs in approximately one third of primary cases.

Membranous glomerulopathy is associated with a higher risk for clotting, particularly when serum albumin is <2.8 g/dL (28 g/L). However, there is no consensus on whether such patients should be offered prophylactic anticoagulation, and most experts in the United States opt for vigilant monitoring rather than prophylactic anticoagulation.

The M-type phospholipase A2 receptor (PLA2R) is the specific podocyte antigen responsible for eliciting immune complex formation with circulating autoantibodies in most cases of primary membranous glomerulopathy. Anti-PLA2R antibodies are detected in approximately 75% of primary cases and rarely found in secondary forms. A negative staining on biopsy for this antigen (which is a more specific test than serum antibody assays) raises suspicion for a secondary form of the disease and does not require serum testing for confirmation.

KEY POINT

- The initial step in the management of newly diagnosed membranous glomerulopathy is to evaluate for secondary forms of the disease, which account for approximately 25% of cases.

Bibliography

Leeaphorn N, Kue-A-Pai P, Thamcharoen N, Ungprasert P, Stokes MB, Knight EL. Prevalence of cancer in membranous nephropathy: a systematic review and meta-analysis of observational studies. Am J Nephrol. 2014;40:29-35. [PMID: 24993974]

Item 16   Answer: B

Educational Objective: Diagnose transitional cell (urothelial) cancer in a patient with Balkan endemic nephropathy.

The most appropriate next step for this patient is an endoscopic urologic evaluation with cystoscopy and upper tract imaging. The patient has Balkan endemic nephropathy (BEN), a slowly progressive tubulointerstitial disease that has been linked to aristolochic acid. Aristolochic acid is a nephrotoxic alkaloid from the plant *Aristolochia clematis*. BEN has a high prevalence rate in southeastern Europe (Serbia, Bulgaria, Romania, Bosnia and Herzegovina, and Croatia) and is the cause of kidney disease in up to 70% of patients receiving dialysis in some of the most heavily affected regions. Aristolochic acid is also sometimes found as a component of herbal therapies used for weight loss. Characteristics of BEN include chronic kidney disease due to tubulointerstitial injury, tubular dysfunction (polyuria and decreased concentrating ability, glucosuria without hyperglycemia, and tubular proteinuria), and anemia. Ultrasound demonstrates small echogenic kidneys. BEN has a familial but not inherited pattern of distribution. It is thought to be caused by exposure to aristolochic acid, and, because it is mutagenic, it is strongly associated with the development of upper tract transitional cell (urothelial) cancers. Therefore, urologic evaluation is indicated.

CT urography is the preferred test for patients with unexplained urologic/nonglomerular hematuria. However, CT urography involves the use of intravenous contrast, which would place this patient at a high risk of developing contrast-induced nephropathy given the severity of his kidney disease. Cystoscopy and retrograde ureteropyelography would be the preferred imaging techniques for this patient.

Kidney biopsy would not explain the nondysmorphic hematuria. Furthermore, kidney biopsy is not indicated in the setting of small echogenic kidneys <9 cm in size, which signifies chronic irreversible disease.

Pyuria, granular casts, and low-grade proteinuria are commonly found in patients with tubulointerstitial nephritis and contrasts with the isolated pyuria associated with most urinary tract infections. In addition, the small, echogenic kidneys, chronic hematuria, and irregular bladder wall are not consistent with a urinary tract infection and more strongly suggest the possibility of a malignancy. Therefore, urine cultures are not indicated.

- Balkan endemic nephropathy is strongly associated with the development of upper tract transitional cell (urothelial) cancers, and urologic evaluation is necessary.

Bibliography
Stefanovic V, Toncheva D, Polenakovic M. Balkan nephropathy. Clin Nephrol. 2015;83:64-9. [PMID: 25725245]

Item 17   Answer: A

Educational Objective: Treat hypernatremia caused by central diabetes insipidus.

In addition to increasing the prednisone, the antidiuretic hormone (ADH) analogue desmopressin acetate is the most appropriate treatment. This patient most likely has central nervous system sarcoidosis and central diabetes insipidus (DI). Nearly half of hypothalamic-pituitary sarcoidosis cases occur in the course of previously treated sarcoidosis. Central DI results from inadequate production of ADH by the posterior pituitary gland. In the presence of ADH, aquaporin water channels are inserted in the collecting tubules and allow water to be reabsorbed. In the absence of ADH, excessive water is excreted by the kidneys. Frank hypernatremia is unusual because patients develop extreme thirst and polydipsia, and with free access to water, can maintain serum sodium in the high normal range. When patients do not drink enough to replace the water lost in the urine, due to poor or absent thirst drive or lack of free access to water, they develop hypernatremia. DI is diagnosed with simultaneous laboratory evidence of inability to concentrate urine (urine osmolality <300 mOsm/kg H_2O) in the face of elevated serum sodium and osmolality. If necessary, a water deprivation test can confirm the diagnosis. A response to exogenous ADH would support a diagnosis of central DI, whereas a lack of response is seen in nephrogenic DI.

Although volume depletion induced by hydrochlorothiazide will help decrease urine output and conserve water, this treatment is reserved for patients with nephrogenic DI and is not necessary in central DI.

The hypernatremia in this case is mild, without symptoms, and can be rapidly treated with the administration of desmopressin acetate; therefore, it is not necessary to administer intravenous 5% dextrose.

Tolvaptan is a vasopressin receptor antagonist sometimes used for the syndrome of inappropriate antidiuretic hormone secretion, which is characterized by normal volume status, hyponatremia, and inappropriately elevated urine osmolality (not present in this patient).

- Diabetes insipidus (DI) is diagnosed with simultaneous laboratory evidence of inability to concentrate urine in the face of elevated serum sodium and osmolality; a water deprivation test can confirm the diagnosis, and response to exogenous antidiuretic hormone supports the diagnosis of central DI.

Bibliography
Langrand C, Bihan H, Raverot G, Varron L, Androdias G, Borson-Chazot F, et al. Hypothalamo-pituitary sarcoidosis: a multicenter study of 24 patients. QJM. 2012;105:981-95. [PMID: 22753675]

Item 18   Answer: B

Educational Objective: Identify heparin as a cause of hyperkalemia.

The most likely cause of this patient's elevated serum potassium level is heparin. Hypoaldosteronism caused by heparin, inhibitors of the renin-angiotensin system, type 4 renal tubular acidosis, or primary adrenal disease can cause hyperkalemia. Both unfractionated and low-molecular-weight heparin use is associated with a decrease in aldosterone synthesis. This occurs more frequently in patients with chronic kidney disease or diabetes mellitus, or in those taking an ACE inhibitor or angiotensin receptor blocker.

Major underlying causes of persistent hyperkalemia are disorders in which urine potassium excretion is impaired. This can be due to a marked decrease in glomerular filtration rate, decreased sodium delivery to the distal potassium secretory sites, and hypoaldosteronism. The most common cause is chronic kidney disease with a glomerular filtration rate <20 mL/min/1.73 m^2 or acute oliguric kidney injury. Except in these cases, the kidney is able to maintain potassium homeostasis. The patient is not oliguric, and the slight increase in serum creatinine postoperatively is not sufficient to cause hyperkalemia.

Extreme elevations in glucose by increasing serum osmolality can directly cause hyperkalemia by pulling water from the intracellular space into the extracellular space, dragging potassium with it. This patient's glucose is only mildly elevated and would have little effect on osmolality and hyperkalemia.

In patients with metabolic acidosis caused by mineral acids (such as hydrochloric acid), buffering of intracellular hydrogen ions leads to potassium movement into the extracellular fluid to maintain electroneutrality. This does not occur with organic acids such as lactate or ketoacids. In most cases of hyperchloremic metabolic acidosis, hyperkalemia typically does not develop because there is concomitant urinary and/or gastrointestinal potassium loss. This is the case in patients with hyperchloremic metabolic acidosis with losses of potassium in the stool as the result of diarrhea or in the urine in patients with renal tubular acidosis.

Topiramate is a carbonic anhydrase inhibitor. Carbonic anhydrase inhibition results in proximal bicarbonate, sodium, and chloride urinary loss. The increased sodium loss causes hypovolemia and triggers secondary hyperaldosteronism, promoting potassium loss and hypokalemia.

- Hypoaldosteronism caused by heparin, inhibitors of the renin-angiotensin system, type 4 renal tubular acidosis, or primary adrenal disease can cause hyperkalemia, especially in patients with chronic kidney disease or diabetes mellitus, or in those taking an ACE inhibitor or angiotensin receptor blocker.

Bibliography

Kovesdy CP. Updates in hyperkalemia: outcomes and therapeutic strategies. Rev Endocr Metab Disord. 2017;18:41-47. [PMID: 27600582]

Item 19   Answer: A

Educational Objective: Select the most appropriate pre-transplant renal replacement therapy.

Due to this patient's full-time occupation and requirement to be present on-site at the workplace, peritoneal dialysis might be the preferred management for his end-stage kidney disease (ESKD). Peritoneal dialysis is a renal replacement therapy (RRT) modality utilizing the peritoneal membrane for diffusion of solutes and osmosis of water against a concentration gradient provided by infused dialysate. Patients exchange the dialysate three to five times per day rather than go to a dialysis center for 4 hours three times per week for hemodialysis. Control over one's dialysis is conducive for patients with full-time obligations, such as school or employment. The peritoneal dialysis exchanges can be performed overnight while the individual is sleeping and allow for greater independence during the day. The patient is otherwise healthy and independent. He has never had abdominal surgery, and his BMI is normal. He is an ideal candidate for peritoneal dialysis, and this modality will also allow him to preserve his independence and more easily transition to a life with ESKD. Planning for the right dialysis modality that best fits the patient's daily routine and lifestyle is important for patient satisfaction and long-term success.

A recent meta-analysis analyzing the effect of peritoneal dialysis versus hemodialysis on renal anemia in patients with ESKD found no significant difference for levels of hemoglobin, ferritin, parathyroid hormone, and transferrin saturation index between the hemodialysis and peritoneal dialysis groups. Both of the two dialysis strategies have a similar effect on renal anemia in patients with ESKD.

Clinical outcomes are similar for patients receiving peritoneal dialysis compared with those receiving hemodialysis, although patients starting RRT with residual kidney function may have better outcomes with peritoneal dialysis. Furthermore, residual kidney function is preserved longer with peritoneal dialysis than with hemodialysis and, although small, helps maintain adequate solute clearance and euvolemia. Finally, patients treated with peritoneal dialysis are more satisfied with their treatment and indicate a more satisfying shared decision-making experience.

Peritonitis is one of the most important complications of peritoneal dialysis and can damage the peritoneum, reducing the efficacy of dialysis. Peritoneal dialysis-associated peritonitis is uncommon, with one episode of peritonitis every 2 to 3 years, usually caused by bacteria from skin introduced by poor sterile technique and often easily treated with antibiotics.

KEY POINT

- In properly selected individuals, peritoneal dialysis allows patients to preserve their independence and offers outcomes similar to those seen with hemodialysis.

Bibliography

Hansson JH, Watnick S. Update on peritoneal dialysis: core curriculum 2016. Am J Kidney Dis. 2016;67:151-64. [PMID: 26376606]

Item 20   Answer: A

Educational Objective: Initiate combination antihypertensive therapy for treatment of stage 2 hypertension.

Combination therapy with amlodipine/benazepril is appropriate treatment for this patient with stage 2 hypertension. The 2017 American College of Cardiology/American Heart Association blood pressure (BP) guideline recommends combination therapy with two first-line antihypertensive drugs of different classes (separately or as a single-dose pill) for adults with stage 2 hypertension and an average BP that is 20/10 mm Hg above their BP target. Stage 2 hypertension is defined as BP ≥140/90 mm Hg. This patient's target BP is <130/80 mm Hg. There are no definitive recommendations for best drug combinations, but some data suggest an ACE inhibitor/calcium channel blocker (CCB) combination may be more efficacious than an ACE inhibitor/thiazide diuretic combination. Using a thiazide diuretic/CCB combination is also an option. It is important to note that in black patients, ACE inhibitors are not as efficacious at reducing BP compared with thiazide diuretics or CCBs.

Specific non-recommended initial agents for the treatment of hypertension include β-blockers (due to higher rate of cardiovascular-related events and mortality compared with angiotensin receptor blockers) and α-blockers (due to higher rate of cardiovascular-related events and mortality compared with thiazides), although compelling clinical indications such as atrial fibrillation or benign prostatic hyperplasia may supersede these recommended restrictions.

Initiation of once-daily dosing of a combination pill simplifies the medication regimen and is appropriate in this patient to ensure adherence. Therefore, initiation of hydralazine is not correct because two-drug therapy is recommended for this patient, and adherence to a thrice-daily medication will be problematic.

Combination therapy with an ACE inhibitor (ramipril) and an angiotensin receptor blocker (telmisartan) is not recommended. Several clinical trials (ONTARGET, NEPHRON-D, ALTITUDE) have revealed more adverse events with these combinations (hyperkalemia, hypotension, acute kidney injury), without additional cardiovascular or renal benefits.

KEY POINT

- The 2017 American College of Cardiology/American Heart Association blood pressure (BP) guideline recommends combination therapy with two first-line antihypertensive drugs of different classes (separately or as a single-dose pill) for adults with stage 2 hypertension and an average BP of 20/10 mm Hg above BP target.

Bibliography

Whelton PK, Carey RM, Aronow WS, Casey DE Jr, Collins KJ, Dennison Himmelfarb C, et al. 2017 ACC/AHA/AAPA/ABC/ACPM/AGS/APhA/ASH/ASPC/NMA/PCNA guideline for the prevention, detection, evaluation, and management of high blood pressure in adults: a report of the American College of Cardiology/American Heart Association Task Force on Clinical Practice Guidelines. Hypertension. 2017. [PMID: 29133356]

Item 21   Answer: A

Educational Objective: Diagnose ANCA-associated glomerulonephritis.

The most likely diagnosis is ANCA-associated glomerulonephritis (pauci-immune crescentic glomerulonephritis). This patient's clinical picture suggests a rapidly progressive glomerulonephritis (RPGN), with an acute and steep rise in serum creatinine accompanied by hematuria and proteinuria. The differential diagnosis for RPGN is classically accounted for by three immunofluorescence findings seen on diagnostic kidney biopsy: pauci-immune staining (for example, ANCA-associated glomerulonephritis), linear staining (for example, anti–glomerular basement membrane glomerulonephritis), and granular staining (for example, lupus nephritis). ANCA-associated glomerulonephritis accounts for more than half of all RPGN cases and has a particularly high prevalence in patients >65 years of age presenting with acute kidney injury and active urine sediment. The patient's clinical presentation of acute onset of flu-like symptoms is a classic presentation for vasculitis, and the lacy or reticular rash on examination is likely related to active ANCA-associated vasculitis. He should be tested for antiproteinase-3 and antimyeloperoxidase ANCA antibodies and undergo kidney biopsy to confirm the diagnosis.

Anti–glomerular basement membrane antibody disease is a far rarer form of RPGN, with peak incidences in young men and older women. More than half of patients present with concomitant alveolar hemorrhage that may progress to life-threatening respiratory failure. These findings are not present in this patient.

Minimal change glomerulopathy is characterized by sudden-onset nephrotic syndrome. It can be associated with acute kidney injury in elderly patients, and the presentation is one of severe nephrotic syndrome without significant hematuria. This is distinctly different from this patient's presentation of rash, hypertension, rapidly progressive kidney failure, and active urine sediment.

Kidney dysfunction is found in 29% of patients with multiple myeloma, often due to cast nephropathy (also termed myeloma kidney), a condition in which excess monoclonal free light chains precipitate in the distal tubules and incite tubulointerstitial damage. Patients will typically have concomitant anemia and hypercalcemia. These findings are absent in this patient.

Proliferative lupus nephritis is a cause of RPGN that is usually limited to the pediatric and young adult patient population.

Bibliography

Bomback AS, Appel GB, Radhakrishnan J, Shirazian S, Herlitz LC, Stokes B, et al. ANCA-associated glomerulonephritis in the very elderly. Kidney Int. 2011;79:757-64. [PMID: 21160463]

Item 22   Answer: C

Educational Objective: Diagnose pyroglutamic acidosis.

The most likely diagnosis is pyroglutamic acidosis. Pyroglutamic acidosis, which presents with mental status changes and an increased anion gap, occurs in selected patients receiving therapeutic doses of acetaminophen on a chronic basis. Susceptible patients are those with critical illness, poor nutrition, liver disease, or chronic kidney disease, as well as those on a strict vegetarian diet. In this context, acetaminophen leads to depletion of glutathione, altering the γ-glutamyl cycle to overproduce pyroglutamic acid (also known as 5-oxoproline). Diagnosis can be confirmed by measuring urine levels of pyroglutamic acid.

D-Lactic acidosis presents with an increased anion gap metabolic acidosis and characteristic neurologic findings of intermittent confusion, slurred speech, and ataxia in patients with short-bowel syndrome. Accumulation of the D-isomer of lactate can occur in patients with short-bowel syndrome following jejunoileal bypass or small-bowel resection. In these patients, excess carbohydrates that reach the colon are metabolized to D-lactate. Laboratory studies show increased anion gap metabolic acidosis with normal plasma lactate levels, because the D-isomer is not measured by conventional laboratory assays for lactate. Diagnosis is confirmed by specifically measuring D-lactate. This patient's lack of short-bowel syndrome rules out this diagnosis.

Propylene glycol, a solvent used to enhance the solubility of various intravenously administered medications, causes an increased anion gap metabolic acidosis through its acid metabolites, L-lactate and D-lactate. An increased osmolal gap accompanies the increased anion gap metabolic acidosis seen with propylene glycol. This patient's clinical history and lack of lactic acidosis are not consistent with propylene glycol toxicity.

Salicylate toxicity most commonly presents in adults as respiratory alkalosis or with features of both respiratory alkalosis and increased anion gap metabolic acidosis. This patient has appropriate respiratory compensation for the metabolic acidosis, not respiratory alkalosis, making salicylate toxicity unlikely.

- Pyroglutamic acidosis occurs in patients receiving therapeutic doses of acetaminophen on a chronic basis in the setting of critical illness, poor nutrition, liver disease, chronic kidney disease, or a strict vegetarian diet; diagnosis can be confirmed by measuring urine levels of pyroglutamic acid.

Bibliography

Fenves AZ, Kirkpatrick HM 3rd, Patel VV, Sweetman L, Emmett M. Increased anion gap metabolic acidosis as a result of 5-oxoproline (pyroglutamic acid): a role for acetaminophen. Clin J Am Soc Nephrol. 2006;1:441-7. [PMID: 17699243]

Item 23   Answer: B

Educational Objective: Diagnose abdominal compartment syndrome.

The most appropriate diagnostic test to perform next is intra-abdominal pressure (IAP) measurement. This patient's findings are consistent with abdominal compartment syndrome, which occurs in the setting of abdominal surgery, large volume fluid resuscitation, and multiple transfusions. It can manifest as a distended abdomen, ascites, and sodium-avid acute kidney injury (AKI). The increased IAP causes direct compression of renal parenchyma and vasculature, resulting in oliguria and decreased glomerular filtration rate. The diagnosis of abdominal compartment syndrome is made by an IAP measurement >20 mm Hg and new organ dysfunction. Indirect measurement of IAP can be with intragastric, intracolonic, intravesical (bladder), or inferior vena cava catheters. Management includes supportive therapy, abdominal compartment decompression, and correction of positive fluid balance.

The increased specific gravity, low urine sodium, and presence of hyaline casts are consistent with a prerenal AKI. The fractional excretion of sodium would not provide any additional information to aid in the diagnosis.

Myoglobin is a heme pigment–containing protein that can cause AKI. The urine is reddish brown, pigmented casts are present, and the urine dipstick is positive for blood in the absence of erythrocytes. Abdominal compartment syndrome is a much more likely cause of this patient's AKI, and urine myoglobin levels do not need to be measured.

The patient is on a cephalosporin, which can cause acute interstitial nephritis (AIN). AIN is characterized by hematuria, pyuria, and/or leukocyte casts. However, the timing is too soon for AIN (unless the patient had been previously exposed), and the urine findings do not support it. Moreover, the urine eosinophil stain is neither sensitive nor specific for the diagnosis of AIN and does not need to be performed.

KEY POINT

- Abdominal compartment syndrome is defined as a sustained intra-abdominal pressure >20 mm Hg associated with at least one organ dysfunction; management includes supportive therapy, abdominal compartment decompression, and correction of positive fluid balance.

Bibliography

Patel DM, Connor MJ Jr. Intra-abdominal hypertension and abdominal compartment syndrome: an underappreciated cause of acute kidney injury. Adv Chronic Kidney Dis. 2016;23:160-6. [PMID: 27113692]

Item 24   Answer: A

Educational Objective: Identify the cause of nonglomerular hematuria.

Cystoscopy is the most appropriate diagnostic test to perform next in this patient. Hematuria is frequently encountered among adults in ambulatory care. For hematuria incidentally discovered on dipstick evaluation, clinicians should confirm the presence of hematuria with microscopic urinalysis that demonstrates ≥3 erythrocytes/hpf before initiating further evaluation in asymptomatic adults. Clinicians should also pursue evaluation of hematuria even if the patient is receiving antiplatelet or anticoagulant therapy. Macroscopic hematuria should prompt urology referral even if self-limited. Hematuria is most often of nonglomerular origin. If a nephrologic cause of hematuria is not suggested, hematuria may indicate a malignancy. Guidelines from the American Urological Association recommend that patients older than 35 years or with risk factors for lower urinary tract malignancy (such as irritative voiding symptoms, smoking, aniline dye exposure, or cyclophosphamide exposure) undergo evaluation for malignancy with imaging. If imaging is negative, cystoscopy should be performed. This male patient is 45 years old without evidence of glomerular disease (no proteinuria or increased serum creatinine) and negative imaging of the upper genitourinary tract. Therefore, it is appropriate to assess for bladder pathology using cystoscopy.

Kidney biopsy in a patient with hematuria is not indicated in the absence of evidence of glomerular disease or change in kidney function. This patient's lack of proteinuria rules out a significant glomerular process, and his normal serum creatinine and lack of systemic symptoms make other kidney disease unlikely.

Kidney ultrasonography will provide no additional information in this patient. Doppler is not indicated because the risk of renal vein thrombosis as a cause of hematuria in this patient is not suspected (normal kidney function, no flank pain, and no risk of thrombosis).

Routine cytologic evaluation of urine is no longer recommended in the initial evaluation of asymptomatic microscopic hematuria, and urine markers approved by the FDA for bladder cancer detection are specifically not recommended for patients with hematuria.

KEY POINT

- Patients with hematuria who are older than 35 years or with risk factors for lower urinary tract malignancy (such as irritative voiding symptoms, smoking, aniline dye exposure, or cyclophosphamide exposure) should undergo evaluation for malignancy with imaging; if imaging is negative, cystoscopy is appropriate to assess for bladder pathology.

Bibliography

Davis R, Jones JS, Barocas DA, Castle EP, Lang EK, Leveillee RJ, et al; American Urological Association. Diagnosis, evaluation and follow-up of asymptomatic microhematuria (AMH) in adults. Available at: http://www.auanet.org/guidelines/asymptomatic-microhematuria-(2012-reviewed-and-validity-confirmed-2016). Accessed December 15, 2017.

Item 25   Answer: B

Educational Objective: Diagnose glomerulonephritis.

This patient likely has glomerulonephritis. Glomerular hematuria typically features brown- or tea-colored urine with dysmorphic erythrocytes (or acanthocytes) and/or erythrocyte casts on urine sediment examination. Erythrocyte casts are recognized by their cylindrical or tubular structure and inclusion of small, agranular spherocytes and, when present, are specific for hematuria of glomerular origin.

Isomorphic erythrocytes are of the same size and shape and usually arise from an extraglomerular urologic process causing bleeding into the genitourinary tract, such as a tumor, stone, or infection. Dysmorphic erythrocytes have varying sizes and shapes. Acanthocytes, a specific form of dysmorphic erythrocytes, are characterized by vesicle-shaped protrusions and suggest a glomerular source of bleeding. Acanthocytes and erythrocyte casts are highly specific for glomerulonephritis and exclude an extraglomerular cause of bleeding such as bladder cancer.

Sterile pyuria and leukocyte casts are hallmarks of tubulointerstitial nephritis, which can present acutely or may progress indolently and present as chronic kidney disease of unclear duration. Mild subnephrotic proteinuria also can be seen with interstitial nephritis. The cells comprising a leukocyte cast are larger than erythrocytes and appear more granular. The presence of erythrocyte casts excludes the diagnosis of tubulointerstitial nephritis.

Although this febrile patient has leukocytes (granular cells larger than erythrocytes) on urinalysis and positive leukocyte esterase on dipstick analysis, the presence of erythrocyte casts is specific for glomerulonephritis. This patient has the nephritic syndrome, which is associated with glomerular inflammation resulting in hematuria, proteinuria, and leukocytes in the urine sediment.

KEY POINT

- Glomerular macroscopic hematuria typically features brown- or tea-colored urine with dysmorphic erythrocytes (or acanthocytes) and/or erythrocyte casts on urine sediment examination.

Bibliography

Simerville JA, Maxted WC, Pahira JJ. Urinalysis: a comprehensive review. Am Fam Physician. 2005;71:1153-62. [PMID: 15791892]

Item 26   Answer: D

Educational Objective: Diagnose vancomycin-induced acute tubular necrosis.

The most likely cause of this patient's acute kidney injury (AKI) is vancomycin. The most common cause of hospital-acquired AKI is acute tubular necrosis (ATN), which represents damage and destruction of the renal tubular epithelial cells and is most commonly caused by ischemia or toxins. A careful evaluation of hemodynamics, volume status, medications, and physical findings of associated illness can help determine the cause of ATN. Most reported cases of vancomycin toxicity are due to acute interstitial nephritis; however, ATN has been reported. ATN is supported by the rapid rise in serum creatinine, fractional excretion of sodium >2%, and urine microscopy with numerous renal tubular epithelial cells and granular casts. Risk factors associated with vancomycin nephrotoxicity include chronic kidney disease, prolonged therapy, vancomycin doses ≥4 g/d, vancomycin trough concentrations >15 mg/L, and concomitant use of loop diuretics. Early recognition and prompt discontinuation of the drug are essential for renal recovery.

Some antibiotics (such as cefepime) and proton pump inhibitors (such as omeprazole) can cause acute interstitial nephritis (AIN). AIN may be associated with drugs, infection, autoimmune diseases, and malignancy. Only 10% to 30% of patients with AIN have the classic triad of fever, rash, and eosinophilia. Urine chemistries will reveal a variable (and unhelpful) fractional excretion of sodium, and urinalysis is characterized by hematuria, pyuria, and/or leukocyte casts and possibly eosinophiluria. Drug-induced AIN is characterized by a slowly increasing serum creatinine 7 to 10 days after exposure; however, it can occur within 1 day of exposure if the patient has been exposed previously. Drug-induced AIN can also occur months after exposure, as seen with NSAIDs and proton pump inhibitors. The patient's urine findings do not support AIN.

Contrast-induced nephropathy (CIN) results in ATN with an increase in serum creatinine within 48 hours of exposure. This patient's serum creatinine was at baseline 48 hours after exposure, making CIN an unlikely diagnosis.

KEY POINT

- Risk factors associated with vancomycin nephrotoxicity include chronic kidney disease, prolonged therapy, doses ≥4 g/d, trough concentrations >15 mg/L, and concomitant use of loop diuretics.

Bibliography

Bamgbola O. Review of vancomycin-induced renal toxicity: an update. Ther Adv Endocrinol Metab. 2016;7:136-47. [PMID: 27293542]

Item 27   Answer: B

Educational Objective: Treat acute hyponatremia in a symptomatic patient with hypertonic saline.

The most appropriate initial treatment is a 100-mL bolus of 3% saline. The hyponatremia in this young woman who presents confused and febrile is most likely due to ingestion of 3,4-methylenedioxymethamphetamine (ecstasy). Ecstasy is associated with hyponatremia both because it stimulates the release of antidiuretic hormone and because users often drink large quantities of water. When treating hyponatremia,

CONT.

the rate of correction of serum sodium concentration must be carefully considered to avoid the osmotic demyelination syndrome. Brain cells adapt to chronic hyponatremia by reducing intracellular concentration of organic osmolytes, such as myoinositol, to cope with hypotonicity. Acute hyponatremia is associated with an increase in brain water and cerebral edema and should be treated rapidly. Because the brain has not adapted to the hypotonic environment by the release of organic osmolytes, the risk of rapid correction and development of osmotic demyelination is absent. Treatment is with a bolus of 3% saline, and a 100-mL bolus should raise the serum sodium level by 2 to 3 mEq/L (2-3 mmol/L). If symptoms persist, this can be repeated one to two times.

In patients with neurologic symptoms, fluid restriction by itself is not an appropriate treatment. The immediate goal is to reduce brain swelling rapidly by the acutely raising the serum sodium level. Even in cases of chronic hyponatremia, the serum sodium can be increased acutely by 2 to 3 mEq/L (2-3 mmol/L) as long as the total change in the serum sodium is <10 mEq/L (10 mmol/L) in a 24-hour period. Except in cases of hypovolemic hyponatremia, the use of 0.9% sodium chloride is not recommended. In patients who are not volume depleted and have syndrome of inappropriate antidiuretic hormone secretion with a fixed urine osmolality, the infused saline can be excreted in the urine in a smaller volume, and thus the serum sodium can actually fall.

Both oral urea and tolvaptan are appropriate treatments for chronic hyponatremia, but they do not raise the serum sodium rapidly enough to reverse neurologic abnormalities and are therefore inappropriate for treatment of acute hyponatremia in this symptomatic patient.

> **KEY POINT**
> - Treatment of acute symptomatic hyponatremia includes a 100-mL bolus of 3% saline to increase the serum sodium level by 2 to 3 mEq/L (2-3 mmol/L).

Bibliography
Sterns RH. Disorders of plasma sodium–causes, consequences, and correction. N Engl J Med. 2015;372:55-65. [PMID: 25551526]

Item 28   Answer: C

Educational Objective: Diagnose fibromuscular dysplasia as the cause of secondary hypertension.

Renal artery imaging is the most appropriate diagnostic test to perform next to evaluate for fibromuscular dysplasia in this young woman with new-onset hypertension. Fibromuscular dysplasia is a nonatherosclerotic form of renovascular disease that usually affects the mid and distal portions of the renal artery. This disorder usually occurs in young persons, particularly young women, and abrupt onset of hypertension in a patient under the age of 35 years is suggestive. The elevation of serum creatinine more than 30% from baseline after the initiation of an ACE inhibitor is a clue that renovascular hypertension may be present. Fibromuscular dysplasia is associated with aneurysm and/or dissection in a variety of

vascular territories (for example, renal artery, carotid artery, and intracranial arteries). This has resulted in a recommendation that patients with fibromuscular dysplasia undergo one-time, head-to-pelvic cross-sectional imaging.

The importance of primary aldosteronism as a cause of hypertension is being increasingly recognized. Testing for primary aldosteronism should be considered in all patients with difficult-to-control hypertension. It should also be performed in patients with hypertension and an incidentally noted adrenal mass, spontaneous hypokalemia, or diuretic-induced hypokalemia. In these cases, the plasma aldosterone concentration/plasma renin activity ratio is obtained. Primary aldosteronism cannot account for this patient's renal bruit or serum creatinine elevation after the initiation of an ACE inhibitor.

Plasma fractionated metanephrines are obtained to screen for a pheochromocytoma. The absence of episodic palpitations, headaches, and tachycardia as well as the presence of an abdominal bruit make pheochromocytoma a less likely diagnosis.

Transthoracic echocardiography can be used for patients with clinical suspicion for white coat hypertension and/or to evaluate for end-organ damage. There are no pertinent findings from the history, physical examination, or electrocardiogram results to raise clinical suspicion for end-organ damage. More importantly, echocardiography will not be helpful in diagnosing the cause of this patient's hypertension or directing its treatment.

> **KEY POINT**
> - Renal artery imaging is the most appropriate diagnostic test to evaluate for fibromuscular dysplasia in a young woman with new-onset hypertension.

Bibliography
Olin JW, Gornik HL, Bacharach JM, Biller J, Fine LJ, Gray BH, et al; American Heart Association Council on Peripheral Vascular Disease. Fibromuscular dysplasia: state of the science and critical unanswered questions: a scientific statement from the American Heart Association. Circulation. 2014;129:1048-78. [PMID: 24548843]

Item 29   Answer: A

Educational Objective: Treat acute coronary syndrome in a patient with chronic kidney disease.

The most appropriate management for this patient with stage G4 chronic kidney disease (CKD) and ST-elevation myocardial infarction is immediate cardiac catheterization. Cardiovascular disease is the leading cause of death among patients with CKD. The risk of cardiovascular-related death in patients with CKD stages G3 and G4 is four to five times higher than the risk of progression to end-stage kidney disease. Mortality risk increases with decreasing estimated glomerular filtration rate and increasing albuminuria. Unfortunately, many clinical trials that guide the prevention or treatment of cardiovascular disease have not included patients with advanced CKD, and the findings may not be generalizable to patients with CKD. However, the recommendation from experts is to

CONT.

offer patients with CKD therapy for cardiovascular disease, including cardiac catheterization, percutaneous coronary intervention, and coronary bypass. The available data suggest that routine invasive management is associated with a statistically significant reduction in death, acute myocardial infarction, and rehospitalization, across most categories of CKD, at the predictable price of a significant increase in major and minor bleeding. Prognosis for patients following myocardial infarction, percutaneous intervention, and coronary artery bypass surgery is worse for patients with CKD than for those without CKD.

Suspected coronary anomalies, such as anomalous coronary origins, can be evaluated by cardiac magnetic resonance (CMR) imaging. CMR imaging is not a practical modality for patients with acute coronary syndrome because of the time necessary to generate the images and inability to provide revascularization therapy. In addition, CMR uses gadolinium contrast, which is associated with the development of nephrogenic systemic fibrosis in patients with CKD.

Studies have examined the potential efficacy of pre-catheterization dialysis to reduce the risk of contrast-induced nephropathy in patients with advanced CKD. The balance of the data suggests no benefit for this invasive maneuver, and it generally is not advocated.

This patient has acute coronary syndrome, and avoiding cardiac catheterization and potential intervention to treat this life-threatening condition in lieu of medical management will not be in the patient's best interest, regardless of the risk for contrast-induced nephropathy.

KEY POINT

- The available data suggest that routine invasive management of coronary artery disease is associated with a statistically significant reduction in death, acute myocardial infarction, and rehospitalization, across most categories of chronic kidney disease.

Bibliography
Lingel JM, Srivastava MC, Gupta A. Management of coronary artery disease and acute coronary syndrome in the chronic kidney disease population-a review of the current literature. Hemodial Int. 2017;21:472-482. [PMID: 28093874]

 Item 30   Answer: A

Educational Objective: Manage large kidney stones with extracorporeal shock wave lithotripsy.

The most appropriate next step in management is extracorporeal shock wave lithotripsy. Acute management of symptomatic nephrolithiasis is aimed at pain management and facilitation of stone passage. Pain can be relieved by NSAIDs and opioids as needed. Combination NSAID and opioid therapy seems more effective than treatment with either one alone. Stone passage decreases with increasing size of the stone. Only 50% of stones >6 mm will pass spontaneously, whereas stones >10 mm are extremely unlikely to pass spontaneously. Urologic intervention is required in all patients with evidence of infection, acute kidney injury, intractable nausea or pain,

and stones that fail to pass or are unlikely to pass. This patient has an 11-mm stone that is at the ureteral pelvic junction. There is associated dilation of the renal calyces suggesting obstruction to urine outflow. It is unlikely that a stone this size will pass. Appropriate management therefore is urology consultation. The patient will most likely require extracorporeal shock wave lithotripsy or percutaneous nephrolithotomy. Extracorporeal shock wave lithotripsy can be used for stones in the renal pelvis and proximal ureter, but it is less effective for stones located in the mid/distal ureter or the lower pole calyx, larger stones (>15 mm), and hard stones (calcium oxalate monohydrate or cystine). Potential complications of extracorporeal shock wave lithotripsy include incomplete stone fragmentation, kidney injury, and possibly increased blood pressure or new-onset hypertension.

Treatment of uncomplicated renal colic with analgesia and maintenance intravenous fluids is just as efficacious as with forced hydration with regard to patient pain perception and opioid use. Moreover, it appears the state of hydration has little impact on stone passage. This patient may require intravenous fluids to avoid dehydration if pain and nausea prevent adequate oral fluid intake, but not as a means to expel the kidney stone.

Stones up to 10 mm can be managed conservatively, although the likelihood of spontaneous passage decreases with increasing size. Medical expulsive therapy with α-blocker therapy (such as tamsulosin) or a calcium channel blocker (such as nifedipine) can aid the passage of small stones (≤10 mm in diameter). This large stone associated with probable obstruction is not a candidate for medical expulsive therapy with either tamsulosin or nifedipine.

KEY POINT

- Urologic intervention is required in all patients with evidence of infection, acute kidney injury, intractable nausea or pain, and stones that fail to pass or are unlikely to pass.

Bibliography
Lawler AC, Ghiraldi EM, Tong C, Friedlander JI. Extracorporeal shock wave therapy: current perspectives and future directions. Curr Urol Rep. 2017;18:25. [PMID: 28247327]

Item 31   Answer: C

Educational Objective: Diagnose sarcoidosis with kidney involvement.

The most likely diagnosis is sarcoidosis, a systemic inflammatory disease that can affect multiple organs. The most common presentations of sarcoidosis are hilar lymphadenopathy and parenchymal lung disease; common extrapulmonary organ involvement includes the skin, joints, and eyes. More than 90% of patients with kidney involvement have thoracic sarcoid identified on chest radiograph. Kidney manifestations in sarcoidosis are common and include nephrocalcinosis from hypercalcemia and hypercalciuria, nephrolithiasis, and chronic interstitial nephritis with granuloma formation. Hypercalcemia occurs due to peripheral conversion of 25-hydroxyvitamin D to 1,25-dihydroxyvitamin D by activated macrophages. Parathyroid hormone is typically suppressed in response to the hypercalcemia. The urinalysis is typical of other chronic tubulointerstitial diseases and can be normal or show only sterile pyuria or mild proteinuria, as in this patient's case. Kidney manifestations of hypercalcemia and interstitial nephritis are treated with glucocorticoids.

Thiazide diuretics can be associated with a mild hypercalcemia but not nephrocalcinosis. Furthermore, they decrease urinary calcium excretion. This patient's urinary calcium excretion is increased.

Primary hyperparathyroidism is characterized by hypercalcemia, hypophosphatemia, and inappropriately normal or elevated parathyroid hormone. This patient's parathyroid hormone is suppressed, making this an unlikely diagnosis.

Increased levels of calcium absorption from the gut can be from markedly high vitamin D levels. Vitamin D intoxication is usually defined as a value >150 ng/mL (374.4 nmol/L). Vitamin D intoxication is not consistent with the laboratory findings because the phosphorus and 25-hydroxyvitamin D levels are normal.

Finally, thiazide diuretic use, primary hyperparathyroidism, or vitamin D intoxication cannot account for the patient's pulmonary findings.

KEY POINT

- Kidney involvement in sarcoidosis can manifest as nephrocalcinosis from hypercalcemia and hypercalciuria, and as tubulointerstitial nephritis with granuloma formation.

Bibliography

Löffler C, Löffler U, Tuleweit A, Waldherr R, Uppenkamp M, Bergner R. Renal sarcoidosis: epidemiological and follow-up data in a cohort of 27 patients. Sarcoidosis Vasc Diffuse Lung Dis. 2015;31:306-15. [PMID: 25591142]

Item 32   Answer: C

Educational Objective: Identify normal physiologic changes in pregnancy as a cause of low serum sodium.

Normal physiologic change in pregnancy is the most likely cause of this patient's low serum sodium level. Mild hyponatremia is common in normal pregnancy due to plasma volume increases with water retention (mediated by an increase in antidiuretic hormone levels) greater than sodium retention. An associated drop in serum osmolality of 8 to 10 mOsm/kg H_2O and serum sodium concentration of 4 to 5 mEq/L (4-5 mmol/L) may occur. As the serum osmolality and sodium concentration decrease, a new set point is maintained, and thirst occurs in response to osmolality (reset osmostat). No treatment is necessary. Other conditions associated with reset osmostat include quadriplegia, tuberculosis, advanced age, psychiatric disorders, and chronic malnutrition.

Primary polydipsia should always be considered in the differential diagnosis of patients with mental illness and hyponatremia, particularly those with schizophrenia who are taking psychotropic drugs. Primary polydipsia presents with hyponatremia, decreased serum osmolality, and decreased urine osmolality, reflecting suppressed antidiuretic hormone (ADH) levels in response to water overload. Primary polydipsia is a rare cause of hyponatremia, and the volume of water intake would need to be very large to induce hyponatremia. This patient is not at risk for primary polydipsia.

Hypovolemia causes stimulation of the sympathetic nervous system, activation of the renin-angiotensin-aldosterone axis, and release of ADH. These adaptive responses allow volume maintenance at the expense of a low serum sodium with excessive water intake. Blood pressure in pregnant women begins to lower in the first trimester and reaches a nadir in the second. Furthermore, she is asymptomatic, and ADH release is therefore not likely to be induced by this level of blood pressure.

The syndrome of inappropriate antidiuretic hormone (SIADH) secretion may be associated with stress and pain; however, hyponatremia does not develop acutely. Although SIADH could have preceded the patient's car accident, she has no risk factors for SIADH (central nervous system disorders, pulmonary disorders, infection, drugs, postoperative status, tumors), and normal pregnancy is a more likely cause of her low serum sodium level.

KEY POINT

- Mild hyponatremia is common in normal pregnancy due to plasma volume increases with water retention greater than sodium retention; no treatment is necessary.

Bibliography

Cheung KL, Lafayette RA. Renal physiology of pregnancy. Adv Chronic Kidney Dis. 2013;20:209-14. [PMID: 23928384]

Item 33   Answer: D

Educational Objective: Treat dyslipidemia in a patient with stage G4 chronic kidney disease.

A statin is appropriate to treat dyslipidemia in this patient with stage G4 chronic kidney disease (CKD). Guidelines from the Kidney Disease: Improving Global Outcomes (KDIGO) group provide a grade 1A recommendation to treat adults aged ≥50 years with an estimated glomerular filtration rate (eGFR) <60 mL/min/1.73 m^2, but not treated with chronic dialysis or kidney transplantation (GFR categories G3a-G5), with a statin or statin/ezetimibe combination. This recommendation largely emanates from results of the Study of Heart and Renal Protection (SHARP) trial, which included 9270 participants with CKD (mean eGFR, 27 mL/min/1.73 m^2) who received simvastatin 20 mg plus ezetimibe 10 mg daily or placebo and were followed for 5 years. Statin plus ezetimibe therapy led to a significant 17% reduction in the relative hazard of the primary outcome of major atherosclerotic events (coronary death, myocardial infarction, nonhemorrhagic stroke, or any revascularization) compared with placebo (HR, 0.83; 95% CI, 0.74-0.94), driven by significant reductions in nonhemorrhagic stroke and coronary revascularization. It should be noted that simvastatin plus ezetimibe did not reduce the risk of progression to end-stage kidney disease.

Hypertriglyceridemia is the primary lipid abnormality in patients with CKD. However, the 2013 KDIGO update states that the evidence supporting the safety and efficacy of fibrates (such as gemfibrozil) is extremely weak, especially in patients with CKD. Therefore, KDIGO does not recommend fibrates for the treatment of hypertriglyceridemia. Finally, in patients taking a statin for dyslipidemia, the addition of a fibrate increases the risk of myalgia, muscle injury, and rhabdomyolysis.

Although niacin raises HDL cholesterol, several trials involving patients with and without CKD have demonstrated no evidence of improvement in cardiovascular events.

Although randomized controlled trials of omega-3 fatty acids have demonstrated a reduction in cardiovascular disease end points in persons with atherosclerotic cardiovascular disease (ASCVD), little to no data demonstrate the role for the benefits of omega-3 fatty acids for the primary prevention of ASCVD in patients at high cardiovascular disease risk.

KEY POINT

- The Kidney Disease: Improving Global Outcomes (KDIGO) guidelines recommend treatment of dyslipidemia with a statin in patients aged ≥50 years with an estimated glomerular filtration rate <60 mL/min/1.73 m^2, but not treated with chronic dialysis or kidney transplantation.

Bibliography

Kidney Disease: Improving Global Outcomes (KDIGO) Lipid Work Group. KDIGO clinical practice guideline for lipid management in chronic kidney disease. Kidney inter., Suppl. 2013;3:259-305. Available at www.kdigo.org.

Item 34   Answer: D

Educational Objective: Diagnose nephrolithiasis with noncontrast helical abdominal CT.

Noncontrast helical abdominal CT is the most appropriate next test for this patient with nephrolithiasis suggested by unilateral flank pain and hematuria. Ultrasonography is an appropriate initial diagnostic test for suspected nephrolithiasis; it is easily available, safe, and relatively inexpensive, and it is the study of choice in pregnant women. Ultrasonography can demonstrate hydronephrosis, kidney size and cortical thickness, echogenicity, and the presence of cysts and tumors. It is useful for uncomplicated nephrolithiasis; a positive ultrasound may be adequate for initial diagnosis. Ultrasonography is less useful in evaluating diseases of the mid or distal ureter, including stones. Furthermore, the

absence of hydronephrosis on ultrasound does not rule out kidney stones. Noncontrast helical CT is the gold standard for diagnosis of nephrolithiasis and is appropriate for evaluating renal colic. Most stones can be detected, including small stones and those in the distal ureter not detected on ultrasound. It may provide information regarding stone composition and, because the entire urinary tract and abdomen are visualized, alternative diagnoses may be suggested.

MRI with contrast is not as sensitive as CT in detecting suspected kidney stones. Due to lack of radiation, MRI may be useful in pregnant women with stone disease if ultrasound is nondiagnostic.

Contrast abdominal CT characterizes renal tumors and cysts, whereas CT urography is the preferred test for patients with unexplained urologic/nonglomerular hematuria. The decision to use contrast depends on the clinical scenario, the patient's risk factors for contrast-induced nephropathy, and the availability and utility of alternative imaging modalities. It is unnecessary in the evaluation of suspected nephrolithiasis and poses greater risk and cost in this situation compared with either ultrasonography or noncontrast helical abdominal CT.

Plain abdominal radiography has limited utility due to its inability to detect radiolucent uric acid stones and does not provide as much anatomic information as other modalities. However, it may be useful in assessing stone burden in patients with known radiopaque stones but is not the initial test of choice for acute nephrolithiasis.

KEY POINT

- Noncontrast helical CT is the gold standard for diagnosis of nephrolithiasis.

Bibliography

Brisbane W, Bailey MR, Sorensen MD. An overview of kidney stone imaging techniques. Nat Rev Urol. 2016;13:654-662. [PMID: 27578040]

Item 35   Answer: C

Educational Objective: Identify increased muscle mass as a cause of an increase in serum creatinine.

Measurement of the serum cystatin C level is appropriate for this patient. Cystatin C may be preferable to creatinine to assess kidney function in individuals with higher muscle mass. An increase in muscle mass would be expected to result in an increase in serum creatinine level in the absence of change in kidney function. This muscular man with a BMI of 29 has increase in muscle mass. Because serum creatinine is derived from the metabolism of creatinine produced by muscle, a significant increase in muscle mass would be expected to increase serum creatinine. An elevation in serum creatinine could also occur with creatine supplements, which he is not taking. This patient has a normal urinalysis and no proteinuria, all of which indicate no evidence of underlying kidney disease. Cystatin C, which is cleared by the kidney, is produced by all nucleated cells; therefore, levels are less dependent on muscle mass. Cystatin C can also be used for more accurate glomerular filtration rate estimation in these patients as a component of the Chronic Kidney Disease Epidemiology Collaboration equation.

Although NSAIDs can cause acute kidney injury, the remote and infrequent use by this patient is unlikely to have any effect on serum creatinine. The hemodynamic effects of NSAIDs will disappear within 24 hours of stopping the medication, and interstitial nephritis from NSAIDs is unlikely to present with occasional dosing and is usually associated with proteinuria. The adverse effects of renal fibrosis associated with NSAIDs are only seen with extensive and long-term use.

Creatine kinase levels can be measured to evaluate for the presence of rhabdomyolysis. Rhabdomyolysis significant enough to cause kidney injury would be expected to result in myoglobinuria reflected by heme-positive urine in the absence of red cells. No blood was seen on urinalysis.

In the absence of other changes suggesting glomerular or interstitial disease, a kidney biopsy is not necessary.

KEY POINT

- Increased muscle mass can result in an increase in serum creatinine level in the absence of change in kidney function.

Bibliography

Baxmann AC, Ahmed MS, Marques NC, Menon VB, Pereira AB, Kirsztajn GM, et al. Influence of muscle mass and physical activity on serum and urinary creatinine and serum cystatin C. Clin J Am Soc Nephrol. 2008;3:348-54. [PMID: 18235143]

Item 36   Answer: B

Educational Objective: Manage recurrent stone disease with hydrochlorothiazide.

The most appropriate next step to decrease this patient's stone recurrence is to add a thiazide diuretic such as hydrochlorothiazide. Hypercalciuria is the most common metabolic risk factor for calcium oxalate stones. In patients with hypercalcemia, increased filtered calcium results in hypercalciuria. However, hypercalciuria is often idiopathic and commonly familial, occurring without associated hypercalcemia. Hypercalciuria due to hypercalcemia is treated by addressing the cause of increased serum calcium. In patients with other forms of hypercalciuria, thiazide diuretics reduce calcium excretion in the urine by inducing mild hypovolemia, triggering increased proximal sodium reabsorption and passive calcium reabsorption. This effect can be enhanced by the addition of sodium restriction.

The patient's evaluation reveals a normal uric acid concentration. In calcium stones that form on a uric acid nidus, allopurinol has been associated with a decrease in stone formation. In this patient, however, stone analysis did not reveal a uric acid core and thus would not be the next step in management.

Urinary citrate inhibits stone formation by binding calcium in the tubular lumen, preventing it from precipitating with oxalate. Hypocitraturia is seen with diets high in animal protein and metabolic acidosis from chronic diarrhea, renal tubular acidosis, ureteral diversion, and carbonic anhydrase inhibitors (including seizure medications such as topiramate). The patient's urine citrate level is in the high-normal range, and the serum bicarbonate level is normal, thus increasing citrate in the urine would not be beneficial.

Although increasing urine volume will reduce the calcium saturation, the present urine volume is acceptable. Urine volume to prevent stone recurrence should be between 2500 and 3000 mL per day.

Recommending a low calcium diet is inappropriate for this patient because reducing calcium in the diet would provide less calcium in the gastrointestinal tract to bind oxalate and would increase oxalate absorption, and thus increase urine oxalate concentration and stone formation.

KEY POINT

- In patients with hypercalciuria and kidney stones, calcium excretion and stone formation can be decreased by the use of thiazide diuretics.

Bibliography

Qaseem A, Dallas P, Forciea MA, Starkey M, Denberg TD; Clinical Guidelines Committee of the American College of Physicians. Dietary and pharmacologic management to prevent recurrent nephrolithiasis in adults: a clinical practice guideline from the American College of Physicians. Ann Intern Med. 2014;161:659-67. [PMID: 25364887]

Item 37   Answer: B

Educational Objective: Screen for intracranial cerebral aneurysms in a patient with autosomal dominant polycystic kidney disease.

MR angiography of the brain is the most appropriate next step in management. This patient has autosomal dominant polycystic kidney disease (ADPKD), a genetic kidney disease characterized by enlarged kidneys with multiple cysts. Intracranial cerebral aneurysms are detected in 5% to 10% of patients with ADPKD and have a strong familial pattern. Guidelines for the Management of Patients with Unruptured Intracranial Aneurysms from the American Heart Association/American Stroke Association recommend that patients with a history of ADPKD, particularly those with a family history of intracranial aneurysm but even those without such history, should be offered screening by CT angiography or MR angiography. This is a class I recommendation (should be performed because benefit greatly exceeds risk) based on level B evidence (data derived from a single randomized trial or nonrandomized studies).

Mitral valve prolapse is an extrarenal manifestation seen in some patients with ADPKD, but screening with echocardiography should be limited to patients with findings of this valvular disorder, including chest pain, shortness of breath, edema, a systolic click(s) that is mobile (timing changes with squatting and standing), and a systolic murmur.

Blood pressure control is recommended to slow progression in ADPKD, but the utility of doing so in someone with low baseline blood pressures is unproven. The agent of choice when blood pressure medications are used in ADPKD is a blocker of the renin-angiotensin system and not a calcium channel blocker.

Vasopressin blockade with tolvaptan in patients with ADPKD has been shown in two randomized clinical trials to delay the need for dialysis from 6 to 9 years. Tolvaptan carries an FDA-mandated safety warning about the possibility of irreversible liver injury. Tolvaptan has not been approved for use in ADPKD in the United States.

> **KEY POINT**
>
> - Screening for intracranial cerebral aneurysms using CT or MR angiography is recommended for patients with autosomal dominant polycystic kidney disease.

Bibliography

Chapman AB, Devuyst O, Eckardt KU, Gansevoort RT, Harris T, Horie S, et al; Conference Participants. Autosomal-dominant polycystic kidney disease (ADPKD): executive summary from a Kidney Disease: Improving Global Outcomes (KDIGO) Controversies Conference. Kidney Int. 2015;88:17-27. [PMID: 25786098]

Item 38   Answer: E

Educational Objective: Manage primary membranous glomerulopathy.

An ACE inhibitor and statin are appropriate for this patient with recently diagnosed primary membranous glomerulopathy. His kidney biopsy findings are consistent with the diagnosis, and the presence of anti-phospholipase A2 receptor (PLA2R) antibodies has been shown to approach 100% specificity for the primary form of this disease. Approximately one third of patients with primary membranous glomerulopathy experience a spontaneous remission of disease over the first 6 to 24 months without immunosuppression. Therefore, within the first 6 months of diagnosis, barring signs of severe complications of the nephrotic syndrome (such as kidney failure, anasarca, or deep vein thrombosis), the recommended strategy is to treat patients with primary membranous glomerulopathy conservatively with renin-angiotensin system blockers, cholesterol-lowering medications (if cholesterol is above goal), and diuretics (for edema). The patient is then monitored with examinations and laboratory studies to gauge for spontaneous remission. If proteinuria increases in 6 to 12 months, a course of immunosuppression should be considered for those with persistent nephrotic-range proteinuria. With the advent of serologic testing for anti-PLA2R antibodies, these titers can now be followed during the observation period alongside traditional clinical parameters, such as proteinuria. Falling anti-PLA2R titers are associated with remission, whereas persistently high titers are associated with ongoing disease activity.

Alternating months of glucocorticoids and alkylating agents is first-line immunosuppressive therapy of choice for primary membranous glomerulopathy, and substituting with a calcineurin inhibitor such as cyclosporine is now considered a viable alternative for patients with contraindications to alkylating agents. However, utilization of such immunosuppressive therapies at this point is premature and runs the risk of treating a patient who may remit spontaneously.

Although hepatitis B and C virus infections, along with lupus, are well-known forms of secondary membranous glomerulopathy in adults, this patient's screening tests are negative and, with PLA2R antibody positivity, further testing is unnecessary.

> **KEY POINT**
>
> - Patients with newly diagnosed primary membranous glomerulopathy are usually observed for 6 to 12 months while on conservative therapy (renin-angiotensin blockade, cholesterol-lowering medication, and edema management) to allow time for possible spontaneous remission before initiating immunosuppression.

Bibliography

Couser WG. Primary membranous nephropathy. Clin J Am Soc Nephrol. 2017;12:983-997. [PMID: 28550082] doi:10.2215/CJN.11761116

Item 39   Answer: A

Educational Objective: Treat hypertension in a patient with atherosclerotic renovascular disease.

The most appropriate next step in management is to begin lisinopril. The patient most likely has atherosclerotic renovascular disease, given his age, diminished pulses, and resistant hypertension despite treatment with four antihypertensive medications, including a diuretic. Most patients with renovascular disease have atherosclerosis (>90%). In this patient, medical therapy should be optimized to include treatment of underlying cardiovascular risk factors such as hypercholesterolemia and addition of an ACE inhibitor or angiotensin receptor blocker (ARB) for blood pressure control. Kidney function should be checked 2 weeks after the addition of an ACE inhibitor or ARB to ensure that the serum creatinine does not increase, and the ACE inhibitor or ARB can be continued if there is not a >25% rise in the serum creatinine from baseline.

Although renal angiography is the gold standard for diagnosis of renovascular disease, it is not recommended as a routine test due to adverse risks such as contrast nephropathy and cholesterol emboli. It is undertaken only if an intervention to correct a discovered stenosis is planned. However, medical therapy is recommended for most adults with atherosclerotic renal artery stenosis.

Three randomized controlled trials (STAR, ASTRAL, and CORAL) failed to show that renal artery angioplasty confers additional benefit above optimal medical therapy for patients with atherosclerotic renovascular disease who have stable kidney function. Patients who may benefit from percutaneous angioplasty and stenting or surgical intervention include those who present with a short hypertension duration; fail medical therapy; or have severe hypertension or recurrent flash pulmonary edema, refractory heart failure, acute kidney injury following treatment with an ACE inhibitor or ARB, or progressive impaired kidney function. In patients who have an indication for renal artery revascularization, surgery is preferred only for those with complex anatomic lesions such as aneurysm or aortoiliac occlusive disease.

KEY POINT

- In most patients with renal artery stenosis, the primary therapeutic intervention is medical management, including correction of modifiable cardiovascular risk factors.

Bibliography

Cooper CJ, Murphy TP, Cutlip DE, Jamerson K, Henrich W, Reid DM, et al; CORAL Investigators. Stenting and medical therapy for atherosclerotic renal-artery stenosis. N Engl J Med. 2014;370:13-22. [PMID: 24245566]

Item 40   Answer: B

Educational Objective: Prevent contrast-induced nephropathy in a patient with chronic kidney disease.

Intravenous isotonic fluid (0.9% sodium chloride or 1.26% sodium bicarbonate) administered before and after cardiac catheterization is the most appropriate preventive measure for this patient with chronic kidney disease (CKD) who is at risk for contrast-induced nephropathy (CIN). CIN is a common cause of acute kidney injury in the hospital. Patients can be exposed to iodinated intravenous contrast during cardiac catheterization, angiography, and CT. Contrast agents are thought to cause acute tubular necrosis through renal vasoconstriction and direct cytotoxicity; however, the mechanisms are not completely understood. Risk factors for CIN include advanced age, diabetic nephropathy, multiple myeloma, concomitant use of nephrotoxins (for example, aminoglycoside antibiotics, NSAIDs), severity of CKD, reduced renal perfusion (due to poor cardiac function or volume depletion), higher dose of contrast, high osmolar contrast (rarely used in industrialized contrast), repeated doses of contrast, and intra-arterial administration. Intravenous isotonic fluids (1-1.5 mL/kg/h 3 to 4 hours before the procedure and continued for 6 to 12 hours) are the mainstay in preventing CIN and perform better than hypotonic fluids. However, among isotonic fluids, evidence does not support the superiority of any one particular fluid when comparing normal saline with sodium bicarbonate. Intravenous fluids should not be given to prevent CIN in patients who are hypervolemic.

Furosemide before catheterization is incorrect because diuresis would induce volume contraction, activate the renal angiotensin-aldosterone system, and increase the risk for CIN.

Oral bicarbonate does not have a role in the prevention of CIN, as studies using alkali therapy looked at intravenous forms only. However, intravenous infusion of 1.26% sodium bicarbonate is as efficacious in preventing CIN as is 0.9% sodium chloride infusion.

This patient has no indications for renal replacement therapy. Hemodialysis does not improve CIN outcomes but rather may exacerbate kidney injury.

KEY POINT

- Intravenous isotonic fluids are the mainstay in preventing contrast-induced nephropathy.

Bibliography

Fähling M, Seeliger E, Patzak A, Persson PB. Understanding and preventing contrast-induced acute kidney injury. Nat Rev Nephrol. 2017;13:169-180. [PMID: 28138128]

Item 41   Answer: B

Educational Objective: Diagnose type 1 (hypokalemic distal) renal tubular acidosis.

The most likely cause of this patient's laboratory findings is type 1 (hypokalemic distal) renal tubular acidosis (RTA). It is due to a defect in urine acidification in the distal nephron and is most commonly caused by decreased activity of the proton pump in collecting duct intercalated-A cells. Because of the inability to excrete hydrogen ions, patients develop a metabolic acidosis with compensatory hyperchloremia, resulting in a normal anion gap, which is 8 mEq/L (8 mmol/L) in this patient, and the inability to acidify urine below a pH of 6.0, even in the context of an acidemia. The urine anion gap (using the equation: [Urine Sodium + Urine Potassium] – Urine Chloride) would be positive in this case, reflecting decreased acid excretion in the form of ammonium and chloride. The same defects also cause potassium wasting, and the increased proximal resorption of citrate that occurs with metabolic acidosis leads to hypocitraturia and increased risk of calcium phosphate kidney stones and nephrocalcinosis. This patient most likely has Sjögren syndrome (arthralgia, sicca, parotid gland enlargement) with concomitant interstitial nephritis (echogenicity seen on kidney ultrasound), one of the most common diseases associated with a distal RTA.

Naproxen, as well as other NSAIDs, can cause an interstitial nephritis usually accompanied by acute kidney injury and proteinuria, neither of which is seen in this case.

Type 2 (proximal) RTA involves a proximal tubular defect in reclaiming bicarbonate and is characterized by a normal anion gap metabolic acidosis, hypokalemia, glycosuria (without hyperglycemia), low-molecular-weight proteinuria, and renal phosphate wasting (known as Fanconi syndrome when all features are present). Because distal urine acidification remains intact, the urine pH is usually <5.5 without alkali therapy, and the urine anion gap should be negative, reflecting increased excretion of acid in the form of ammonium and chloride. This patient's high urine pH and absence of other characteristic features make type 2 (proximal) RTA unlikely.

Type 4 (hyperkalemic distal) RTA due to aldosterone deficiency or resistance is associated with hyperkalemia and a urine pH <5.5, neither of which is seen in this patient.

KEY POINT

- Type 1 (hypokalemic distal) renal tubular acidosis is due to a defect in urine acidification in the distal nephron and is characterized by a normal anion gap metabolic acidosis, positive urine anion gap, inability to acidify urine below a pH of 6.0, and potassium wasting.

Bibliography

Rastegar M, Nagami GT. Non-anion gap metabolic acidosis: a clinical approach to evaluation. Am J Kidney Dis. 2017;69:296-301. [PMID: 28029394]

H **Item 42** **Answer: B**

Educational Objective: Treat alcoholic ketoacidosis.

The most appropriate treatment is 5% dextrose in 0.9% saline for this patient who most likely has alcoholic ketoacidosis. Alcoholic ketoacidosis occurs in patients with chronic ethanol abuse, frequently with associated liver disease, and develops following an episode of acute intoxication. This patient has an increased anion gap metabolic acidosis (with an anion gap of 31), and ketoacidosis due to acute ethanol intoxication is the most likely cause. The ethanol level may be low or normal at the time of presentation because ingested ethanol may have already been extensively metabolized. Decreased insulin secretion (as a result of starvation) and increased counter-regulatory hormones cause lipolysis and generation of ketones, such as acetoacetate, which result in the anion gap. The urine in this case shows ketones, although ketone test results may be falsely negative in some cases because the nitroprusside reagent in the ketone assay detects only acetoacetate and the ketone β-hydroxybutyrate may predominate. Treatment with dextrose will increase insulin and decrease glucagon secretion, while saline will repair any volume deficit; the combination will correct ketoacidosis. In patients with alcoholism, thiamine should be administered before any glucose-containing solutions to decrease the risk of precipitating Wernicke encephalopathy.

Saline alone will correct the volume deficit, but glucose is needed to stimulate insulin secretion to correct the ketoacidosis.

Although dextrose with sodium bicarbonate may correct the underlying acidosis, there is no indication for additional bicarbonate in treating the ketoacidosis. In addition, alcoholic ketoacidosis may be associated with metabolic alkalosis due to concurrent vomiting. To determine if there is a concomitant metabolic alkalosis present, the corrected bicarbonate can be calculated. The corrected bicarbonate is the difference between the normal bicarbonate concentration and the delta anion gap. The delta anion gap is the difference between the measured anion gap and the normal anion gap. In this case the corrected bicarbonate concentration is 5 mEq/L (5 mmol/L) [24 − (31 − 12)]. Because the measured bicarbonate concentration (10 mEq/L [10 mmol/L]) is greater than the corrected, or expected, bicarbonate concentration, a concomitant metabolic alkalosis is present. Treatment with bicarbonate would be inappropriate.

Insulin treatment is not necessary because dextrose alone will increase insulin levels in patients who do not have diabetes mellitus.

KEY POINT

- For patients with alcoholic ketoacidosis, 5% dextrose in 0.9% saline is appropriate treatment.

Bibliography

Palmer BF, Clegg DJ. Electrolyte disturbances in patients with chronic alcohol-use disorder. N Engl J Med. 2017;377:1368-1377. [PMID: 28976856]

Item 43 **Answer: A**

Educational Objective: Treat edema associated with the nephrotic syndrome.

Addition of the thiazide diuretic metolazone is the most appropriate treatment. Edema management in a patient with newly diagnosed nephrotic syndrome generally starts with a salt-restricted diet and an oral loop diuretic, with a goal weight loss of 1 to 2 kg (2.2-4.4 lb) per week. Loop diuretics should be uptitrated toward this weight loss goal until a maximal dose is achieved, with close monitoring of electrolytes. It is appropriate for blood urea nitrogen, serum creatinine, and serum urate to rise slightly (≤10%) with effective diuresis. When oral loop diuretics have been maximally uptitrated, and weight loss and edema control are insufficient, it is often necessary to add a second oral diuretic (a thiazide diuretic and/or potassium-sparing diuretic) that works distal to the loop of Henle, which in this case can be accomplished via the addition of metolazone in this patient taking maximal-dose furosemide.

Loop diuretics are similarly effective when administered at equipotent doses. All loop diuretics have a similar dose-response curve characterized by an increased diuresis as more of the drug is renally excreted and flattening of the curve, at which further increases in dose are not associated with increased drug excretion and resultant diuresis.

Hospitalization for intravenous diuresis should be reserved for patients who have not responded to maximal doses of oral diuretics (that is, loop diuretic *and* thiazide diuretic) or for patients with severe symptoms of anasarca such as shortness of breath, swelling of genital regions, or gastrointestinal discomfort from ascites.

Repeating lower extremity Doppler ultrasonography is not indicated at this time given this patient's prior negative test results; serum albumin level >2.8 g/dL (28 g/L) (clotting risk in membranous glomerulopathy rises when albumin is ≤2.8 g/dL [28 g/L]); and the symmetric nature of his edema.

KEY POINT

- Edema management in a patient with newly diagnosed nephrotic syndrome starts with a salt-restricted diet and an oral loop diuretic; when loop diuretics have been maximally uptitrated and weight loss/edema control is insufficient, it is often necessary to add a thiazide and/or potassium-sparing diuretic.

Bibliography
Kodner C. Diagnosis and management of nephrotic syndrome in adults. Am Fam Physician. 2016;93:479-85. [PMID: 26977832]

Item 44   Answer: D

Educational Objective: Diagnose secondary focal segmental glomerulosclerosis.

Secondary focal segmental glomerulosclerosis (FSGS) is the most likely diagnosis. FSGS is the most common form of the nephrotic syndrome in black persons. In the United States, FSGS currently accounts for up to 40% of idiopathic (primary) nephrotic syndromes in adults. The pathogenesis of FSGS stems from podocyte injury due to immunologic, genetic, and/or hyperfiltration causes. A large and growing proportion of FSGS cases are considered secondary forms of FSGS due to hyperfiltration injury in the setting of relatively reduced renal mass. The overworking of the glomerulus in this setting leads to adaptive podocyte injury and segmental sclerosis. This hyperfiltration form of FSGS is classically seen in obese patients but also can manifest in patients with a history of premature birth or solitary kidney. This patient has two risk factors for the secondary form of FSGS: obesity and a history of premature birth. In addition, her presentation is more typical of a secondary FSGS lesion, with subnephrotic proteinuria and no associated clinical findings. Electron microscopy of her kidney biopsy would be expected to show only mild to moderate effacement of the podocyte's foot processes. An immunologic route to injury is considered the main pathogenic mechanism behind primary forms of FSGS, with leukocytes producing a soluble circulating factor that directly targets podocytes. In such cases, proteinuria tends to be heavy (nephrotic range) with associated hypoalbuminemia, and edema is usually present on physical examination. Electron microscopy of a kidney biopsy with primary FSGS will typically show extensive effacement of the podocyte's foot process.

Diabetic nephropathy is the sequelae of chronic glycemic-induced damage to the glomerulus. On average, it occurs 8 years after the diagnosis of overt diabetes mellitus and is typically associated with other microvascular or macrovascular complications of diabetes. This patient's short history of prediabetes and lack of other microvascular/macrovascular findings makes diabetic nephropathy an unlikely diagnosis.

Lipoprotein glomerulopathy is a rare kidney disease characterized by moderate to severe proteinuria, progressive kidney failure, and distinct histopathologic findings of glomerular capillary dilatation by lipoprotein thrombi. To date, less than 100 cases have been reported in the medical literature, nearly all of which are from East Asian countries (predominantly Japan and China). This patient does not fit the profile for lipoprotein glomerulopathy.

Minimal change glomerulopathy typically presents with the full nephrotic syndrome (proteinuria >3500 mg/24 h, serum albumin usually <3.0 g/dL [30 g/L], hypercholesterolemia,

and edema on examination). These findings do not fit this patient's mild presentation.

KEY POINT
- Secondary focal segmental glomerulosclerosis is due to hyperfiltration injury in the setting of relatively reduced renal mass; it is classically seen in obese patients but also can manifest in those with a history of premature birth or solitary kidney.

Bibliography
D'Agati VD, Kaskel FJ, Falk RJ. Focal segmental glomerulosclerosis. N Engl J Med. 2011;365:2398-411. [PMID: 22187987] doi:10.1056/NEJMra1106556

Item 45   Answer: D

Educational Objective: Identify the risk of venous thromboembolism in the nephrotic syndrome.

The nephrotic syndrome can be complicated by clotting manifestations due to a secondary hypercoagulable state. Of all the nephrotic syndromes, membranous glomerulopathy carries the greatest risk for clotting abnormalities, with some series reporting thrombotic complications in up to 35% of the most severe membranous glomerulopathy cases. The etiology for the hypercoagulable state in membranous glomerulopathy and other forms of heavy nephrosis is multifactorial. In response to the hypoalbuminemia induced by nephrotic-range proteinuria, the liver overproduces proteins. This is most classically seen in the form of hyperlipidemia. In addition, hepatic overproduction of proteins in response to hypoalbuminemia can also lead to increased levels of procoagulant proteins such as factor V, factor VIII, and fibrinogen. Urinary loss of albumin in high volume is also accompanied by similar urinary losses of low-molecular-weight anticoagulants (notably, antithrombin III and protein S) and fibrinolytics (such as plasminogen). In a large retrospective cohort of clotting complications in membranous glomerulopathy, >70% of the clots occurred within 2 years of diagnosis, and the risk of clotting markedly increased once albumin levels dropped below 2.8 g/dL (28 g/L) (OR, 2.53; $P = 0.02$, compared with albumin ≥2.8 g/dL [28 g/L]).

Chronic kidney disease is a risk factor for hyperuricemia and acute gout due to underexcretion of urate by the kidneys. In these patients, hyperuricemia may be due to impaired glomerular filtration and/or defects of urate handling in the renal proximal tubule. This patient's current kidney function does not place her at increased risk for gout.

Patients with membranous glomerulopathy have an increased risk of malignancy. Most cancers are diagnosed in men ≥65 years of age and are often solid tumors of the prostate, lung, or gastrointestinal tract. The risk for malignancy seems to be reduced in patients with anti-phospholipase A2 receptor (PLA2R) antibody. Taking into account her negative age- and sex-appropriate cancer screening, young age, and anti-PLA2R antibody status, this patient's risk of malignancy is low.

Patients with end-stage kidney disease have a markedly increased risk for renal cell carcinoma. Although current guidelines do not support routine screening for renal cell carcinoma in all patients with chronic kidney disease, a high level of suspicion is warranted in patients with symptoms such as new-onset gross hematuria or unexplained flank pain. In the absence of end-stage kidney disease, this patient is not at increased risk for renal cell carcinoma.

KEY POINT

- The nephrotic syndrome can be complicated by clotting manifestations due to a secondary hypercoagulable state, and risk is related to the degree of hypoalbuminemia.

Bibliography

Gyamlani G, Molnar MZ, Lu JL, Sumida K, Kalantar-Zadeh K, Kovesdy CP. Association of serum albumin level and venous thromboembolic events in a large cohort of patients with nephrotic syndrome. Nephrol Dial Transplant. 2017;32:157-164. [PMID: 28391310]

Item 46   Answer: B

Educational Objective: Treat hypertension in a patient with chronic kidney disease using an ACE inhibitor or angiotensin receptor blocker.

The addition of losartan is the most appropriate management. This patient has chronic kidney disease (CKD), given the presence of albuminuria, as well as uncontrolled hypertension. His antihypertensive medication regimen needs to be modified to control his blood pressure to target, given that uncontrolled hypertension will lead to CKD progression. The best option for this patient is to add an angiotensin receptor blocker (ARB) (such as losartan) or an ACE inhibitor, which are antihypertensive agents of choice in patients with CKD. Several studies have shown that use of an ARB or ACE inhibitor can result in decreased progression of albuminuria and CKD. Addition of losartan will also likely increase his serum potassium back to within normal range.

Adding amlodipine, a calcium channel blocker, is not the most appropriate next step in hypertension management for this patient and should be reserved if treatment with a maximum-tolerated dose of an ACE inhibitor or ARB does not result in blood pressure control.

Adding a low-dose aldosterone antagonist (such as spironolactone or eplerenone) may improve blood pressure control in patients with resistant hypertension. Treatment-resistant hypertension is defined as blood pressure that remains above goal despite concurrent use of three antihypertensive agents of different classes, one of which is a diuretic. Spironolactone is typically the fourth drug added to a three-drug regimen. This patient does not meet the definition of resistant hypertension.

Failure to act on this patient's blood pressure and albuminuria and reevaluating in 3 months misses the opportunity to slow the progression of CKD and albuminuria. In addition, guidelines recommend that adults initiating a new or adjusted drug regimen for hypertension should have a follow-up evaluation of adherence and response to treatment at monthly intervals until control is achieved.

KEY POINT

- An ACE inhibitor or angiotensin receptor blocker is an agent of choice for treatment of hypertension in a patient with chronic kidney disease.

Bibliography

Whelton PK, Carey RM, Aronow WS, Casey DE Jr, Collins KJ, Dennison Himmelfarb C, et al. 2017 ACC/AHA/AAPA/ABC/ACPM/AGS/APhA/ASH/ASPC/NMA/PCNA guideline for the prevention, detection, evaluation, and management of high blood pressure in adults: a report of the American College of Cardiology/American Heart Association Task Force on Clinical Practice Guidelines. Hypertension. 2017. [PMID: 29133356]

Item 47   Answer: E

Educational Objective: Diagnose preeclampsia.

The most likely diagnosis is preeclampsia. Preeclampsia is defined by new-onset hypertension and proteinuria (≥300 mg/24 h from a timed collection or ≥300 mg/g by urine protein-creatinine ratio) that occurs after 20 weeks of pregnancy. New-onset hypertension with new-onset end-organ damage (such as liver or kidney injury, pulmonary edema, cerebral or visual symptoms, or thrombocytopenia) is also diagnostic of preeclampsia. Severe preeclampsia is identified by persistent systolic blood pressure >160 mm Hg or diastolic blood pressure >110 mm Hg and end-organ damage. Thrombocytopenia, liver enzyme elevation, and kidney involvement are all present in this pregnant patient with new-onset hypertension, making preeclampsia the most likely diagnosis.

Chronic hypertension is defined as a systolic blood pressure ≥140 mm Hg or diastolic pressure ≥90 mm Hg starting before pregnancy or before 20 weeks of gestation or persisting longer than 12 weeks' postpartum. In this case, the patient had normal blood pressures earlier in pregnancy.

Eclampsia is the presence of generalized tonic-clonic seizures in women with preeclampsia, which are not present in this patient.

Gestational hypertension first manifests after 20 weeks of pregnancy without proteinuria or other end-organ damage. Seen in 6% of pregnancies, gestational hypertension resolves within 12 weeks of delivery. Hypertension that persists beyond the 12 weeks is considered chronic hypertension. Of those who develop gestational hypertension, 15% to 25% progress to preeclampsia, and the rate increases to up to 50% in women who develop hypertension before 30 weeks. End-organ involvement in this case is inconsistent with gestational hypertension.

HELLP (hemolysis, elevated liver enzymes, and low platelets) syndrome is a life-threatening state that complicates 10% to 20% of cases of preeclampsia. The cause of HELLP syndrome is unknown, but it may be related to placental factors. However, it likely represents a separate disorder from preeclampsia. The diagnosis requires the presence of microangiopathic hemolytic anemia, which is excluded by the normal bilirubin level and peripheral blood smear.

KEY POINT

- Preeclampsia is defined by new-onset hypertension and proteinuria that occurs after 20 weeks of pregnancy; new-onset hypertension with new-onset end-organ damage (such as liver or kidney injury, pulmonary edema, cerebral or visual symptoms, or thrombocytopenia) are also diagnostic.

Bibliography
American College of Obstetricians and Gynecologists. Hypertension in pregnancy. Report of the American College of Obstetricians and Gynecologists' Task Force on Hypertension in Pregnancy. Obstet Gynecol. 2013;122:1122-31. [PMID: 24150027]

Item 48   Answer: A
Educational Objective: **Diagnose Fabry disease.**

The most likely disease is Fabry disease, an X-linked recessive inborn error of glycosphingolipid metabolism caused by deficiency of α-galactosidase A. The enzyme deficiency leads to defective storage of sphingolipid and progressive endothelial accumulation, causing abnormalities in the skin, eye, kidney, heart, brain, and peripheral nervous system. Typically, the disease begins in childhood with episodes of pain and burning sensations in the hands and feet. These painful episodes can be brought on by exercise, fever, fatigue, or other stressors. In addition, young patients often develop angiokeratomas (violaceous papules with overlying scale), decreased perspiration, and corneal and lens opacities of the eyes. The disease is progressive, and symptoms of kidney, heart, and/or neurologic involvement usually occur between the ages of 30 and 45 years. As an X-linked disorder, males who inherit a mutation in the gene responsible for α-galactosidase always display the disease phenotype. Females, on the other hand, who inherit only one copy of a disease-causing mutation, can show a wide range of clinical manifestations, ranging from asymptomatic carriers to severe heart and kidney failure no different from a hemizygous male's phenotype. This variability is likely due to varying degrees of random inactivation of one copy of the X chromosome in each cell (lyonization). The most common finding of Fabry disease seen in heterozygous females is corneal dystrophy, which occurs in more than half of females. Fabry disease should be considered as a cause of chronic kidney disease of unknown etiology in young adulthood, especially when there is a family history of early end-stage kidney disease or cardiovascular-related death (via myocardial infarction or cerebrovascular accident). Diagnosis can be made via kidney biopsy but also noninvasively with measurement of leukocyte enzymatic activity and subsequent genetic confirmation. Screening for the disease is recommended for family members of affected patients. Enzyme replacement therapy with recombinant human α-galactosidase A is available.

Hereditary nephritis (Alport syndrome), like Fabry disease, can present with kidney failure if diagnosed late but is not associated with abnormalities in the skin or peripheral nervous system.

Medullary cystic kidney disease is a familial form of kidney disease with no known extrarenal symptomatology and usually presents with bland urinary findings.

This degree of kidney failure in a patient with tuberous sclerosis complex would be associated with abnormal kidney imaging, such as angiomyolipomas and cysts, and the classic skin lesions in this condition are hamartoma formations, not angiokeratomas.

KEY POINT

- Fabry disease should be considered as a cause of chronic kidney disease of unknown etiology in young adulthood.

Bibliography
Pisani A, Visciano B, Imbriaco M, Di Nuzzi A, Mancini A, Marchetiello C, et al. The kidney in Fabry's disease. Clin Genet. 2014;86:301-9. [PMID: 24645664]

Item 49   Answer: C
Educational Objective: **Manage a patient with a struvite stone.**

In addition to starting antibiotics, stone removal should be considered to decrease future episodes of urinary tract infections in this patient who has a struvite stone. Struvite stones occur most frequently in older women with chronic urinary tract infections. These stones occur in the presence of urea-splitting bacteria such as *Proteus*, *Klebsiella*, or, less frequently, *Pseudomonas*. These bacteria split urea into ammonium, which markedly increases urine pH (>7.5) and results in the precipitation of magnesium ammonium phosphate (struvite). Struvite stones can form rapidly and commonly produce staghorn calculi (stones that bridge two or more renal calyces). Because bacteria can live within the interstices of the stone, limiting antibiotic access, the only intervention that will decrease recurrent infections is removal of the stone. Although this may be accomplished by means of shock wave lithotripsy, patients often require percutaneous nephrolithotomy and breakup of the stone. A percutaneous nephrostomy tube is often inserted to allow for irrigation and to ensure complete removal of all fragments.

Although antibiotics are needed to treat infection, chronic antibiotic suppression is rarely successful as a primary treatment. Continued use of antibiotics increases the risk of the development of antibiotic resistance.

Pure struvite stones often occur in women who have upper urinary tract infections, but oftentimes other components such as calcium oxalate serve as the initial nidus. Because this nidus may not be among the stone fragments submitted for analysis, it may be missed. It is therefore important that a metabolic evaluation be performed in all patients. If the evaluation reveals decreased levels of urine citrate, potassium citrate can be added. Potassium citrate should not, however, be used empirically.

The urease inhibitor acetohydroxamic acid can decrease stone growth; however, it is associated with significant side effects (nausea, vomiting, diarrhea, headache, hallucinations, rash, abdominal discomfort, anemia) and is therefore not recommended as a primary treatment.

The use of acidifying agents such as ammonium chloride rarely is able to achieve acidic urine in patients with urea-splitting bacteria and therefore is not recommended.

KEY POINT

• Patients with struvite stones require stone removal.

Bibliography

Marien T, Miller NL. Treatment of the infected stone. Urol Clin North Am. 2015;42:459-72. [PMID: 26475943]

Item 50   Answer: A

Educational Objective: Diagnose adynamic bone disease in a patient with chronic kidney disease.

The most likely bone pathology is adynamic bone disease in this patient with end-stage kidney disease and normal serum calcium and phosphorus and relatively suppressed parathyroid hormone (PTH) and alkaline phosphatase levels. Adynamic bone disease can occur in patients with chronic kidney disease (CKD) or those on dialysis. It is typically associated with significant vascular calcifications. The gold standard for the diagnosis of adynamic bone disease is bone biopsy; however, this is rarely performed. Adynamic bone disease has no specific markers, but a constellation of findings may suggest this diagnosis. Patients with adynamic bone disease may present with fracture or bone pain. The latter has been attributed to the inability to repair microdamage because of low turnover. Serum calcium may be normal or elevated because the bone is unable to take up calcium. High PTH and alkaline phosphatase would exclude adynamic bone disease; in this disorder, both are typically normal. Treatment is targeted at factors that allow PTH secretion to rise. This includes avoiding calcium-based binders, conservative use of vitamin D, and decreasing the dialysate calcium concentration. It is important to note that, as with the general population, patients with CKD may also develop osteoporosis, particularly if they received glucocorticoid therapy for the primary kidney disorder or for immunosuppression in the setting of a kidney transplant.

β_2-Microglobulin–associated amyloidosis is usually seen in patients who have been on dialysis for at least 5 years. This disorder involves osteoarticular sites, and patients may present with carpal tunnel syndrome or shoulder pain. Bone cysts may be visible on radiograph.

Osteitis fibrosa cystica is the classic pathology associated with kidney disease. This disorder is associated with increased bone turnover and elevated PTH and alkaline phosphatase levels. Mixed uremic osteodystrophy has elements of both high and low bone turnover.

Osteomalacia refers to a defect with both low turnover and abnormal mineralization of bone. This disorder can be seen by vitamin D deficiency, but in the past, it was a common complication of aluminum toxicity. This patient's vitamin D level is in the "sufficient range," and there is no history of aluminum exposure.

KEY POINT

• Adynamic bone disease can occur in patients with chronic kidney disease or those on dialysis and is associated with fracture or bone pain; parathyroid hormone and alkaline phosphatase levels are typically normal.

Bibliography

Carvalho C, Alves CM, Frazão JM. The role of bone biopsy for the diagnosis of renal osteodystrophy: a short overview and future perspectives. J Nephrol. 2016;29:617-26. [PMID: 27473148]

Item 51   Answer: C

Educational Objective: Treat cardiorenal syndrome.

Increasing the furosemide dose is the most appropriate treatment in this patient with cardiorenal syndrome type 1 (CRS1). CRS is a disorder of the heart and kidneys in which acute or long-term dysfunction in one organ induces acute or long-term dysfunction in the other. CRS is characterized by the triad of concomitant decreased kidney function, diuretic-resistant heart failure with congestion, and worsening kidney function during heart failure therapy. CRS1 is defined as a worsening kidney function in patients with acute worsening of cardiac function (decompensated heart failure, acute coronary syndrome, cardiogenic shock). Management is challenging because treatment directed toward improving cardiac function can worsen kidney function. For this patient, an increase to his loop diuretic dose to a sufficient dose to induce a diuresis is appropriate. Among patients with decompensated heart failure, the best outcomes may occur with aggressive fluid removal even if associated with mild to moderate worsening of kidney function. An elevated blood urea nitrogen (BUN)-creatinine ratio should not discourage the use of diuretic therapy in patients with evidence of congestion. The decline in his kidney function with relative increase in BUN-creatinine ratio reflects the CRS1 physiology, rather than volume depletion due to diuresis.

Vasopressin receptor antagonists such as conivaptan can be used for the treatment of patients with hypervolemic or euvolemic hyponatremia. However, there is no evidence that treatment of hyponatremia improves clinical outcomes in patients with severe chronic heart failure.

Dobutamine, as well as milrinone, is used in the management of cardiogenic shock or decompensated acute heart failure with severe impaired left ventricular function and would not be indicated for a patient with preserved ejection fraction.

Ultrafiltration therapy is reserved for patients with severe volume overload refractory to medical management.

CONT.

In the Cardiorenal Rescue Study in Acute Decompensated Heart Failure (Caress-HF) study, the use of a stepwise pharmacologic therapy algorithm was superior to ultrafiltration for the preservation of kidney function at 96 hours, with a similar weight loss between the two strategies.

KEY POINT

- In cardiorenal syndrome type 1, loop diuretics are first-line therapy for managing volume overload in patients with decompensated heart failure with evidence of peripheral and/or pulmonary edema.

Bibliography

Verbrugge FH, Grieten L, Mullens W. Management of the cardiorenal syndrome in decompensated heart failure. Cardiorenal Med. 2014;4:176-88. [PMID: 25737682]

Item 52   Answer: D

Educational Objective: Treat anemia associated with chronic kidney disease using iron supplementation.

Iron supplementation is the most appropriate treatment for this patient with anemia associated with stage G4 chronic kidney disease (CKD). The prevalence of anemia increases as CKD progresses due to several factors, including impaired erythropoietin production, erythropoietin resistance, and reduced erythrocyte life span. Initial evaluation for the cause of anemia in patients with CKD includes laboratory studies as would be appropriate for patients without CKD. All patients with CKD and anemia should have iron profiles assessed, including total transferrin saturation (serum iron ÷ total iron-binding capacity × 100) and serum ferritin levels. The Kidney Disease: Improving Global Outcomes (KDIGO) recommendations suggest maintaining transferrin saturation levels of >30% and serum ferritin levels of >500 ng/mL (500 µg/L) using either oral or intravenous iron supplementation. Patients with stage G3 or G4 CKD can be treated with oral iron supplements but may need parenteral administration if oral iron is not effective. Patients with stage G5 CKD generally do not respond well to oral iron due to impaired gastrointestinal absorption and therefore often need intravenous administration. This patient with stage G4 CKD has iron deficiency and should have iron repletion.

Although blood transfusions are effective at acutely raising the hemoglobin, they are associated with adverse side effects. Specific to the advanced CKD population, blood transfusions should be avoided if possible to prevent HLA sensitization to foreign antigens, which may increase waiting time for kidney transplantation.

A bone marrow biopsy is not indicated because there is no evidence to suggest bone marrow dysfunction. Platelet count and leukocyte count are normal. The low hemoglobin and erythrocyte reticulocyte count reflect the inadequate iron stores. A brisk reticulocytosis should be observed within days of starting iron therapy.

Although many patients with advanced CKD and end-stage kidney disease require an erythropoietin-stimulating agent (ESA), its use is indicated only when the patient has adequate iron stores. Iron deficiency is a common reason for ESA resistance. ESAs take several weeks to achieve full effect and are sometimes started at the same time as parenteral iron. Current KDIGO guidelines recommend consideration of ESAs for patients with CKD and hemoglobin concentrations <10 g/dL (100 g/L). However, it is premature to consider ESA in this patient for she may respond to supplemental iron administration alone with an increase in hemoglobin level.

KEY POINT

- All patients with chronic kidney disease and anemia should have iron profiles assessed, including transferrin saturation and ferritin levels; treatment target levels are a transferrin saturation level >30% and a serum ferritin level >500 ng/mL (500 µg/L) using either oral or intravenous iron supplementation.

Bibliography

Panwar B, Gutiérrez OM. Disorders of iron metabolism and anemia in chronic kidney disease. Semin Nephrol. 2016;36:252-61. [PMID: 27475656]

Item 53   Answer: B

Educational Objective: Evaluate for primary hyperaldosteronism as the underlying cause of hypokalemia and resistant hypertension.

The most appropriate diagnostic test to perform next is plasma aldosterone concentration (PAC)/plasma renin activity (PRA) ratio. The patient presents with a triad of resistant hypertension, metabolic alkalosis, and hypokalemia following the addition of a thiazide diuretic, which raises suspicion for primary hyperaldosteronism. Primary hyperaldosteronism, in which aldosterone production cannot be suppressed with sodium loading, is the most common cause of secondary hypertension in middle-aged adults and an important cause of resistant hypertension. Testing for primary hyperaldosteronism is recommended if any of the following are present: resistant hypertension, hypokalemia (spontaneous or substantial, if diuretic induced), incidentally discovered adrenal mass, family history of early-onset hypertension, or stroke at age <40 years. Diuretics should be discontinued prior to testing to assure euvolemia. Calculation of the PAC/PRA ratio is used for screening, with a very high ratio of PAC/PRA suggestive of diagnosis. A positive screening test would reveal a reduced or undetectable PRA or concentration and an inappropriately high (usually >15 ng/dL) PAC, which results in a high PAC/PRA ratio of >20. Confirmatory testing is performed except when initial testing is diagnostic, as in cases of spontaneous hypokalemia with undetectable PRA and PAC (>30 ng/dL [828 pmol/L]). Confirmatory tests include oral and intravenous salt loading and the fludrocortisone suppression and captopril challenge tests.

Kidney ultrasonography with Doppler is performed to diagnose renovascular disease, which can be a secondary cause of hypertension. However, no clinical trials have

CONT.

demonstrated that percutaneous intervention results in improvement of hypertension or lessens kidney deterioration; therefore, diagnostic testing is reserved for patients with otherwise strong indications for this study, such as a young woman with possible fibromuscular dysplasia, but not this patient.

Plasma fractionated metanephrines are obtained to screen for a pheochromocytoma, which could result in hypertension; however, this is a relatively rare diagnosis that cannot explain the patient's current findings, and there are no symptoms or signs (episodic headaches, palpitations) in this patient to indicate pheochromocytoma.

Polysomnography is used to diagnose obstructive sleep apnea, another secondary cause of hypertension. However, clinical suspicion for this diagnosis is low given that it cannot explain the patient's metabolic findings, and the patient is not obese and does not present with snoring and daytime sleepiness.

KEY POINT

- Calculation of the plasma aldosterone concentration/ plasma renin activity ratio is used to diagnose primary hyperaldosteronism.

Bibliography

Braam B, Taler SJ, Rahman M, Fillaus JA, Greco BA, Forman JP, et al. Recognition and management of resistant hypertension. Clin J Am Soc Nephrol. 2017;12:524-535. [PMID: 27895136]

Item 54 Answer: D

Educational Objective: Diagnose surreptitious vomiting as a cause of metabolic alkalosis.

The most likely cause of this patient's metabolic alkalosis is surreptitious vomiting. Metabolic alkalosis is diagnosed by an elevation in serum bicarbonate concentration. This disorder is caused either by a loss of acid or administration or retention of bicarbonate. Conditions that contribute to the maintenance of metabolic alkalosis include volume contraction, ineffective arterial blood volume, hypokalemia, chloride depletion, and decreased glomerular filtration. Laboratory evaluation of metabolic alkalosis is based on urine chloride concentration. Metabolic alkalosis is considered saline responsive when associated with true hypovolemia and responds to correction of the volume deficit with isotonic saline. Saline-responsive metabolic alkalosis presents with a low urine chloride of <15 mEq/L (15 mmol/L); the most common causes are vomiting, nasogastric suction, and diuretic use. Hypokalemia occurs secondarily due to aldosterone elevation and cation loss as the kidney attempts to lose bicarbonate. Although these patients are usually hypovolemic or normovolemic (with normal or low blood pressures), patients with preexisting chronic hypertension may present with high to normal blood pressures.

For those who have a high urine chloride (>15 mEq/L [15 mmol/L]) with elevated blood pressure and hypokalemia and do not appear to be overtly volume overloaded,

a mineralocorticoid excess disorder must be considered (saline-resistant metabolic alkalosis). Examples include Cushing syndrome and primary aldosteronism. Neither is a likely diagnosis based on the low urine chloride and absence of hypertension. Rarely, patients with metabolic alkalosis may appear to have clinical features consistent with saline-responsive metabolic alkalosis (normal/low extracellular fluid status, normal/low blood pressure) but have a urine chloride of >15 mEq/L (15 mmol/L). Diuretic use and inherited kidney disorders of sodium and chloride handling, such as Bartter and Gitelman syndromes, can mimic this presentation. These two autosomal recessive genetic disorders of renal sodium and chloride transporters clinically mimic loop diuretic and thiazide diuretic use, respectively. These diagnoses should be considered only after urine diuretic screening.

KEY POINT

- Saline-responsive metabolic alkalosis typically presents with hypovolemia and a low urine chloride of <15 mEq/L (15 mmol/L); the most common causes are vomiting, nasogastric suction, and diuretic use.

Bibliography

Soifer JT, Kim HT. Approach to metabolic alkalosis. Emerg Med Clin North Am. 2014;32:453-63. [PMID: 24766943]

Item 55 Answer: A

Educational Objective: Diagnose IgG4-related disease.

The patient's decline in kidney function is most likely due to IgG4-related disease, a syndrome that mostly affects middle-aged or older men. Plasma cell–rich tubulointerstitial nephritis (TIN) is the most common kidney manifestation. Other manifestations can include autoimmune pancreatitis, allergic rhinitis, submandibular gland swelling, an elevated antinuclear antibody (ANA) titer, low serum complement levels, elevated serum IgG, elevated serum IgE, and peripheral eosinophilia. Kidney imaging may show enlarged kidneys or renal masses that may present as small peripheral cortical nodules. This patient's urinalysis findings of trace protein and pyuria with progressive decline of kidney function are consistent with TIN. Definitive diagnosis of IgG4-related disease requires a tissue biopsy to demonstrate an infiltrate with IgG4-positive plasma cells. IgG4-related disease is readily treatable with glucocorticoids.

Although elevated ANA titers and hypocomplementemia are seen in lupus, lupus nephritis is usually characterized by proteinuria and a more active urine sediment (dysmorphic erythrocytes and cellular casts). Furthermore, lupus is more common in women and usually manifests at a much earlier age than in this patient.

Sarcoidosis can affect multiple organs and cause TIN. However, sarcoidosis is not associated with autoimmune pancreatitis, hypocomplementemia, elevated serum immunoglobulin levels, or cortical nodules on kidney ultrasound.

Although Sjögren syndrome can affect lacrimal and salivary glands and cause TIN, this patient's constellation of symptoms is more consistent with IgG4-related disease. Dryness of the eyes and mouth is extremely common in Sjögren but not in IgG4-related disease. Allergy symptoms, such as asthma or allergic rhinitis, are rarely seen in Sjögren but are common in IgG4-related disease. Hypocomplementemia and the presence of cortical nodules on kidney ultrasound also favor the diagnosis of IgG4-related disease.

> **KEY POINT**
>
> - Tubulointerstitial nephritis is the most common kidney manifestation of IgG4-related disease and typically presents with pyuria, proteinuria, and elevated serum IgG and IgE levels; kidney imaging may show enlarged kidneys or renal masses.

Bibliography

Zhang P, Cornell LD. IgG4-related tubulointerstitial nephritis. Adv Chronic Kidney Dis. 2017;24:94-100. [PMID: 28284385]

Item 56   Answer: A

Educational Objective: Identify NSAIDs as a cause of acute kidney injury in a patient with chronic kidney disease.

Discontinuation of naproxen is the most appropriate management for this patient with chronic kidney disease (CKD) who has developed acute kidney injury. NSAIDs are one of the most frequently used over-the-counter medications and a mainstay in many pain and inflammatory conditions. However, NSAIDs inhibit cyclooxygenase-1 and cyclooxygenase-2, which decrease vasodilatory prostaglandin production. In patients who are prostaglandin dependent (volume depleted, heart failure, CKD), this decreases renal blood flow and leads to decreased glomerular filtration rate. Patients with CKD are sensitive to the nephrotoxic effects of NSAIDs; therefore, these medications are a frequent cause of acute kidney injury in this patient population. The nephrotoxic effect of NSAIDs is augmented by concomitant use of renin-angiotensin system inhibitors due to concomitant effects on afferent and efferent vascular tone. Discontinuation of naproxen is the best treatment for this patient's acute kidney injury. The American Society of Nephrology recommends the avoidance of NSAIDs, including cyclooxygenase-2 inhibitors, in patients with CKD due to the risk of worsening kidney function. There are safer treatment alternatives for osteoarthritis (OA). Exercise is among the most important nonpharmacologic treatments for most patients with OA, and evidence for its efficacy is most convincing for knee OA. Because excessive weight contributes to both knee OA risk and symptomatology, measures to promote weight loss are appropriate for overweight patients with knee OA. Topical NSAIDs may be a safer, effective alternative to oral NSAIDs in this patient population.

CT angiography of the renal arteries with iodinated contrast is contraindicated in the setting of acute kidney injury.

There is no evidence to suggest that renal artery stenosis is contributing to this patient's acute kidney injury.

Kidney biopsy can be performed to diagnosis glomerulonephritis. Although NSAIDs can cause glomerulonephritis, there are no signs to suggest acute glomerulonephritis because the patient's urinalysis does not show blood or significant protein.

Starting furosemide would help with the new peripheral edema that has developed but would not reverse the acute kidney injury; in fact, it may worsen the acute kidney injury by decreasing intravascular volume and further decreasing renal blood flow.

> **KEY POINT**
>
> - In patients with chronic kidney disease, NSAIDs are potentially nephrotoxic and a frequent cause of acute kidney injury and should be avoided.

Bibliography

Zhang X, Donnan PT, Bell S, Guthrie B. Non-steroidal anti-inflammatory drug induced acute kidney injury in the community dwelling general population and people with chronic kidney disease: systematic review and meta-analysis. BMC Nephrol. 2017;18:256. [PMID: 28764659]

Item 57   Answer: A

Educational Objective: Treat calcineurin inhibitor–induced hypertension and hyperkalemia in a kidney transplant recipient.

The most appropriate treatment for calcineurin inhibitor–induced hypertension and hyperkalemia in this kidney transplant recipient is a thiazide or thiazide-like diuretic such as chlorthalidone. Patients with kidney transplants must receive immunosuppressive medications to prevent their immune system from rejecting the kidney allograft. Doses are typically highest immediately after transplant and are tapered gradually over several months to minimize toxicities associated with these medications while maintaining adequate immunosuppression. The most commonly used immunosuppressants in the immediate posttransplant period for immunosuppression induction are anti–T-cell and interleukin-2 receptor–blocking antibodies. The most commonly prescribed medications for chronic maintenance immunosuppression include calcineurin inhibitors (tacrolimus or cyclosporine), antimetabolites (mycophenolate mofetil or azathioprine), and glucocorticoids. Although these medications are usually well tolerated, they can have significant side effects. Calcineurin inhibitors activate the sodium chloride cotransporter in the distal convoluted tubule, which reabsorbs sodium and chloride to cause hypertension. Decreased distal tubular flow impairs potassium secretion in the connecting tubule and collecting duct, leading to hyperkalemia. Calcineurin inhibitor–induced hypertension and hyperkalemia share the same phenotype as Gordon syndrome (familial hyperkalemic hypertension), which is due to a dysregulation of the WNK kinases in the distal convoluted tubule. Thiazide and thiazide-like diuretics such as chlorthalidone address the underlying mechanism of calcineurin inhibitor–induced hypertension and hyperkalemia by inhibiting the sodium chloride cotransporter.

Although fludrocortisone, a synthetic mineralocorticoid, would treat the hyperkalemia, this medication would exacerbate sodium retention and raise blood pressure in this patient with already uncontrolled hypertension. Sodium polystyrene sulfonate would also treat the hyperkalemia but provides a significant sodium load with each dose and may also raise the blood pressure. These medications do not address the underlying mechanism and are therefore not indicated.

Spironolactone may lower the blood pressure but would raise serum potassium and is therefore contraindicated in this patient who is already hyperkalemic.

KEY POINT

- Treatment using thiazide diuretics is appropriate for calcineurin inhibitor–induced hypertension and hyperkalemia in kidney transplant recipients.

Bibliography

Moes AD, Hesselink DA, Zietse R, van Schaik RH, van Gelder T, Hoorn EJ. Calcineurin inhibitors and hypertension: a role for pharmacogenetics? Pharmacogenomics. 2014;15:1243-51. [PMID: 25141899]

Item 58   Answer: B

Educational Objective: Treat hypermagnesemia using intravenous calcium.

In addition to administration of 0.9% saline and furosemide, intravenous calcium is appropriate treatment for this patient with hypermagnesemia. Because the kidney can efficiently eliminate magnesium, hypermagnesemia occurs infrequently and most commonly results from excessive intake in the setting of decreased kidney function. Numerous medications such as antacids and laxatives contain magnesium, and magnesium sulfate is the treatment of choice for prevention of eclampsia. Hypermagnesemia is usually not associated with significant symptoms until the level is >7.2 mg/dL (2.9 mmol/L). Symptoms include somnolence, headache, loss of deep tendon reflexes, bradycardia, hypotension, and hypocalcemia. At levels >12 mg/dL (4.9 mmol/L), flaccid paralysis, respiratory failure, and complete heart block can occur. Hypermagnesemia is usually self-limited. Magnesium-containing medications should be discontinued, and magnesium excretion can be enhanced with saline diuresis. In patients with hypotension and significant neuromuscular deficits, treatment is aimed at direct antagonism of the effects of hypermagnesemia, which is accomplished by intravenous administration of calcium. After this, efforts to lower the serum level should be instituted. If kidney function is adequate, a trial of 0.9% saline and furosemide will increase kidney excretion. Magnesium-containing agents should be limited or avoided in individuals with kidney disease.

If kidney failure is advanced, hemodialysis will effectively lower magnesium levels. However, this would require access to the central venous system and mobilization of the dialysis team, which can take several hours, and in the interim patients with symptomatic hypermagnesemia should be given intravenous calcium.

There is no role for either intravenous potassium or sodium bicarbonate other than correcting preexisting metabolic abnormalities.

Although sodium polystyrene sulfonate will bind a small amount of magnesium, this effect is minimal and not advocated as a treatment.

KEY POINT

- Management of hypermagnesemia includes discontinuation of magnesium-containing medications, administration of saline diuresis to enhance magnesium excretion, and administration of intravenous calcium to treat severe symptoms.

Bibliography

Van Hook JW. Endocrine crises. Hypermagnesemia. Crit Care Clin. 1991;7:215-23. [PMID: 2007216]

Item 59   Answer: A

Educational Objective: Diagnose the cause of acute kidney injury.

The most appropriate next step is examination of the urine sediment for cells and casts. This patient has developed oliguric acute kidney injury (AKI). He has multiple risk factors for AKI, including type 2 diabetes mellitus, recent coronary arteriography, hypotension, and cardiac surgery. The main consideration is whether the AKI is due to renal hypoperfusion (prerenal AKI) or whether the AKI is due to acute tubular necrosis (ATN). In the setting of diuretics, the fractional excretion of urea (FE_{Urea}) is more accurate than the fractional excretion of sodium because urea excretion is not promoted by diuretics and is still retained in volume-depleted states. FE_{Urea} is calculated using the equation:

$$FE_{Urea} = (U_{Urea} \times P_{Creatinine})/(U_{Creatinine} \times P_{Urea}) \times 100\%$$

FE_{Urea} <35% is suggestive of a prerenal state. The presence of granular casts and/or renal epithelial cells has strong predictive value for ATN. Urine microscopy can also help differentiate other causes of AKI, such as acute interstitial nephritis and glomerulonephritis.

The fractional excretion of sodium (FE_{Na}) is calculated as follows:

$$FE_{Na} = (U_{Sodium} \times P_{Creatinine})/(U_{Creatinine} \times P_{Sodium}) \times 100\%$$

FE_{Na} <1% indicates prerenal AKI but can also be seen in contrast-induced nephropathy, acute interstitial nephritis, rhabdomyolysis, glomerulonephritis, and early obstruction because the tubular handling of sodium is intact in these conditions. FE_{Na} >2% indicates ATN but is also seen in patients who are prerenal and are on diuretics or who have adrenal insufficiency, bicarbonaturia, or chronic kidney disease due to the increased distal tubular delivery of sodium in these conditions.

CONT.

Kidney ultrasonography should be performed to rule out obstructive uropathy as the cause of AKI. However, the patient already has a urinary catheter, so the likelihood of obstruction as the cause of AKI is low.

Central venous pressure is not a reliable indicator of organ perfusion and would not be able to differentiate prerenal AKI from ATN or other causes of AKI.

> **KEY POINT**
> - The presence of granular casts and/or renal epithelial cells on urine microscopy has strong predictive value for acute tubular necrosis.

Bibliography

Perazella MA, Coca SG, Kanbay M, Brewster UC, Parikh CR. Diagnostic value of urine microscopy for differential diagnosis of acute kidney injury in hospitalized patients. Clin J Am Soc Nephrol. 2008;3:1615-9. [PMID: 18784207]

Item 60   Answer: A

Educational Objective: Diagnose masked hypertension using ambulatory blood pressure monitoring.

The most appropriate test to perform next is 24-hour ambulatory blood pressure monitoring (ABPM) in this patient who has a strong family history of hypertension with cardiovascular complications. According to the American College of Cardiology/American Heart Association (ACC/AHA) blood pressure guideline, the patient has elevated blood pressure (BP), defined as systolic BP between 120-129 mm Hg and diastolic BP <80 mm Hg, and is at risk for development of hypertension (defined as systolic BP ≥130 mm Hg or diastolic BP ≥80 mm Hg). In addition, she has left ventricular hypertrophy on electrocardiogram, which raises concern for underlying long-standing hypertension. Therefore, masked hypertension, defined as BP that is normal in the office but elevated in the ambulatory setting, should be ruled out. Masked hypertension is associated with an increased risk of sustained hypertension and cardiovascular disease. The diagnostic test of choice is 24-hour ABPM; home blood pressure monitoring is an alternative strategy. Up to 10% to 40% of patients who are normotensive by clinic measurement may be hypertensive by ABPM or home blood pressure monitoring, which should be performed in patients referred for hypertension but with normal office BP and in those with end-organ damage such as left ventricular hypertrophy. Finally, the ACC/AHA notes that it is reasonable to evaluate for masked hypertension in patients with elevated BP, even in the absence of a strong family history of cardiovascular disease or evidence of sustained hypertension (for example, left ventricular hypertrophy on electrocardiogram).

A plasma aldosterone concentration/plasma renin activity ratio is often obtained in the evaluation of hyperaldosteronism. Such patients present with hypertension and often hypokalemia and metabolic alkalosis. It is premature to evaluate the patient for secondary causes of hypertension without first establishing the diagnosis of hypertension with ABPM or home blood pressure monitoring.

Disordered breathing events such as obstructive sleep apnea are associated with autonomic instability, increased vascular tone, hypertension, and alterations in heart rate. However, this patient has no symptoms to suggest obstructive sleep apnea (frequent awakenings, dry mouth, snoring, daytime sleepiness, nonrestorative sleep), and testing with polysomnography is not indicated at this time.

Measurement of thyroid-stimulating hormone levels is not the next best diagnostic test because the patient does not manifest any symptoms or signs concerning for hyperthyroidism, such as tachycardia, heat intolerance, palpitations, dyspnea, tremulousness, weight loss, fatigue, insomnia, and mood disturbances.

> **KEY POINT**
> - Suspected masked hypertension (defined as blood pressure that is normal in the office but elevated in the ambulatory setting) should be confirmed with ambulatory blood pressure monitoring or home blood pressure monitoring.

Bibliography

Whelton PK, Carey RM, Aronow WS, Casey DE Jr, Collins KJ, Dennison Himmelfarb C, et al. 2017 ACC/AHA/AAPA/ABC/ACPM/AGS/APhA/ASH/ASPC/NMA/PCNA guideline for the prevention, detection, evaluation, and management of high blood pressure in adults: a report of the American College of Cardiology/American Heart Association Task Force on Clinical Practice Guidelines. Hypertension. 2017. [PMID: 29133356]

Item 61   Answer: A

Educational Objective: Treat hypertension in a black patient using a thiazide diuretic and a calcium channel blocker.

Addition of the calcium channel blocker (CCB) amlodipine is the most appropriate next step in management. A landmark trial (ALLHAT) revealed that in black patients, a thiazide diuretic was more effective in improving cardiovascular outcomes compared with an ACE inhibitor, and there was a higher risk of stroke with use of an ACE inhibitor as initial therapy compared with a CCB. For these reasons, initial antihypertensive treatment in black patients, including those with diabetes mellitus, should include a thiazide diuretic or CCB, or combination of the two. However, if chronic kidney disease (CKD) is present, initial or add-on therapy should include an ACE inhibitor or angiotensin receptor blocker, especially in those with proteinuria, as illustrated by the AASK study. There is no evidence of CKD in this patient, given the normal serum creatinine and absence of an elevated urine albumin-creatinine ratio. Although hydrochlorothiazide was initiated 1 month ago, his blood pressure is still not at the target. Addition of the CCB amlodipine is therefore appropriate.

This patient is already on an adequate dose of hydrochlorothiazide, and his serum potassium level is borderline low at 3.5 mEq/L (3.5 mmol/L). Increasing the hydrochlorothiazide dose may further decrease his serum potassium and may be associated with adverse side effects, such as orthostasis and erectile dysfunction.

According to the American College of Cardiology/American Heart Association (ACC/AHA) blood pressure guideline, target blood pressure for most patients with hypertension, with or without coronary artery disease, diabetes, or CKD is <130/80 mm Hg. This patient is substantially above target, and reassessing in 3 months' time would not be adequate management. In addition, the ACC/AHA guideline recommends that adults initiating a new or adjusted drug regimen for hypertension should have a follow-up evaluation of adherence and response to treatment at monthly intervals until control is achieved. Waiting 3 months to reevaluate the patient is too long.

> **KEY POINT**
>
> - Initial antihypertensive treatment in black patients without chronic kidney disease should include a thiazide diuretic or calcium channel blocker, or combination of the two.

Bibliography

ALLHAT Officers and Coordinators for the ALLHAT Collaborative Research Group. The Antihypertensive and Lipid-Lowering Treatment to Prevent Heart Attack Trial. Major outcomes in high-risk hypertensive patients randomized to angiotensin-converting enzyme inhibitor or calcium channel blocker vs diuretic: the Antihypertensive and Lipid-Lowering Treatment to Prevent Heart Attack Trial (ALLHAT). JAMA. 2002;288:2981-97. [PMID: 12479763]

Item 62   Answer: A

Educational Objective: Diagnose chronic hypertension in a pregnant patient.

The most likely diagnosis in this pregnant patient is chronic hypertension. Hypertension first recognized during pregnancy at <20 weeks' gestation usually indicates chronic hypertension. The American College of Obstetricians and Gynecologists (ACOG) defines chronic hypertension as a systolic blood pressure ≥140 mm Hg or diastolic blood pressure ≥90 mm Hg starting before pregnancy or before 20 weeks of gestation or persists longer than 12 weeks' postpartum. In normal pregnancy, the blood pressure declines during the first trimester, reaches its lowest level in the second trimester, and rises slowly thereafter. A patient with hypertension in the first trimester suggests that the hypertension predates the pregnancy. To avoid overtreatment of hypertension and associated fetal risk, the 2013 ACOG guidelines recommend treating persistent systolic blood pressure ≥160 mm Hg or diastolic blood pressure ≥105 mm Hg in women with chronic hypertension. Blood pressure goals with medications are 120 to 160/80 to 105 mm Hg. Antihypertensive treatment reduces the risk of progression to severe hypertension by 50% compared with placebo but has not been shown to prevent preeclampsia, preterm birth, small size for gestational age, or infant mortality.

Gestational hypertension first manifests after 20 weeks of pregnancy without proteinuria or other end-organ damage and resolves within 12 weeks of delivery. This patient's early presentation is not consistent with gestational hypertension.

Normal physiologic changes in pregnancy are usually associated with decreased blood pressure in the first trimester with a nadir blood pressure in the second. In this patient, the high blood pressure is inconsistent with normal pregnancy changes.

Preeclampsia is defined clinically by new-onset hypertension and proteinuria that occur after 20 weeks of pregnancy. In addition to blood pressure criteria, there must be proteinuria or new-onset end-organ damage, including liver or kidney injury, pulmonary edema, cerebral or visual symptoms, or thrombocytopenia. This patient's early presentation in the first trimester and lack of end-organ involvement is not consistent with preeclampsia.

> **KEY POINT**
>
> - The American College of Obstetricians and Gynecologists defines chronic hypertension as a systolic blood pressure ≥140 mm Hg or diastolic blood pressure ≥90 mm Hg starting before pregnancy or before 20 weeks of gestation or persists longer than 12 weeks' postpartum.

Bibliography

American College of Obstetricians and Gynecologists. Hypertension in pregnancy. Report of the American College of Obstetricians and Gynecologists' Task Force on Hypertension in Pregnancy. Obstet Gynecol. 2013;122:1122-31. [PMID: 24150027]

Item 63   Answer: B

Educational Objective: Diagnose anti–glomerular basement membrane antibody disease.

The most appropriate diagnostic test to perform next is anti–glomerular basement membrane (GBM) antibodies. This patient presents with a rapidly progressive glomerulonephritis (RPGN), an acute and steep rise in serum creatinine accompanied by hematuria and proteinuria. The differential diagnosis for RPGN is divided histologically into three patterns on immunofluorescence microscopy of the kidney biopsy: pauci-immune staining (for example, ANCA-associated glomerulonephritis), linear staining (for example, anti-GBM antibody disease), and granular staining (for example, lupus nephritis). The patient's positive antimyeloperoxidase (MPO) antibodies predict that she will have pauci-immune staining on the biopsy, but the linear staining on her biopsy is more consistent with anti-GBM antibody disease. Therefore, testing for anti-GBM antibodies is required to confirm this diagnosis, although treatment for her condition should not be delayed while awaiting results. One in three patients with anti-GBM antibody disease will have positive ANCA serologies, usually MPO antibodies (or p-ANCA in older assays). This combined seropositivity is most commonly seen in the subset of anti-GBM patients who are older women, as in this case. Diagnosing anti-GBM antibody disease could affect treatment decisions in this case, particularly whether to pursue plasmapheresis, which is indicated for all cases of anti-GBM antibody disease. For ANCA-associated glomerulonephritis, plasmapheresis is reserved for those with alveolar hemorrhage and/or severe kidney failure (defined as requiring dialysis or a serum creatinine >5.8 mg/dL [512.7 µmol/L]).

This patient has negative antinuclear antibody testing and a biopsy not consistent with lupus nephritis, making testing for anti–double-stranded DNA antibodies unnecessary.

Anti–phospholipase A2 receptor (PLA2R) antibodies can be checked in patients suspected of having primary membranous glomerulopathy, which typically presents with the nephrotic syndrome and preserved kidney function, not RPGN.

Antihistone antibodies are measured if drug-induced vasculitis or drug-induced lupus erythematosus is suspected. This patient was not taking any medications, making this test unnecessary.

KEY POINT

- Serologic testing for anti–glomerular basement membrane antibodies and kidney biopsy can confirm the diagnosis of anti–glomerular basement membrane antibody disease as the cause of rapidly progressive glomerulonephritis.

Bibliography

Sethi S, Haas M, Markowitz GS, D'Agati VD, Rennke HG, Jennette JC, et al. Mayo Clinic/Renal Pathology Society consensus report on pathologic classification, diagnosis, and reporting of GN. J Am Soc Nephrol. 2016;27:1278-87. [PMID: 26567243]

Item 64   Answer: C

Educational Objective: Diagnose white coat hypertension using ambulatory blood pressure monitoring.

The most appropriate next step is to evaluate for white coat hypertension using 24-hour ambulatory blood pressure monitoring (ABPM). ABPM uses a continuously worn device that can be programmed to measure blood pressure every 15 to 20 minutes during the day and every 30 to 60 minutes at night. White coat hypertension refers to elevated blood pressure measured in the office, but normal out-of-office blood pressure averages. According to the American College of Cardiology/American Heart Association blood pressure guideline, in adults with untreated systolic blood pressure >130 mm Hg but <160 mm Hg or diastolic blood pressure >80 mm Hg but <100 mm Hg, it is reasonable to screen for white coat hypertension using either ABPM (the gold standard) or home blood pressure monitoring. Before white coat hypertension is diagnosed, it needs to be confirmed that the out-of-office measurements are reliable; for example, the patient's home blood pressure monitor should be calibrated against the office sphygmomanometer or, preferably, blood pressure should be measured by ABPM. If white coat hypertension is con-

firmed, lifestyle modification and careful monitoring are indicated because there is risk for future development of hypertension.

Before initiating hydrochlorothiazide, 24-hour ABPM or home blood pressure monitoring should be performed to rule out white coat hypertension.

Screening echocardiography is not the correct next step in diagnosis, although it may be considered if the diagnosis of hypertension remains in doubt in order to evaluate for left ventricular hypertrophy. The presence of confirmed left ventricular hypertrophy will necessitate treatment with antihypertensive medication.

The patient's blood pressure has been elevated in the office on three different occasions, and it is unlikely that another measurement in 3 months' time will produce a different result. The issue at hand is the diagnosis of white coat hypertension, which will require out-of-office blood pressure measurements.

KEY POINT

- White coat hypertension refers to elevated blood pressure measured in the office, but normal out-of-office blood pressure averages; diagnosis requires confirmation using 24-hour ambulatory blood pressure monitoring (gold standard) or home blood pressure monitoring.

Bibliography

Pierdomenico SD, Cuccurullo F. Prognostic value of white-coat and masked hypertension diagnosed by ambulatory monitoring in initially untreated subjects: an updated meta analysis. Am J Hypertens. 2011;24:52-8. [PMID: 20847724]

Item 65   Answer: B   H

Educational Objective: Treat hyperkalemia in a patient with acute kidney injury using hemodialysis.

Intermittent hemodialysis (IHD) is the most efficient way to correct this patient's hyperkalemia in the setting of anuric-oliguric acute kidney injury (AKI). IHD, typically delivered 3 to 6 times a week for 3 to 5 hours per session, allows for rapid correction of electrolyte disturbances and rapid removal of drugs or toxins. This patient has severe hyperkalemia with electrocardiographic changes, which should be corrected urgently to prevent lethal cardiac arrhythmias. Calcium, insulin, and dextrose are only temporizing measures and will not result in potassium removal from the body. Only dialysis will result in potassium removal from the body.

Continuous renal replacement therapy (CRRT) is a type of dialysis that is performed in critically ill patients who are hemodynamically unstable. CRRT provides hemodynamic stability by removing fluid and solutes at a much slower rate than IHD. As a result, CRRT would not be able to clear potassium rapidly but may be considered if the patient cannot tolerate IHD.

Furosemide can induce urinary potassium loss by increasing urine flow and delivery of sodium to the distal nephron for exchange with potassium. However, this patient

CONT.

is nearly anuric with acute tubular necrosis based on urine microscopy and unlikely to respond to furosemide.

Sodium bicarbonate causes a shift of hydrogen ion from the intracellular fluid compartment to the extracellular compartment, causing an opposing net intracellular potassium shift to maintain electroneutrality. The effect of bicarbonate is transient and ineffective in end-stage kidney disease or severe AKI.

Sodium polystyrene sulfonate is a cation exchange resin that removes potassium through the gastrointestinal tract. The onset of action is hours to days, and its effectiveness is disputed. It is contraindicated in patients with recent bowel surgery because of an increased risk for intestinal necrosis.

KEY POINT

- In the setting of anuric-oliguric acute kidney injury, intermittent hemodialysis allows for rapid correction of electrolyte disturbances and rapid removal of drugs or toxins.

Bibliography

Rossignol P, Legrand M, Kosiborod M, Hollenberg SM, Peacock WF, Emmett M, et al. Emergency management of severe hyperkalemia: guideline for best practice and opportunities for the future. Pharmacol Res. 2016;113:585-591. [PMID: 27693804]

 Item 66   Answer: D

Educational Objective: Diagnose type 4 (hyperkalemic distal) renal tubular acidosis.

The most likely diagnosis is type 4 (hyperkalemic distal) renal tubular acidosis (RTA), which is caused by aldosterone deficiency or resistance. Primary adrenal insufficiency (Addison disease) may cause aldosterone deficiency, although hyporeninemic hypoaldosteronism is a more common cause and may occur in the presence of various kidney diseases, most often diabetes mellitus. Aldosterone resistance is seen in patients with tubulointerstitial disease, including urinary obstruction, sickle cell disease, medullary cystic kidney disease, and kidney transplant rejection. Drug-induced type 4 (hyperkalemic distal) RTA can be caused by numerous drugs that reduce aldosterone production, including ACE inhibitors, angiotensin receptor blockers, heparin, and NSAIDs. Patients with type 4 (hyperkalemic distal) RTA have a positive urine anion gap (using the equation: [Urine Sodium + Urine Potassium] – Urine Chloride), indicating a reduced excretion of acid in the form of ammonium and chloride, but a urine pH <5.5. Hyperkalemia decreases ammonia production with consequent lower ammonium excretion and therefore results in the positive urine anion gap. Due to the inadequate amount of ammonia available to buffer protons, the few protons that are secreted distally will result in the low urine pH (<5.5). Treatment is focused on correcting the underlying cause if possible. Fludrocortisone is used to replace mineralocorticoids in adrenal insufficiency and should be considered in hyporeninemic hypoaldosteronism in those without hypertension or heart failure.

Although chronic kidney disease may result in hyperkalemia and metabolic acidosis, the acidosis does not usually develop until later progression (glomerular filtration rate <40-45 mL/min/1.73 m^2), and hyperkalemia is usually not present until the glomerular filtration rate is at even lower levels (usually stage 4 or worse).

The normal anion gap of type 1 (hypokalemic distal) RTA results from a distal tubular defect and associated impaired excretion of hydrogen ions by the distal nephron. It is usually associated with hypokalemia and a negative urine anion gap, which are not present in this patient.

Type 2 (proximal) RTA results from failure of the proximal tubule to adequately reclaim filtered bicarbonate, driving the development of a normal anion gap metabolic acidosis and a positive urine anion gap. Type 2 (proximal) RTA is usually accompanied by other evidence of proximal tubular dysfunction (hypokalemia, glycosuria, and hypophosphatemia), none of which is present in this patient.

KEY POINT

- Type 4 (hyperkalemic distal) renal tubular acidosis is characterized by hyperkalemia, a normal anion gap metabolic acidosis, impaired urine acidification (positive urine anion gap), and a urine pH <5.5.

Bibliography

Yaxley J, Pirrone C. Review of the diagnostic evaluation of renal tubular acidosis. Ochsner J. 2016;16:525-530. [PMID: 27999512]

Item 67   Answer: D

Educational Objective: Diagnose lupus nephritis.

The most appropriate next step is a kidney biopsy. The presence of hematuria, dysmorphic erythrocytes, and proteinuria in a patient with known systemic lupus erythematosus (SLE) is highly suggestive of lupus nephritis; when serologies are positive and serum complement levels are low, this diagnosis is even more likely. Commonly cited indications for kidney biopsy include increasing serum creatinine without explanation, proteinuria >500 mg/24 h, or active urine sediment (dysmorphic erythrocytes, erythrocyte casts). Patients meeting these criteria are more likely to have focal or diffuse proliferative lupus nephritis or lupus membranous nephropathy requiring immunosuppressive therapy. Patients with proteinuria <500 mg/24 h and inactive urine sediment are more likely to have milder kidney involvement and may be followed with urinalysis, urine protein-creatinine ratio, and serum creatinine every 3 to 6 months.

Unless absolutely contraindicated (for example, bleeding diathesis or inability to stop anticoagulation), both rheumatology and nephrology guidelines support performing a kidney biopsy in patients with SLE who develop evidence of significant kidney involvement to establish the diagnosis and, of equal importance with regard to treatment decisions, to identify the International Society of Nephrology/Renal Pathology Society (ISN/RPS) class of lupus nephritis.

This patient's kidney biopsy could show a proliferative lupus nephritis (class III or IV), in which case treatment with glucocorticoids and mycophenolate mofetil or cyclophosphamide would be indicated (mycophenolate mofetil would likely be preferred given this patient's age). However, her biopsy could also conceivably show a milder, mesangial proliferative lupus nephritis (class II) or membranous lupus nephritis (class V), neither of which would require immunosuppression at this stage. Therefore, empiric therapy in this setting is substandard to biopsy-guided therapy according to ISN/RPS class of nephritis.

KEY POINT

- A kidney biopsy should be performed in patients with known systemic lupus erythematosus with suspected significant kidney involvement to establish the diagnosis and to identify the class, which will guide treatment decisions.

Bibliography

Hahn BH, McMahon MA, Wilkinson A, Wallace WD, Daikh DI, Fitzgerald JD, et al; American College of Rheumatology. American College of Rheumatology guidelines for screening, treatment, and management of lupus nephritis. Arthritis Care Res (Hoboken). 2012;64:797-808. [PMID: 22556106]

Item 68   Answer: D

Educational Objective: Treat hypertension associated with volume expansion in chronic kidney disease.

Stopping chlorthalidone and beginning furosemide is the most appropriate treatment for this patient's hypertension. Hypertension is a risk factor for cardiovascular morbidity and mortality. The most common cause of death in patients with chronic kidney disease (CKD) is cardiovascular disease. Therefore, blood pressure control is critical for preventing disease and death. Diuretics are central to the management of hypertension. Although thiazide diuretics (such as chlorthalidone) are recommended first-line agents for hypertension, efficacy decreases with advanced stages of CKD. Therefore, loop diuretics (furosemide, bumetanide, torsemide) are a cornerstone of blood pressure management in patients with advanced CKD. Sodium retention and impaired natriuresis lead to volume expansion and an increase in blood pressure. Loop diuretics are effective natriuretics and retain their activity even at low glomerular filtration rate (GFR); however, doses need to be increased as GFR declines to maintain appropriate urine output and negative fluid balance. Loop diuretics are equally effective if given in equipotent doses. The loop diuretic furosemide would effectively treat this patient's volume expansion and therefore reduce blood pressure. Additional benefit would include increased urine potassium and acid excretion to treat the mild hyperkalemia and metabolic acidosis associated with CKD. The most common side effects of loop diuretics are electrolyte and fluid abnormalities, hypersensitivity, and ototoxicity.

Hydralazine is not indicated for this patient who has volume expansion and needs diuresis; this drug is also relatively contraindicated in coronary artery disease.

Losartan is an angiotensin receptor blocker, which should not be combined with an ACE inhibitor due to the risk of hyperkalemia and acute kidney injury.

Although spironolactone can help reduce blood pressure and edema through its anti-aldosterone effects and blockade of sodium reabsorption in the cortical collecting duct, it would be contraindicated in this patient with advanced CKD and hyperkalemia.

KEY POINT

- Loop diuretics are a cornerstone of blood pressure management in patients with advanced chronic kidney disease.

Bibliography

Valika A, Peixoto AJ. Hypertension management in transition: from CKD to ESRD. Adv Chronic Kidney Dis. 2016;23:255-61. [PMID: 27324679]

Item 69   Answer: D

Educational Objective: Select the most appropriate venous access for a patient with advanced chronic kidney disease.

A tunneled internal jugular central venous catheter is the most appropriate venous access strategy for this patient. In patients with osteomyelitis, 6 weeks of antimicrobial therapy after surgical débridement is the preferred treatment course, and for most patients this requires long-term reliable venous access. However, this patient's advanced degree of kidney disease, relatively young age, and type 2 diabetes mellitus put her at high risk for progressing to end-stage kidney disease, and the upper extremity veins should be protected for future hemodialysis access creation. The American Society of Nephrology recommends nephrology consultation first before placing peripherally inserted central catheter (PICC) lines in patients with stage G3 to G5 CKD. PICCs are long catheters that are inserted peripherally and terminate in the central veins. PICCs are popular because of their ease of insertion and use. However, a national, population-based analysis revealed that PICCs placed before or after hemodialysis initiation were independently associated with lower likelihoods of transition to any working fistula or graft. PICC lines can lead to significant vein trauma and venous stenosis in the veins that may be used for arteriovenous fistula creation. This could impair blood flow through the fistula, impair maturation, and even lead to primary nonfunctioning of the hemodialysis access. Although central lines are associated with central venous stenosis, a central line is a better alternative than a PICC for long-term parenteral antibiotics because central lines are not inserted into a peripheral vein, which would be used for the creation of a hemodialysis site.

Arteriovenous fistula or graft creation is inappropriate due to the presence of active infection. Additionally, inserting a PICC line in the arm next to the fistula may also still cause damage to the access itself or damage one of the branching veins, which could impair the maturation of the access.

KEY POINT

- Peripherally inserted central catheter placement before or after hemodialysis initiation is associated with adverse vascular access outcomes in patients with chronic kidney disease.

Bibliography

McGill RL, Ruthazer R, Meyer KB, Miskulin DC, Weiner DE. Peripherally inserted central catheters and hemodialysis outcomes. Clin J Am Soc Nephrol. 2016;11:1434-40. [PMID: 27340280]

Item 70   Answer: C

Educational Objective: Treat hypertension in a patient with diabetes mellitus and albuminuria using an ACE inhibitor or angiotensin receptor blocker.

In addition to lifestyle modifications, initiation of the angiotensin receptor blocker (ARB) losartan is the most appropriate treatment for this patient with newly diagnosed hypertension. She has a normal serum creatinine level but has moderately increased albuminuria. Her blood pressure has been elevated at two office visits and confirmed with home blood pressure monitoring, and she needs to be treated to target, given that uncontrolled hypertension will lead to progression of albuminuria and chronic kidney disease (CKD). A reasonable target blood pressure for this patient is <130/80 mm Hg. The 2017 high blood pressure guideline from the American College of Cardiology (ACC), American Heart Association (AHA), and nine other organizations recommends a treatment goal of <130/80 mm Hg. The ACC/AHA guideline notes that ACE inhibitors or ARBs may be considered as initial treatment choices in the presence of albuminuria. The American Diabetes Association (ADA) Standards of Medical Care in Diabetes 2018 recommends that most patients with diabetes mellitus and hypertension should be treated to a systolic blood pressure goal of <140 mm Hg and a diastolic blood pressure goal of <90 mm Hg. Lower systolic and diastolic blood pressure targets, such as 130/80 mm Hg, may be appropriate for individuals at high risk of cardiovascular disease if they can be achieved without undue treatment burden. In nonpregnant patients with diabetes and hypertension, the ADA recommends either an ACE inhibitor or an ARB for those with albuminuria. Several large randomized controlled trials and systematic reviews have shown that use of an ARB or ACE inhibitor can result in decreased progression of albuminuria and CKD in patients with diabetes.

The ACC/AHA blood pressure guideline recommends the following lifestyle modifications for individuals with elevated blood pressure or hypertension: weight loss in adults who are overweight or obese; a heart-healthy diet, such as DASH (Dietary Approaches to Stop Hypertension), that facilitates achieving a desirable weight; sodium reduction; potassium supplementation, preferably in dietary modification, unless contraindicated by the presence of CKD or use of drugs that reduce potassium excretion; increased physical activity with a structured exercise program; and limiting alcohol consumption of standard drinks to two (men) and one (women) per day. Although these recommendations are appropriate for this patient, it is not the only recommended intervention to control hypertension in this patient with diabetes and albuminuria. Therefore, simply asking the patient to return in 2 months for a blood pressure measurement after initiating lifestyle changes is not sufficient.

Calcium channel blockers (such as amlodipine) and thiazide diuretics (such as chlorthalidone) are not initial choices for treating hypertension in patients with diabetes and albuminuria. If this patient's blood pressure is still not controlled to target after maximizing the dose of the ARB, then one of these agents can be added.

KEY POINT

- An ACE inhibitor or angiotensin receptor blocker is the initial treatment of choice for hypertension in patients with diabetes mellitus and albuminuria.

Bibliography

Palmer SC, Mavridis D, Navarese E, Craig JC, Tonelli M, Salanti G, et al. Comparative efficacy and safety of blood pressure-lowering agents in adults with diabetes and kidney disease: a network meta-analysis. Lancet. 2015;385:2047-56. [PMID: 26009228]

Item 71   Answer: C

Educational Objective: Identify medication as a cause of an increase in serum creatinine.

Reassessing this patient's serum creatinine level in 1 week is the most appropriate next step in management. Some medications (such as cimetidine, trimethoprim, cobicistat, dolutegravir, bictegravir, and rilpivirine) reduce proximal tubule secretion of creatinine, resulting in increases in serum creatinine that are nonprogressive. This patient has chronic kidney disease (CKD), long-standing hypertension, and HIV infection. His antiretroviral medication regimen was recently adjusted to a once-a-day dosing, with the integrase inhibitor raltegravir discontinued and dolutegravir started 3 weeks ago. Dolutegravir is known to interfere with creatinine secretion without affecting glomerular filtration rate. Slight increases in serum creatinine of 0.2 to 0.3 mg/dL (17.7-26.5 µmol/L) may occur. This is more pronounced in those with preexisting CKD, in which creatinine secretion may contribute proportionately more to creatinine clearance. In patients with HIV taking the integrase inhibitors dolutegravir or bictegravir, the non-nucleoside reverse transcriptase inhibitor rilpivirine, or the pharmacokinetic enhancer (CYP3A inhibitor) cobicistat, serum creatinine elevations are nonprogressive and will remain unchanged within 1 to 2 weeks of initiation. Therefore, in the absence of other signs of kidney disease (hematuria, pyuria, or increasing proteinuria), reassessment of the serum creatinine level in 1 week will confirm the drug's effect in this patient.

Answers and Critiques

Further increases in serum creatinine levels will require additional evaluation.

Discontinuation of the ACE inhibitor lisinopril is not necessary. This patient has long-standing hypertension and is likely benefiting from the lisinopril for his CKD and moderate albuminuria. It is unlikely to have caused this acute increase in serum creatinine because the hemodynamic effects of ACE inhibitors on glomerular filtration occur within days of initiating the medication and then stabilize.

A 24-hour urine creatinine clearance will be decreased in this case (due to drug-related lower creatinine secretion) and will not provide additional diagnostic information.

Should a repeat serum creatinine level be stable, no further evaluation will be necessary.

KEY POINT

- Some medications (such as cimetidine, trimethoprim, cobicistat, dolutegravir, bictegravir, and rilpivirine) reduce proximal tubule secretion of creatinine, resulting in increases in serum creatinine that are nonprogressive; repeat serum creatinine measurement is required to confirm stable levels.

Bibliography

Milburn J, Jones R, Levy JB. Renal effects of novel antiretroviral drugs. Nephrol Dial Transplant. 2017;32:434-439. [PMID: 27190354]

Item 72   Answer: B

Educational Objective: Identify calcium phosphate as the composition of a kidney stone in a patient taking topiramate.

The most likely composition of this patient's kidney stone is calcium phospate. Approximately 80% of kidney stones contain calcium oxalate, calcium phosphate, or both. Calcium stones are radiopaque on plain radiograph. Hypercalciuria, hyperoxaluria, and hypocitraturia are risk factors for calcium stones. Calcium phosphate stones occur when there is persistently elevated urine pH. These stones are therefore commonly associated with distal renal tubular acidosis and hyperparathyroidism. This patient is taking topiramate for migraine prophylaxis, a carbonic anhydrase inhibitor that is associated with calcium phosphate stones. Carbonic anhydrase promotes proximal tubule sodium, bicarbonate, and chloride reabsorption. Inhibitors of carbonic anhydrase produce both sodium chloride and bicarbonate urinary loss. The resultant mild metabolic acidosis causes decreased citrate excretion, and the persistent alkaline urine favors the precipitation of calcium phosphate.

Although calcium oxalate is the most common cause of kidney stones, there are no calcium oxalate crystals noted on this patient's urinalysis. The most common crystal formations of calcium oxalate in the urine are the dumbbell-shaped calcium oxalate monohydrate crystals and envelope-shaped calcium oxalate dihydrate crystals. She has amorphous crystals in alkaline urine, which are usually calcium phosphate crystals.

Cystine stones occur with cystinuria, which is a genetic disease. This patient has no family history of kidney stones, and the characteristic hexagonal-shaped crystals are not seen on urine microscopy.

Struvite stones occur in the presence of urea-splitting bacteria (*Proteus, Klebsiella,* or, less frequently, *Pseudomonas*). These bacteria split urea into ammonium, which markedly increases urine pH and results in the precipitation of magnesium ammonium phosphate (struvite). The pH of the urine will be >7.5. Struvite stones commonly produce staghorn calculi (stones that bridge two or more renal calyces) and occur most frequently in older women with chronic urinary infections. Coffin lid–shaped crystals may be seen in the urine. This patient does not demonstrate these findings.

Uric acid stones are uncommon (10% of stones), but the incidence increases in hotter, arid climates due to low urine volumes. The main risk factor is low urine pH, which decreases the solubility of uric acid. Hyperuricosuria is not a consistent finding. Comorbid risk factors for uric acid stones include gout, diabetes mellitus, the metabolic syndrome, and chronic diarrhea. Because uric acid stones occur in persistently acidic urine, this is an unlikely diagnosis for this patient.

KEY POINT

- Topiramate, a carbonic anhydrase inhibitor, causes a decrease in urinary citrate excretion and formation of alkaline urine that favor the creation of calcium phosphate stones.

Bibliography

Dell'Orto VG, Belotti EA, Goeggel-Simonetti B, Simonetti GD, Ramelli GP, Bianchetti MG, et al. Metabolic disturbances and renal stone promotion on treatment with topiramate: a systematic review. Br J Clin Pharmacol. 2014;77:958-64. [PMID: 24219102]

Item 73   Answer: C

Educational Objective: Diagnose proton pump inhibitor-induced tubulointerstitial nephritis.

The proton pump inhibitor omeprazole is the most likely cause of this patient's kidney findings. Nonspecific symptoms of tubulointerstitial disease include polyuria, malaise, and anorexia, as well as progressive kidney dysfunction. Urinary findings can range from minimal findings to the presence of sterile pyuria, proteinuria, and hematuria. Chronic tubulointerstitial diseases most commonly result from previous injury due to acute interstitial nephritis. Therefore, the history and physical examination should focus on conditions associated with acute tubulointerstitial disease and other potential treatable causes with a careful review of medications. Proton pump inhibitors are the most commonly prescribed drugs worldwide. The occurrence of interstitial nephritis is not dose related, and disease can recur with reexposure. The median time from drug initiation to interstitial nephritis diagnosis is variable but can exceed 6 months to 9 months, with 10 to 11 weeks the most common interval. There is also emerging

CONT.

literature that proton pump inhibitors may contribute to the development and progression of chronic kidney disease.

Although large amounts of aspirin and NSAIDs can cause tubulointerstitial nephritis, a daily dose of low-dose aspirin (81 mg) is unlikely to cause interstitial nephritis. It is unlikely that therapeutic doses of aspirin alone cause chronic kidney disease in patients with normal underlying kidney function.

Fenofibrate nephrotoxicity is characterized by a rise in serum creatinine typically occurring ≥6 months after initiation of therapy. The sediment is bland, and there is usually no significant proteinuria. The mechanism of increase in creatinine is unknown. This patient has been taking fenofibrate for only 2 months, making this drug an unlikely cause of his interstitial nephritis.

St. John's wort (*Hypericum perforatum*) is most commonly used to treat depression. Adverse effects are uncommon but the following have been reported: gastrointestinal symptoms, dizziness, confusion, tiredness, sedation, photosensitivity, dry mouth, urinary frequency, anorgasmia, and swelling. St. John's wort has not been associated with tubulointerstitial nephritis.

KEY POINT

- Chronic tubulointerstitial nephritis can be caused by proton pump inhibitors, and the median time from drug initiation to diagnosis may exceed 6 to 9 months.

Bibliography

Moledina DG, Perazella MA. PPIs and kidney disease: from AIN to CKD. J Nephrol. 2016;29:611-6. [PMID: 27072818]

Item 74 Answer: C

Educational Objective: Diagnose pseudohyperkalemia.

The most appropriate next step in management is a repeat plasma potassium measurement. This patient has an elevated serum potassium level of 6.4 mEq/L (6.4 mmol/L) in the setting of leukocytosis likely due to acute leukemia. Hyperkalemia is defined as a serum potassium level >5.0 mEq/L (5.0 mmol/L). Any level >6.0 mEq/L (6.0 mmol/L) can be life-threatening. Because of the potential cardiac effects of hyperkalemia, immediate electrocardiography (ECG) is indicated. The earliest ECG changes of hyperkalemia are peaking of the T waves and shortening of the QT interval. As hyperkalemia progresses, there is prolongation of the PR interval, loss of P waves, and eventual widening of the QRS complexes with a "sine-wave" pattern that can precede asystole. This patient has no ECG evidence of hyperkalemia. Pseudohyperkalemia is therefore the most likely cause of his elevated serum potassium level. Pseudohyperkalemia occurs with a false rise in potassium values from cellular release of potassium during venipuncture due to hemolysis or prolonged tourniquet use. It also occurs with significant leukocytosis or thrombocytosis. During the clotting process, these cells are disrupted with the release of intracellular potassium, and pseudohyperkalemia may occur in serum specimens when there are extreme

elevations of leukocytes or platelets. The next step is to obtain a plasma specimen and rapidly separate the plasma from the cells. Normally, the serum potassium is 0.3 to 0.4 mEq/L (0.3-0.4 mmol/L) greater than a plasma specimen obtained at the same time. In extreme cases of leukocytosis or thrombocytosis, the serum potassium can be more than 1.0 mEq/L (1.0 mmol/L) higher. In cases of pseudohyperkalemia, a rapidly processed plasma specimen will be normal.

In patients with normal kidney function, intravenous saline, usually with the concomitant administration of a loop diuretic, can increase potassium excretion. Intravenous calcium should be reserved for cases of hyperkalemia exhibiting ECG changes. The effect of calcium on stabilizing the cardiac membrane is a transient event that lasts only 30 minutes. Inhaled albuterol lowers potassium by shifting it into cells. However, this patient has no indication to rapidly reduce potassium levels or stabilize the cardiac membrane because his ECG is normal.

The use of sodium bicarbonate in hyperkalemia has fallen out of favor. It has minimal effects on potassium levels and is usually reserved for patients with metabolic acidosis.

KEY POINT

- Pseudohyperkalemia may occur in serum specimens when there are extreme elevations of leukocytes or platelets; repeat plasma potassium measurements can confirm a normal potassium level.

Bibliography

Meng QH, Wagar EA. Pseudohyperkalemia: a new twist on an old phenomenon. Crit Rev Clin Lab Sci. 2015;52:45-55. [PMID: 25319088]

Item 75 Answer: C

Educational Objective: Treat anemia associated with chronic kidney disease using an erythropoiesis-stimulating agent.

An erythropoiesis-stimulating agent (ESA) is appropriate to treat anemia in this patient with stage G4 chronic kidney disease (CKD). The prevalence of anemia increases as CKD progresses due to several factors, including impaired erythropoietin production, erythropoietin resistance, and reduced erythrocyte life span. Iron deficiency may contribute to erythropoietin resistance. The Kidney Disease: Improving Global Outcomes (KDIGO) recommendations suggest maintaining transferrin saturation levels of >30% and serum ferritin levels of >500 ng/mL (500 μg/L). The patient's iron stores are adequate based on the patient's transferrin saturation and ferritin levels, and the next step in treatment is to start an ESA. ESAs are highly effective in raising hemoglobin concentrations and alleviating symptoms, and can avoid the need for transfusion. ESAs should not be used in patients with active malignancy, history of malignancy, or history of stroke. ESAs should be started in symptomatic patients with CKD who have a hemoglobin concentration <10 g/dL (100 g/L), and the dose should be titrated to avoid hemoglobin concentrations increasing above 11.5 g/dL (115 g/L).

CONT.

ACE inhibitors and angiotensin receptor blockers (ARBs) inhibit erythropoiesis, and patients on maintenance dialysis taking either ACE inhibitors or ARBs may have increased erythropoietin requirements. However, the mechanisms by which this occurs are poorly defined. Discontinuing losartan is incorrect because renin-angiotensin system blockade in CKD is beneficial in delaying the progression of CKD to end-stage kidney disease, which outweighs any potential interaction with anemia. However, discontinuing the medication could be considered if the patient demonstrated signs of erythropoietin resistance or refractory anemia.

Packed red blood cell transfusion is not indicated at this time and would expose the patient to transfusion-related risks and side effects. Additionally, blood transfusions can cause allosensitization, which can lead to antibody formation, and may prolong transplant waiting times.

Starting iron is incorrect because the patient is iron replete. Iron repletion is recommended if the transferrin saturation is ≤30% and the ferritin is ≤500 ng/mL (500 µg/L).

KEY POINT

- The Kidney Disease: Improving Global Outcomes (KDIGO) guidelines recommend consideration of erythropoiesis-stimulating agents to treat anemia in patients with chronic kidney disease and adequate iron stores who have hemoglobin concentrations <10 g/dL (100 g/L); the dose should be titrated to avoid hemoglobin concentrations increasing above 11.5 g/dL (115 g/L).

Bibliography
Kidney Disease: Improving Global Outcomes (KDIGO) Anemia Work Group. KDIGO clinical practice guideline for anemia in chronic kidney disease. Kidney inter., Suppl. 2012;2:279–335. Available at www.kdigo.org.

Item 76   Answer: C

Educational Objective: Identify hypomagnesemia as a cause of hypokalemia.

The most likely cause of this patient's hypokalemia is hypomagnesemia. Symptoms of hypokalemia include weakness or paralysis; decreased gastrointestinal motility or ileus with nausea; and cardiac arrhythmias. This patient has symptomatic hypokalemia, presenting with lower extremity weakness and nausea. Hypokalemia can be caused by renal losses or nonrenal losses. In this case, the urine potassium is inappropriately high, pointing toward renal potassium wasting. Renal losses of potassium can occur with renal tubular acidosis; renal excretion of non-reabsorbable anions such as bicarbonate, hippurate, and ketones; drugs such as aminoglycosides or cisplatinum; Gitelman and Bartter syndromes; or hypomagnesemia. Hypomagnesemia is common, occurring in up to 12% of hospitalized patients. Chronic alcohol abuse results in excessive urinary excretion of magnesium and appears to reflect a reversible alcohol-induced tubular dysfunction. Intracellular magnesium is necessary to modulate the excretion of potassium through the potassium channel in the

cortical collecting tubule. Hypomagnesemia results in loss of potassium through this channel. Importantly, the hypokalemia will be refractory to therapy until magnesium is repleted. Target levels for magnesium replacement are at least 2 mg/dL (0.83 mmol/L).

Unlike calcium and magnesium, which have substantial binding to albumin, potassium levels are not affected by the concentration of albumin.

Low levels of magnesium (due to alcohol abuse or malnutrition) activate G-proteins that stimulate calcium-sensing receptors and decrease parathyroid hormone (PTH) secretion and are a cause of hypocalcemia. Low magnesium levels are also associated with resistance to PTH activity at the level of bone, further contributing to hypocalcemia. Hypocalcemia and hypokalemia in this patient are a direct result of chronic magnesium loss due to the patient's alcoholism. Hypocalcemia has no significant effect on potassium concentration.

Because the kidneys can reduce urine potassium excretion to <20 mEq/24 h (20 mmol/24 h), hypokalemia from inadequate intake is uncommon. Urinary or gastrointestinal losses of potassium are most common. Assessment of urine potassium excretion is critical to establish renal potassium wasting. Urine potassium loss >20 mEq/24 h (20 mmol/24 h), a spot urine potassium >20 mEq/L (20 mmol/L), or a spot urine potassium-creatinine ratio >13 mEq/g (1.5 mEq/mmol) suggests excessive urinary losses. Conversely, urine potassium loss <20 mEq/24 h (20 mmol/24 h) suggests cellular shift, decreased intake, or extrarenal losses of potassium. This patient's high urinary potassium suggests urinary loss rather than poor nutrition as the cause of hypokalemia.

KEY POINT

- Hypomagnesemia can cause symptomatic hypokalemia via renal losses of potassium; importantly, the hypokalemia will be refractory to therapy until magnesium is repleted.

Bibliography
Rodan AR, Cheng CJ, Huang CL. Recent advances in distal tubular potassium handling. Am J Physiol Renal Physiol. 2011;300:F821-7. [PMID: 21270092]

Item 77   Answer: A

Educational Objective: Identify *Staphylococcus aureus* as a cause of infection-related glomerulonephritis.

Staphylococcus aureus is the most likely cause of this patient's infection-related glomerulonephritis (IRGN). This patient has acute kidney injury in the setting of cellulitis, with active urine sediment and low serum complement levels. The biopsy shows a proliferative glomerulonephritis on light microscopy with immunofluorescence of C3 and IgA and subepithelial hump-like deposits on electron microscopy, confirming a diagnosis of IRGN. In the developed world, the epidemiology of IRGN has drastically shifted over the past few decades, moving away from streptococcal-associated glomerulonephritides to infections caused primarily by *S. aureus* and, at a significantly lower rate, gram-negative bacteria. In this patient with cellulitis and IRGN occurring at the time of infection, *S. aureus* is the most likely culprit pathogen.

In patients with poststreptococcal glomerulonephritis (group A *Streptococcus*, or *Streptococcus pyogenes*), there is a latent period between the resolution of the streptococcal infection and the acute onset of the nephritic syndrome, usually 7 to 10 days after oropharyngeal infections and 2 to 4 weeks after skin infections. In adults with non-poststreptococcal IRGN, the glomerulonephritis often coexists with the triggering infection. Sites of infection can include the upper and lower respiratory tract, skin/soft tissue, bone, teeth/oral mucosa, heart, deep abscesses, shunts, and indwelling catheters. Notably, this patient's kidney failure has occurred at the same time as the cellulitis, consistent with a staphylococcal-mediated form of IRGN.

Streptococcus pneumoniae is an uncommon cause of cellulitis, and *Streptococcus agalactiae* (group B *Streptococcus*) is capable of causing cellulitis in nonpregnant adults in special circumstances (lymphedema, vascular insufficiency, chronic dermatitis, or radiation-induced cutaneous injury). *S. pyogenes* and *S. aureus* are much more common causes of cellulitis, and the co-occurrence of the infection and IRGN points to *S. aureus* as the most likely culprit.

KEY POINT

- In adults, most cases of infection-related glomerulonephritis are no longer poststreptococcal, and the glomerulonephritis often coexists with the triggering infection.

Bibliography

Glassock RJ, Alvarado A, Prosek J, Hebert C, Parikh S, Satoskar A, et al. Staphylococcus-related glomerulonephritis and poststreptococcal glomerulonephritis: why defining "post" is important in understanding and treating infection-related glomerulonephritis. Am J Kidney Dis. 2015; 65:826-32. [PMID: 25890425]

Item 78   Answer: D

Educational Objective: Recognize differing guideline recommendations for blood pressure targets in older patients.

According to target blood pressure goals recommended by the American College of Physicians and the American Academy of Family Physicians, this 72-year-old woman's blood pressure is at target, and no changes are necessary. This guideline recommends that antihypertensive drugs be initiated in patients ≥60 years old if blood pressure is >150/90 mm Hg, with a goal of reducing systolic blood pressure to <150 mm Hg to reduce the risk for mortality, stroke, and cardiac events. The guideline further recommends that physicians consider initiating or intensifying pharmacologic treatment in patients ≥60 years of age with a history of stroke or transient ischemic attack to achieve a target systolic blood pressure <140 mm Hg to reduce the risk for recurrent stroke. The guideline also recommends

considering the initiation or intensification of pharmacologic treatment in some patients ≥60 years of age at high cardiovascular risk, based on individualized assessment, to achieve a target systolic blood pressure <140 mm Hg to reduce the risk for stroke or cardiac events. These recommendations are based on evidence that demonstrates the greatest absolute benefit of antihypertensive therapy is seen in patients with the highest blood pressure and cardiovascular risk.

On the other hand, the 2017 American College of Cardiology/American Heart Association blood pressure guideline recommends a target systolic blood pressure goal of <130 mm Hg for noninstitutionalized, ambulatory community-dwelling patients ≥65 years of age. In those with a high burden of comorbidity and limited life expectancy, clinical judgment, patient preference, and an assessment of risk-benefit ratio should be considered for decisions about the intensity of blood pressure control and antihypertensive medication choice. This recommendation is based upon randomized controlled trials of antihypertensive therapy that have included large numbers of older persons, which demonstrated that more intensive treatment safely reduced the risk of cardiovascular disease for those ≥65 years of age.

KEY POINT

- Based on evidence that the greatest absolute benefit of antihypertensive therapy is seen in patients with the highest blood pressure and cardiovascular risk, the American College of Physicians and American Academy of Family Physicians recommend that antihypertensive drugs be initiated in patients ≥60 years old if blood pressure is >150/90 mm Hg, with a goal of reducing systolic blood pressure to <150 mm Hg; the American College of Cardiology/American Heart Association recommends a systolic blood pressure target of <130 mm Hg in patients ≥65 years old.

Bibliography

Kansagara D, Wilt TJ, Frost J, Qaseem A. Pharmacologic treatment of hypertension in adults aged 60 years or older. Ann Intern Med. 2017;167:291-292. [PMID: 28806807]

Item 79   Answer: D

Educational Objective: Treat hyperphosphatemia in a patient with stage G4 chronic kidney disease.

Sevelamer is the most appropriate treatment for this patient with secondary hyperparathyroidism and hyperphosphatemia associated with stage G4 chronic kidney disease (CKD). Increased plasma parathyroid hormone (PTH) occurring as a result of CKD is referred to as secondary hyperparathyroidism. Increased PTH levels result in reduced calcium excretion and increased phosphorus excretion by the kidneys. Early in CKD, the PTH-induced increase in renal phosphorus excretion enables normal serum phosphorus levels despite reduced renal excretory capacity. However, as CKD progresses, the kidney is unable to compensate for the increased phosphorus, and

CONT.

phosphorus levels rise. This results in a vicious cycle as phosphorus stimulates PTH production. Initial treatment of secondary hyperparathyroidism in CKD stages G3 through G5 is correction of serum calcium, phosphorus, and vitamin D levels. Current Kidney Disease: Improving Global Outcomes (KDIGO) guidelines recommend that elevated phosphorus levels should be lowered *toward* the normal range, not into the normal range, because there is an absence of data showing that efforts to maintain phosphorus in the normal range are of benefit to CKD stage G3a to G4. Thus, treatment should be aimed at overt hyperphosphatemia, and decisions to start phosphate-lowering treatment should be based solely on progressively or persistently elevated serum phosphorus levels. KDIGO guidelines also recommend avoiding hypercalcemia. In this patient, treatment of hyperphosphatemia with a phosphate binder and a low phosphorus diet is indicated. Sevelamer is a non–calcium-containing binder that might improve bone turnover, limit vascular calcification, and reduce all-cause mortality, compared with calcium-containing binders, although these potential benefits have not been consistently proven.

Aluminum hydroxide is an effective phosphate binder and is still used for very short-term treatment of severe secondary hyperparathyroidism. However, it would not be recommended in the chronic setting due to the toxic effects of aluminum (myalgia, weakness, osteomalacia, iron-resistant microcytic anemia, dementia), particularly because non–calcium-containing binders are now available.

This patient's 25-hydroxyvitamin D level is in the "sufficient" range. However, calcitriol may be warranted if hyperparathyroidism persists after normalization of serum calcium and phosphorus levels even in the setting of normal 25-hydroxyvitamin D levels, as impaired hydroxylation at the 1 position by the kidney can lead to functional deficiency.

Cinacalcet, a calcimimetic that decreases PTH levels, is currently FDA approved only for use in patients who are undergoing dialysis, although it has been used off-label for secondary hyperparathyroidism associated with hypercalcemia in cases in which use of vitamin D analogues has led to hypercalcemia.

> **KEY POINT**
>
> - Initial treatment of secondary hyperparathyroidism in chronic kidney disease stages G3 through G5 is correction of serum calcium, phosphorus, and vitamin D levels.

Bibliography

Patel L, Bernard LM, Elder GJ. Sevelamer versus calcium-based binders for treatment of hyperphosphatemia in CKD: a meta-analysis of randomized controlled trials. Clin J Am Soc Nephrol. 2016;11:232-44. [PMID: 26668024]

Item 80   Answer: C

Educational Objective: Discontinue NSAIDs in a patient with elevated blood pressure.

The most appropriate management is to discontinue ibuprofen and measure the blood pressure (BP) in 1 month.

The American College of Cardiology/American Heart Association BP guideline defines stage 1 hypertension as a systolic BP of 130 to 139 mm Hg or diastolic BP of 80 to 89 mm Hg. This change is based on epidemiologic studies that indicate systolic BP >115 mm Hg and diastolic BP >75 mm Hg are associated in a linear fashion with cardiovascular events. In the initial assessment of a patient with elevated BP, before a diagnosis of hypertension is made, it is imperative that a complete history with a list of prescription, nonprescription (including complementary and alternative medications such as herbals), and illicit drugs is elicited. NSAIDs are one of the medication classes that can result in reversible elevations in BP, the mechanism for which is increased sodium retention. Therefore, ibuprofen, an NSAID, should be discontinued and BP remeasured. If the patient has ongoing pain, an alternative pain management strategy that does not result in BP elevation, such as nondrug interventions, topical analgesics (if appropriate), or acetaminophen, should be prescribed because pain can also result in BP elevation.

This patient's elevated BP would need to be confirmed 1 month after discontinuation of ibuprofen before antihypertensive medications such as amlodipine or hydrochlorothiazide are started in this otherwise healthy young individual.

Antihistamines such as loratadine generally do not result in BP elevation; therefore, loratadine does not need to be discontinued in this patient.

> **KEY POINT**
>
> - Many medications, such as NSAIDS, can result in reversible elevations in blood pressure; discontinuation of the drug and a reassessment of blood pressure 1 month later are necessary to confirm a return to normal blood pressure measurement.

Bibliography

Weir MR. In the clinic: hypertension. Ann Intern Med. 2014;161:ITC1-15; quiz ITC16. [PMID: 25437425]

Item 81   Answer: C

Educational Objective: Identify hepatitis C virus infection as the cause of membranoproliferative glomerulonephritis.

The most appropriate test to perform next is measurement of hepatitis C antibodies. This patient presents with glomerulonephritis (elevated serum creatinine level, hematuria, and subnephrotic proteinuria), which shows a membranoproliferative (MPGN) pattern on kidney biopsy. The new approach to MPGN lesions is a bifurcation based on the pattern of staining on immunofluorescence microscopy. The more common pattern, as seen in this patient, is immune-complex deposition with the presence of both immunoglobulin (IgG, IgM, and/or IgA) and complement (C1q and/or C3) on immunofluorescence, which infers that the classical pathway has been activated by an inciting cause or event that generally falls into one of three major categories: infectious, autoimmune, or malignancy associated. The most common is infectious, specifically infection with hepatitis C virus (HCV).

When an MPGN lesion on immunofluorescence microscopy shows only C3 staining (that is, without immunoglobulin or C1q staining), this extremely rare finding is suggestive of an antibody-independent means of complement activation and points to hyperactivity of the alternative complement pathway. In these C3 glomerulopathies, named based on the isolated C3 staining pattern seen on immunofluorescence, screening for genetic abnormalities in alternative complement pathway proteins is an appropriate part of the diagnostic evaluation.

Hepatitis B virus infection and HIV infection have been linked to glomerular diseases, but these are classically associated with the nephrotic syndrome, specifically membranous glomerulopathy with hepatitis B virus infection and focal segmental glomerulosclerosis with HIV infection.

> **KEY POINT**
>
> - An immune-complex membranoproliferative glomerulonephritis is the classic form of kidney involvement seen in patients with hepatitis C virus infection.

Bibliography

Sethi S, Fervenza FC. Membranoproliferative glomerulonephritis–a new look at an old entity. N Engl J Med. 2012;366:1119-31. [PMID: 22435371]

Item 82   Answer: D

Educational Objective: Diagnose lead nephropathy.

The most likely diagnosis is lead nephropathy, which causes a chronic tubulointerstitial disease after years of continuous or intermittent lead exposure. Lead nephropathy can occur in patients with occupational exposure to lead or exposure to lead in water, soil, paint, or food products. Chronic lead nephropathy is frequently associated with hyperuricemia, hypertension, and recurrent gouty attacks. This patient's lead exposure is likely due to lead-contaminated moonshine. Contamination occurs when lead-containing car radiators are used to condense the alcohol during the distilling process. The initial diagnostic test is measurement of blood lead levels, although lead levels may have normalized if exposure has been reduced or stopped.

Analgesic nephropathy occurs in patients with long-term excessive ingestion of analgesics such as aspirin, acetaminophen, and phenacetin, usually in combination. Patients frequently present with nocturia, sterile pyuria, hypertension, anemia, and chronic tubulointerstitial disease. This patient has no history of prolonged analgesic exposure.

Balkan nephropathy is a form of chronic tubulointerstitial disease that progresses to end-stage kidney disease in patients from southeastern Europe (Serbia, Bulgaria, Romania, Bosnia and Herzegovina, and Croatia). This patient is not from this region.

Cadmium nephropathy occurs in patients with prolonged exposure to plastic, metal, alloys, and electrical equipment manufacturing industries. Early manifestations are those of tubular dysfunction, including low-molecular-weight tubular proteinuria (for example, β_2-microglobulin), aminoaciduria, renal glucosuria, and hypercalciuria. Patients can develop osteomalacia and nephrolithiasis. Clinically, patients present with hypertension, bone pain, and chronic kidney disease. This patient does not give any history of an occupation that would result in cadmium exposure.

> **KEY POINT**
>
> - Lead nephropathy can occur in patients with occupational exposure to lead or exposure to lead in water, soil, paint, or food products; it is frequently associated with hyperuricemia, hypertension, and recurrent gouty attacks.

Bibliography

Lin JL, Lin-Tan DT, Li YJ, Chen KH, Huang YL. Low-level environmental exposure to lead and progressive chronic kidney diseases. Am J Med. 2006;119:707.e1-9. [PMID: 16887418]

Item 83   Answer: A

Educational Objective: Identify laxative abuse as a cause of a normal anion gap metabolic acidosis.

Laxative abuse is the most likely cause of this patient's normal anion gap metabolic acidosis. Normal anion gap metabolic acidosis can be caused by gastrointestinal bicarbonate loss, renal loss of bicarbonate, or the inability of the kidney to excrete acid. The normal physiologic response to systemic acidosis is an increase in urine acid excretion. Therefore, an initial diagnostic step in normal anion gap metabolic acidosis is to determine whether the kidney is appropriately excreting acid or whether impaired kidney acid excretion is the cause of the metabolic acidosis. Increased acid excretion by the kidney is reflected as a marked increase in urine ammonium. However, urine ammonium is difficult to measure directly. Because ammonium carries a positive charge, chloride is excreted into the urine in equal amounts with ammonium to maintain electrical neutrality. Therefore, the amount of chloride in the urine reflects the amount of ammonium present, and the urine anion gap can be used as an indicator of the ability of the kidney to excrete acid. The urine anion gap is calculated as follows:

$$\text{Urine Anion Gap} = (\text{Urine Sodium} + \text{Urine Potassium}) - \text{Urine Chloride}$$

In the context of increased urinary ammonium excretion, therefore, the urine anion gap will be negative. The negative urine anion gap in this patient (-6 mEq/L [-6 mmol/L]) suggests a gastrointestinal cause of the normal anion gap metabolic acidosis, and laxative abuse is a possible, even likely explanation. In addition, the low urine potassium indicates appropriate renal compensation in context of laxative-induced hypokalemia.

Vomiting and gastric acid loss result in metabolic alkalosis, not metabolic acidosis.

CONT.

Renal causes of normal anion gap metabolic acidosis are due to specific defects in renal handling of bicarbonate reclamation (type 2/proximal RTA) or in hydrogen ion secretion (type 1/hypokalemic distal RTA). Type 1 (hypokalemic distal) RTA is caused by a defect in hydrogen secretion and a consequent decrease in ammonium excretion, and is therefore associated with a positive urine anion gap; it is also characterized by high urine potassium secretion and hypokalemia. Type 4 (hyperkalemic distal) RTA is usually caused by aldosterone deficiency or resistance and is characterized by a high serum potassium and positive urine anion gap.

> **KEY POINT**
>
> - Normal anion gap metabolic acidosis can be caused by gastrointestinal bicarbonate loss, renal loss of bicarbonate, or the inability of the kidney to excrete acid.

Bibliography

Rastegar M, Nagami GT. Non-anion gap metabolic acidosis: a clinical approach to evaluation. Am J Kidney Dis. 2017;69:296-301. [PMID: 28029394]

Item 84   Answer: B

Educational Objective: Diagnose the cause of acute kidney injury with a kidney biopsy.

The most appropriate next step in the evaluation of this patient's acute kidney injury (AKI) is a kidney biopsy. This patient with sepsis has developed AKI that has continued to worsen despite discontinuation of antibiotics 4 days ago. His urinalysis is notable for hematuria, pyuria, and proteinuria. The differential diagnosis includes ischemic or toxic acute tubular necrosis in the setting of hypotension, acute interstitial nephritis (AIN) from antibiotics or a proton pump inhibitor, and infection-associated glomerulonephritis. Given multiple potential contributing factors, a kidney biopsy is necessary to differentiate.

Glucocorticoids would be indicated if AIN is identified on biopsy, but empiric therapy is not justified because other causes may be contributing to his AKI. Moreover, glucocorticoids can cause significant adverse side effects, including worsening glycemic control in a patient with diabetes mellitus. If AIN is confirmed on kidney biopsy, a trial of glucocorticoids can be considered.

Prerenal AKI results from decreased renal perfusion and will typically respond to restoration of effective arterial circulation. However, the patient has no findings of hypoperfusion, and the elevated fractional excretion of sodium argues against this diagnosis (typically <1%) and the need for a fluid challenge. Such an intervention may be deleterious in a patient with oliguric AKI.

Postrenal AKI results from urinary tract obstruction. Bladder outlet obstruction should be suspected in patients with prostate enlargement or in the setting of diabetes mellitus (neurogenic bladder), pain medications, or anticholinergic medications. This patient's kidney ultrasound does not show obstruction; therefore, placement of a urinary catheter is not appropriate and would increase his risk of catheter associated urinary tract infection.

> **KEY POINT**
>
> - Kidney biopsy should be considered in patients with acute kidney injury from no apparent or unclear cause, suspected glomerulonephritis, or unexplained systemic disease.

Bibliography

Levey AS, James MT. Acute kidney injury. Ann Intern Med. 2017;167:ITC66-ITC80. [PMID: 29114754]

Item 85   Answer: B

Educational Objective: Recognize the role of genetic counseling in the diagnosis and management of hereditary nephritis.

Genetic counseling potentially followed by genetic testing for hereditary nephritis (Alport syndrome) is appropriate for this patient. Hereditary nephritis is a familial form of glomerulonephritis that affects approximately 0.4% of U.S. adults. The earliest presentation is microscopic hematuria, with or without proteinuria. Heavier proteinuria, hypertension, and chronic kidney disease usually develop over time, with end-stage kidney disease occurring between the late teenage years and the fourth decade of life. There are three genetic variants: X-linked (80%), autosomal recessive (15%), and autosomal dominant (5%). This patient's family history fits the X-linked version of disease. Her mother and maternal grandmother are asymptomatic carriers; each has a 50% chance of passing the affected gene to male offspring (in this family, the maternal uncle and the patient's older brother), and their daughters likewise have a 50% chance of carrying the gene. Almost all female heterozygotes have some degree of hematuria. Females with the X-linked variant can develop kidney disease depending on activity of the X chromosome in somatic renal cells (lyonization), but that does not appear to be the case in this family. Given widespread access to genetic testing, in patients with a clearly documented family history and abnormal urinary findings, the diagnosis of hereditary nephritis is now increasingly being made by the noninvasive route using genetic testing. Genetic testing is the only way to diagnose a female with a family history of X-linked hereditary nephritis, such as this patient.

Hereditary nephritis is accompanied by sensorineural hearing loss that can be subtle and only picked up by audiometry, but this complication would not be expected in an asymptomatic carrier, such as this patient.

The diagnosis of hereditary nephritis for affected patients has traditionally been made by the more invasive route of kidney biopsy, with electron microscopy required for the hallmark finding of prominent thickening and lamellation of the glomerular basement membrane (a basket-weave appearance). Other than the expected microscopic hematuria, this patient has normal kidney function and does not require a kidney biopsy.

A diagnostic skin biopsy can be performed when X-linked hereditary nephritis is suspected. Type IV collagen alpha-5 chain (COL4A5) is normally present in the skin, and approximately 60% to 80% of patients with X-linked hereditary nephritis will show abnormal staining for COL4A5 in the skin biopsy, although these findings would not be expected in an asymptomatic carrier.

KEY POINT

- The diagnosis of hereditary nephritis is confirmed with kidney biopsy, skin biopsy, or molecular genetic analysis.

Bibliography

Gross O, Kashtan CE, Rheault MN, Flinter F, Savige J, Miner JH, et al. Advances and unmet needs in genetic, basic and clinical science in Alport syndrome: report from the 2015 International Workshop on Alport Syndrome. Nephrol Dial Transplant. 2017;32:916-924. [PMID: 27190345]

Item 86   Answer: A

Educational Objective: Identify the composition of a kidney stone in a patient with Crohn disease.

The most likely composition of this patient's kidney stone is calcium oxalate. This patient has classic symptoms of renal colic, including flank pain that radiates to the groin. Stone movement may result in pain migration to the genitalia. Nausea, vomiting, and dysuria may also be present. Microscopic hematuria is usually noted, although its absence does not exclude a stone. Patients with diarrhea who are volume depleted and have a metabolic acidosis are at increased risk for developing a kidney stone, particularly stones composed of calcium oxalate and uric acid. In this patient with Crohn disease and chronic diarrhea, the most likely composition of the stone is calcium oxalate because the chronic metabolic acidosis (suggested by the low serum bicarbonate concentration and relatively low urine pH) increases calcium loss from bone and decreases citrate excretion. Citrate is the major inhibitor of calcium crystallization in the urine. In addition, if there is concomitant fat malabsorption, a common occurrence in inflammatory bowel disease, calcium will bind to fat in the gut, allowing increased absorption of oxalate.

Struvite stones are composed of magnesium ammonium phosphate (struvite) and calcium carbonate-apatite and occur in the presence of urea-splitting bacteria, such as *Proteus* or *Klebsiella*, in the upper urinary tract. These organisms convert urea to ammonium, which alkalinizes the urine, decreases the solubility of phosphate, and leads to struvite precipitation. Struvite stones can rapidly enlarge to fill the entire renal pelvis within weeks to months, taking on a characteristic "staghorn" shape. Calcium phosphate stones also form in alkaline urine. The low urine pH and absence of signs of infection on urinalysis make these diagnoses unlikely.

Cystine stones are caused by cystinuria, a rare autosomal recessive disorder of proximal tubular transport of dibasic amino acids such as cystine that presents at a young age.

The main risk factor for uric acid stones is low urine pH, usually ≤5.0, which decreases the solubility of uric acid. Hyperuricosuria is not a consistent finding. Comorbid risk factors for uric acid stones include gout, diabetes mellitus, the metabolic syndrome, and chronic diarrhea.

KEY POINT

- Patients with diarrhea who are volume depleted and have a metabolic acidosis are at increased risk for developing kidney stones, particularly calcium oxalate stones and, less commonly, uric acid stones.

Bibliography

Worcester EM, Coe FL. Clinical practice. Calcium kidney stones. N Engl J Med. 2010;363:954-63. [PMID: 20818905]

Item 87   Answer: A

Educational Objective: Diagnose D-lactic acidosis.

The most likely diagnosis is D-lactic acidosis. D-lactic acidosis is an unusual cause of lactic acidosis that presents with an increased anion gap metabolic acidosis in patients with short-bowel syndrome, mostly in the context of small-bowel resection or jejunoileal bypass. D-lactate may accumulate when excess carbohydrates reach the colon and are metabolized to D-lactate by bacteria. Therefore, it is sometimes manifested after a large carbohydrate load. D-lactate is the stereoisomer of L-lactate, the isomer usually responsible for lactic acidosis. The conventional lactate assay measures the L-lactate isomer, and therefore lactic acid levels in this case are normal. Characteristic symptoms include intermittent confusion, slurred speech, and ataxia. The diagnosis should therefore be considered in a patient with characteristic neurologic findings who presents with an increased anion gap metabolic acidosis, normal lactate level, negative ketones, and short-bowel syndrome or other forms of malabsorption; it is confirmed by measuring a D-lactate level.

Ethylene glycol or methanol intoxication also presents with an increased anion gap metabolic acidosis and neurologic symptoms. However, they are usually accompanied by a serum osmolal gap >10 mOsm/kg H_2O (6 mOsm/kg H_2O in this case) and a serum bicarbonate level <10 mEq/L (10 mmol/L). The serum osmolal gap is calculated as the difference between the measured osmolality and calculated osmolality, which is determined as follows:

$$\text{Serum Osmolality (mOsm/kg } H_2O) = (2 \times \text{Serum Sodium [mEq/L])} + \text{Plasma Glucose (mg/dL)}/18 + \text{Blood Urea Nitrogen (mg/dL)}/2.8$$

Pyroglutamic acidosis also manifests as mental status changes in the context of an increased anion gap. This acidosis occurs in patients chronically receiving therapeutic doses of acetaminophen. Susceptible patients are those with critical illness, poor nutrition, liver disease, and chronic kidney

CONT.

disease, as well as those on a strict vegetarian diet. Diagnosis can be confirmed by measuring urine levels of pyroglutamic acid. This patient's history does not include acetaminophen ingestion and is more consistent with a D-lactic acidosis.

> **KEY POINT**
>
> - D-lactic acidosis is characterized by an increased anion gap metabolic acidosis in patients with short-bowel syndrome or other forms of malabsorption; diagnosis is confirmed by measuring the D-lactate level rather than the conventional L-lactate level.

Bibliography

Seheult J, Fitzpatrick G, Boran G. Lactic acidosis: an update. Clin Chem Lab Med. 2017;55:322-333. [PMID: 27522622]

Item 88   Answer: B

Educational Objective: Manage chronic hypertension prior to conception.

Discontinuation of the angiotensin receptor blocker (ARB) losartan is necessary for this patient who anticipates pregnancy. The renin-angiotensin system agents (ACE inhibitors, ARBs, and direct renin inhibitors) are contraindicated in pregnancy and should be stopped prior to conception. Exposure during the second and third trimesters of pregnancy has been associated with neonatal kidney failure and death. Although the level of risk for first trimester exposure is controversial, studies have suggested an association with cardiac abnormalities, and consensus is to stop these drugs prior to pregnancy. In patients with chronic hypertension, the 2013 American College of Obstetricians and Gynecologists guidelines recommend a goal blood pressure during pregnancy of 120-160/80-105 mm Hg. Antihypertensive treatment reduces the risk of progression to severe hypertension by 50% compared with placebo but has not been shown to prevent preeclampsia, preterm birth, small size for gestational age, or infant mortality. This patient's blood pressure is well below this goal of therapy, and her blood pressure would be expected to decline during pregnancy. Therefore, monitoring her blood pressure after discontinuation of losartan is a reasonable approach. If her blood pressure rises, initiation of a drug that is safe during pregnancy is recommended. Candidate drugs include methyldopa, nifedipine, and/or labetalol. No specific agent is first choice because no data support one over another. Therapeutic classes are not recommended because potential toxicity differs among agents within classes.

Diuretics may be continued in pregnancy, particularly if the woman is already taking them prior to pregnancy. If blood pressure remains low through the first trimester of pregnancy, the dose of the diuretic may be lowered. Although one could consider discontinuation of the diuretic if the patient's blood pressure remains within at or below target, there is no contraindication to its use.

Because ARBs and ACE inhibitors are contraindicated in pregnancy and carry similar risk, switching to the ACE inhibitor lisinopril is not recommended.

Although risks are less during the first trimester, recent data regarding first trimester risk of exposure suggest that the safest approach is to discontinue a renin-angiotensin system agent prior to conception. Waiting until the patient is pregnant is not recommended.

> **KEY POINT**
>
> - The renin-angiotensin system agents (ACE inhibitors, angiotensin receptor blockers, and direct renin inhibitors) are contraindicated in pregnancy and should be stopped prior to conception.

Bibliography

Whelton PK, Carey RM, Aronow WS, Casey DE Jr, Collins KJ, Dennison Himmelfarb C, et al. 2017 ACC/AHA/AAPA/ABC/ACPM/AGS/APhA/ASH/ASPC/NMA/PCNA guideline for the prevention, detection, evaluation, and management of high blood pressure in adults: a report of the American College of Cardiology/American Heart Association Task Force on Clinical Practice Guidelines. Hypertension. 2017. [PMID: 29133356]

Item 89   Answer: A

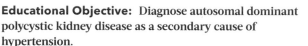

Educational Objective: Diagnose autosomal dominant polycystic kidney disease as a secondary cause of hypertension.

Kidney ultrasonography is the most appropriate diagnostic test to perform in this patient. The presence of hypertension, microhematuria, and a positive family history of chronic kidney disease requiring dialysis, as well as a brain aneurysm, raises clinical suspicion for autosomal dominant polycystic kidney disease (ADPKD). Clinical manifestations of ADPKD include gradual kidney enlargement, which may cause persistent abdominal pain and/or early satiety. Hypertension is common in patients with ADPKD, often preceding chronic kidney disease. Kidney cyst enlargement leads to stimulation of the intrarenal and circulating renin-angiotensin-aldosterone system. More than 50% of patients with ADPKD develop recurrent flank or back pain; causes include kidney stones, cyst rupture or hemorrhage, or infection. Nephrolithiasis occurs in approximately 20% of patients. A ruptured intracranial cerebral aneurysm resulting in a subarachnoid or intracerebral hemorrhage is the most serious extrarenal complication of ADPKD. Kidney ultrasonography is the most common and least costly screening and diagnostic method for ADPKD; it would reveal bilaterally enlarged kidneys with multiple cysts.

Calculation of the plasma aldosterone concentration/plasma renin activity ratio is used to screen for primary hyperaldosteronism, characterized by a triad of resistant hypertension, metabolic alkalosis, and hypokalemia. Although <50% of patients with primary hyperaldosteronism manifest hypokalemia, this diagnosis cannot account for the patient's flank fullness on palpation and hematuria or his family history of kidney failure.

Plasma fractionated metanephrines are obtained to screen for a pheochromocytoma, which could result in hypertension, but this patient has no symptoms or signs (for example, resistant hypertension, headaches, sweating) to indicate the presence of this tumor, and this diagnosis cannot account for the patient's flank fullness and hematuria.

CONT.

Although hyperthyroidism can be a secondary cause of hypertension, the patient does not manifest any symptoms or signs (heat intolerance, resting tachycardia, thyromegaly) to suggest this, making measurement of thyroid-stimulating hormone unnecessary.

> **KEY POINT**
>
> - Hypertension is common in patients with autosomal dominant polycystic kidney disease (ADPKD), often preceding chronic kidney disease; kidney ultrasonography is the most common and least costly screening and diagnostic method for ADPKD.

Bibliography

Krishnappa V, Vinod P, Deverakonda D, Raina R. Autosomal dominant polycystic kidney disease and the heart and brain. Cleve Clin J Med. 2017;84:471-481. [PMID: 28628430]

Item 90   Answer: B

Educational Objective: Discontinue mycophenolate mofetil in a woman who is planning pregnancy.

The most appropriate management for this kidney transplant recipient who is planning pregnancy is to discontinue mycophenolate mofetil and begin azathioprine. Fertility increases after kidney transplantation, although fertility rates remain lower and pregnancy complications are higher compared with the general population. Pregnancy planning for a kidney transplant recipient is essential to improve outcomes and includes adjusting medications and optimizing clinical status. Kidney transplant recipients should wait 1 to 2 years with a stable allograft before attempting conception. Other comorbid conditions (such as systemic lupus erythematosus) should also be stable prior to conception. Outcomes are improved with better allograft function (serum creatinine <1.5 mg/dL [132.6 µmol/L]) and stable immunosuppression. Mycophenolate mofetil (as well as sirolimus and everolimus) is teratogenic and needs to be replaced 3 to 6 months prior to conception with azathioprine, which is generally safer and well tolerated in pregnancy.

Calcineurin inhibitors (both tacrolimus and cyclosporine) have been used safely in pregnancy. Therefore, tacrolimus does not need to be discontinued and replaced with cyclosporine in this patient.

Although this would constitute a high-risk pregnancy, the success rate of pregnancies in patients with kidney transplants is high; with stable allograft function, a normotensive patient and her fetus have favorable prognoses, and therefore the patient could proceed with pregnancy following modification of her maintenance immunosuppression regimen.

> **KEY POINT**
>
> - In kidney transplant recipients who are planning pregnancy, mycophenolate mofetil, sirolimus, and everolimus must be discontinued 3 to 6 months prior to conception and replaced with azathioprine, which is generally safer and well tolerated in pregnancy.

Bibliography

Hou S. Pregnancy in renal transplant recipients. Adv Chronic Kidney Dis. 2013;20:253-9. [PMID: 23928390]

Item 91   Answer: A

Educational Objective: Diagnose light chain cast nephropathy in a patient with multiple myeloma.

The most likely diagnosis is light chain cast nephropathy in this patient with multiple myeloma. In multiple myeloma, acute kidney injury from light chain cast nephropathy is the most common type of kidney disease. Cast nephropathy is characterized by intratubular obstruction with light chain casts that can result in acute tubular injury. A clinical clue to the diagnosis is the presence of an elevated urine protein-creatinine ratio, with minimal proteinuria detected by dipstick urinalysis (dipstick urinalysis detects albumin but not light chains). Other supporting findings are the presence of anemia and hypercalcemia (when calcium measurement is corrected for albumin).

Exposure to NSAIDs can cause tubular injury. However, NSAIDs do not cause a discrepancy in proteinuria between urinalysis and urine protein-creatinine ratio.

Renal sarcoidosis can result in tubulointerstitial dysfunction. Other kidney manifestations include direct ureteral involvement, retroperitoneal fibrosis, and, more commonly, hypercalcemia, hypercalciuria, nephrolithiasis, and nephrocalcinosis via excessive production of 1,25-dihydroxyvitamin D in granulomas. However, renal sarcoidosis is rare in patients without thoracic sarcoidosis and cannot account for the discrepancy in proteinuria between urinalysis and urine protein-creatinine ratio.

Uric acid nephropathy is unlikely given the modest elevation in the serum urate level. Furthermore, an elevated urine protein-creatinine ratio is not consistent with uric acid nephropathy.

> **KEY POINT**
>
> - Clinical clues to the diagnosis of light chain cast nephropathy from multiple myeloma include an elevated urine protein-creatinine ratio with minimal proteinuria by urine dipstick, anemia, and hypercalcemia.

Bibliography

Heher EC, Rennke HG, Laubach JP, Richardson PG. Kidney disease and multiple myeloma. Clin J Am Soc Nephrol. 2013;8:2007-17. [PMID: 23868898]

Item 92   Answer: B

Educational Objective: Diagnose IgA nephropathy.

IgA nephropathy is the most likely diagnosis. Recurrent gross hematuria, in which macroscopic hematuria occurs concomitantly or within days after an upper respiratory infection (synpharyngitic nephritis) or physical exertion, is a classic presentation of IgA nephropathy, particularly in younger patients.

This nephritic presentation usually follows a benign clinical course without associated kidney insufficiency, although in a minority of cases intraluminal obstructive erythrocyte casts can be a cause of moderate to severe acute kidney injury that typically responds to supportive care measures. The diagnosis of IgA nephropathy can only be made by kidney biopsy, but some clinicians will make an empiric diagnosis for young patients with a classic history of recurrent gross hematuria, negative imaging for masses/stones, and normal kidney function with little to no proteinuria.

IgA vasculitis (Henoch-Schönlein purpura) is the most common childhood vasculitis and tends to appear after upper respiratory infections. IgA vasculitis is rarer among adults. Characteristic symptoms are abdominal pain and palpable purpura. Gastrointestinal ischemia may be severe enough to cause intestinal bleeding. Arthritis is common, other organ systems may be involved, and patients may present with glomerulonephritis. The patient's recurrent symptoms, lack of additional findings, benign clinical course, and urine findings are not compatible with a diagnosis of IgA vasculitis.

Lupus nephritis and postinfectious glomerulonephritis can present with macroscopic glomerular hematuria, but these disease states usually induce low complement levels (low C3 with or without low C4). Postinfectious glomerulonephritis, when associated with upper respiratory infections caused by streptococcal organisms, usually occurs 2 to 3 weeks after the resolution of the streptococcal infection. In the developed world, it is more common to see peri-infectious glomerulonephritis associated with staphylococcal infections (usually skin infections), with onset at the time of infection, but these are not usually associated with gross hematuria or a recurrent history of such episodes.

KEY POINT

- A classic presentation of IgA nephropathy is recurrent gross hematuria that occurs concomitantly or within days after an upper respiratory infection or physical exertion and usually follows a benign course.

Bibliography

Lai KN, Tang SC, Schena FP, Novak J, Tomino Y, Fogo AB, et al. IgA nephropathy. Nat Rev Dis Primers. 2016;2:16001. [PMID: 27189177]

Item 93   Answer: D

Educational Objective: Diagnose a complex mixed acid-base disorder.

The most likely diagnosis is a complex mixed acid-base disorder consisting of respiratory alkalosis, increased anion gap metabolic acidosis, and metabolic alkalosis. Interpretation of acid-base disorders requires the identification of the likely dominant acid-base disorder, followed by an assessment of the compensatory response. When measured values fall outside the expected compensatory range, a mixed acid-base disorder is considered present. Multiple acid-base disturbances may coexist, as seen in this patient.

Because the blood pH is 7.56, the patient's dominant acid-base disorder is an alkalosis. The low P_{CO_2} indicates a respiratory component to the alkalosis. The expected metabolic compensation for chronic respiratory alkalosis is a reduction in the serum bicarbonate of 4 to 5 mEq/L (4-5 mmol/L) for each 10 mm Hg (1.3 kPa) decrease in the P_{CO_2} (in this case, the decrease in P_{CO_2} is 20 mm Hg [2.7 kPa]). The expected serum bicarbonate concentration in this patient is calculated as follows:

Normal Bicarbonate - Expected Compensation
24 − (8-10) mEq/L (mmol/L) = 14-16 mEq/L
(14-16 mmol/L)

Because the measured bicarbonate of 20 mEq/L (20 mmol/L) is higher than expected, this suggests coexistence of a metabolic alkalosis.

An elevated anion gap is also present, indicating the presence of an increased anion gap metabolic acidosis. Assessing the ratio of the change in the anion gap (Δ anion gap) to the change in bicarbonate level (Δ bicarbonate), or the "delta-delta (Δ-Δ) ratio," may indicate the presence of a coexistent acid-base disturbance. A ratio of <0.5 to 1 may reflect the presence of concurrent normal anion gap metabolic acidosis, whereas a ratio >2 may indicate the presence of metabolic alkalosis. This patient's Δ-Δ ratio is 2.5 [Δ anion gap/Δ bicarbonate = (22 - 12)/(24 - 20) = 2.5], confirming the coexistence of the metabolic alkalosis.

The clinical situation most likely to present with this acid-base disorder is salicylate toxicity. Central hyperventilation from salicylate will cause the respiratory alkalosis; salicylate itself will cause the anion gap metabolic acidosis; and vomiting will cause the metabolic alkalosis.

KEY POINT

- Interpretation of acid-base disorders requires the identification of the likely dominant acid-base disorder, followed by an assessment of the compensatory response; when measured values fall outside the range of the predicted compensatory response, a mixed acid-base disorder is considered present.

Bibliography

Seifter JL, Chang HY. Disorders of acid-base balance: new perspectives. Kidney Dis (Basel). 2017;2:170-186. [PMID: 28232934]

Item 94   Answer: D

Educational Objective: Evaluate proteinuria in the absence of albuminuria.

The most appropriate next step in management is to obtain a urine protein electrophoresis. Albumin is the predominant protein detected on urine dipstick, which detects albumin excretion graded as trace (10-30 mg/dL), 1+ (30 mg/dL), 2+ (100 mg/dL), 3+ (300 mg/dL), and 4+ (>1000 mg/dL). Highly alkaline urine specimens can produce false-positive results on dipstick testing for protein. The sulfosalicylic acid (SSA) test can be used to detect the presence of not only albumin

CONT.

but also other proteins that are not detected with the urine dipstick, such as urine light chains or immunoglobulins. The possibility of cast nephropathy should be raised in patients with acute kidney injury and anemia when the urine dipstick reads negative or trace for protein, but the urine shows increased positivity for protein by the SSA test or by measuring the urine protein-creatinine ratio. Although these findings are most concerning for myeloma cast nephropathy, light chains are associated with other renal findings such as proximal tubulopathy. Proximal tubule involvement may be associated with hypophosphatemia and glucosuria (Fanconi syndrome).

Omeprazole and other proton pump inhibitors are well-described causes of acute interstitial nephritis. Although this is possible, this patient's proteinuria patterns are far more consistent with multiple myeloma.

Although a 24-hour urine collection is likely to provide a more accurate assessment of the total urine protein, the urine protein-creatinine ratio is sufficiently accurate to determine the presence of proteinuria.

Noncontrast helical abdominal CT may be helpful if the presence of a stone or mass in the kidney is suspected; however, in the absence of flank pain or hematuria, this imaging study is unlikely to provide additional diagnostic information.

KEY POINT

- The presence of significant measured proteinuria in the context of minimal proteinuria on urine dipstick suggests the presence of Bence-Jones (light chain) proteinuria, which can be confirmed by a urine protein electrophoresis.

Bibliography
Simerville JA, Maxted WC, Pahira JJ. Urinalysis: a comprehensive review. Am Fam Physician. 2005;71:1153-62. [PMID: 15791892]

Item 95   Answer: D

Educational Objective: Refer a patient with chronic kidney disease for kidney transplant evaluation.

Kidney transplant evaluation is the most appropriate management for this patient with stage G4 chronic kidney disease (CKD). Referral to a kidney transplant center is indicated when the estimated glomerular filtration rate (eGFR) is <20 mL/min/1.73 m^2. Kidney transplantation is the preferred treatment for patients with end-stage kidney disease, because it improves life expectancy and quality of life. It also provides a significant cost savings to the health care system compared with maintaining a patient on dialysis. Early referral allows adequate time to identify suitable living donors. If no living donor is available, early listing is essential to begin the waiting process for a deceased-donor kidney. Patients undergo an extensive health screening to identify potential issues that may affect the safety and/or outcome of the transplant. In the potential recipient, these include active malignancy, coronary ischemia, or active infections. An adequate social support system and financial resources also are important to ensure

medication adherence and long-term survival of the transplanted allograft.

Patients with stage G4 chronic kidney disease should be seen at least every 3 months, not 6 months. More importantly, clinical follow-up alone does not address the immediate problem of planning for renal replacement therapy, ideally with kidney transplantation.

Fistulography is not indicated because physical examination findings suggest that the fistula is mature and may be ready to use for hemodialysis. Invasive imaging is not required to confirm patency unless physical examination findings suggest a problem. Additionally, fistulography exposes the patient to nephrotoxic iodinated contrast and may reduce residual kidney function.

Although this patient has an arteriovenous fistula, hemodialysis is not indicated at this time because she has normal serum potassium and bicarbonate levels, does not have significant volume overload, and does not have uremic symptoms. Several recent studies have demonstrated no benefit in starting dialysis in asymptomatic patients early based upon an arbitrary eGFR cutoff compared with waiting until patients develop very low eGFR (<8-10 mL/min/1.73 m^2) or clinical indications for dialysis are present.

KEY POINT

- Referral for kidney transplant evaluation is indicated when the estimated glomerular filtration rate is <20 mL/min/1.73 m^2 to allow for adequate time to identify suitable living donors or to be put on an early listing if no living donor is available.

Bibliography
Educational Guidance on Patient Referral to Kidney Transplantation-Organ Procurement and Transplantation Network, US Department of Health and Human Services. Available at: https://optn.transplant.hrsa.gov/resources/guidance/educational-guidance-on-patient-referral-to-kidney-transplantation/. Accessed October 30, 2017.

Item 96   Answer: C

Educational Objective: Treat type 1 hepatorenal syndrome.

Vasoconstrictor therapy with octreotide and oral midodrine is appropriate for this patient with type 1 hepatorenal syndrome (HRS). Type 1 HRS is a clinical diagnosis made after exclusion of other causes of kidney dysfunction. It is characterized by a rise in serum creatinine of at least 0.3 mg/dL (26.5 µmol/L) and/or ≥50% from baseline within 48 hours, bland urinalysis, and normal findings on kidney ultrasound. It is also supported by a lack of improvement in kidney function after withdrawal of diuretics and 2 days of volume expansion with intravenous albumin. Often, patients also have low urine sodium, low fractional excretion of sodium, and oliguria. Type 2 HRS is defined as a more gradual decline in kidney function associated with refractory ascites. General management of type 1 HRS includes discontinuing diuretics, restricting sodium, restricting water in hyponatremic patients, and searching for precipitating factors. Initial therapeutic interventions include

CONT.

treatment with vasoconstrictors in conjunction with intravenous albumin.

Dialysis should be initiated only if the patient does not respond to HRS medical therapy with midodrine and octreotide and/or if indications for dialysis develop. Absolute indications for dialysis include hyperkalemia, metabolic acidosis, and pulmonary edema refractory to medical therapy; uremic symptoms; uremic pericarditis; and certain drug intoxications. Currently, this patient has no acute indications for dialysis.

The patient was volume expanded with intravenous albumin, which should have corrected hypovolemia. Furthermore, she is not volume depleted on physical examination, has edema and ascites, and has stable blood pressure without tachycardia. Therefore, intravenous fluids are not indicated.

The transjugular intrahepatic portosystemic shunt is primarily used to treat variceal hemorrhage and ascites. It has been used as a last resort in the treatment of refractory ascites in highly selected patients with HRS who do not respond to medical therapy and who are awaiting liver transplantation. Complications include an increase in the rate of hepatic encephalopathy and risk of kidney injury associated with intravenous contrast. This procedure is not indicated at this time.

KEY POINT

- General management of type 1 hepatorenal syndrome includes discontinuing diuretics, volume replacement with albumin, and use of vasoconstrictors.

Bibliography
Colle I, Laterre PF. Hepatorenal syndrome: the clinical impact of vasoactive therapy. Expert Rev Gastroenterol Hepatol. 2018;12:173-188. [PMID: 29258378]

Item 97   **Answer:**   **D**
Educational Objective: Identify urea osmotic diuresis as a cause of hypernatremia.

Urea osmotic diuresis is the most likely cause of this patient's hypernatremia. This patient is recovering from acute kidney injury and is having a urea diuresis, with an elevated urine osmolality of 420 mOsm/kg H_2O. In osmotic diuresis, urine osmolality is usually between 300 and 600 mOsm/kg H_2O. The majority of the osmolality of the urine is made up of nonelectrolytes. This loss of electrolyte-free water is causing her serum sodium level to increase. The two major nonelectrolytes found in urine are urea and glucose. Her glucose is only 136 mg/dL (7.5 mmol/L), below the threshold for glucose appearing in the urine; therefore, the likely cause is excretion of urea. This can be confirmed by measuring urea in the urine.

Hyponatremia is found in 70% to 80% of patients with adrenal insufficiency and is a consequence of sodium loss and volume depletion caused by mineralocorticoid deficiency and increased vasopressin secretion caused by cortisol deficiency. In addition, hyperkalemia and hyperchloremic acidosis is found in approximately 50% of patients with adrenal insufficiency. Hypernatremia and hypokalemia would be unusual manifestations of adrenal insufficiency.

In the absence of antidiuretic hormone, excessive water is excreted by the kidneys, and the urine osmolality is low. The patient's urine osmolality is 420 mOsm/kg H_2O, making diabetes insipidus unlikely. In addition, there is no reason to suspect diabetes insipidus in this woman. Nevertheless, it would not be possible to rule out partial nephrogenic diabetes insipidus until her urea normalized.

Glycosuria is not the cause of this patient's hypernatremia because her glucose level is below the tubular threshold for reabsorption, approximately 180 mg/dL (10 mmol/L). A urine dipstick would verify the lack of glycosuria.

KEY POINT

- Hypernatremia may be caused by osmotic diuresis, in which the urine osmolality is usually between 300 and 600 mOsm/kg H_2O.

Bibliography
Lindner G, Schwarz C, Funk GC. Osmotic diuresis due to urea as the cause of hypernatraemia in critically ill patients. Nephrol Dial Transplant. 2012;27:962-7. [PMID: 21810766]

Item 98   **Answer:**   **D**
Educational Objective: Perform a kidney biopsy to evaluate a decline in kidney function.

A kidney biopsy is appropriate for this patient with a decline in kidney function. Clinical and laboratory features are often insufficient for definitive diagnosis of kidney disease. Kidney biopsy may therefore be essential for diagnosis and management. Indications include glomerular hematuria, severely increased albuminuria, acute or chronic kidney disease of unclear cause, and kidney transplant dysfunction or monitoring. In this case, the patient has an elevated serum creatinine without clear cause. Although further serologic testing may be done to guide diagnosis, a kidney biopsy will provide definitive diagnosis.

Due to preferential dilation of the efferent arteriole, the ACE inhibitor lisinopril may reduce glomerular filtration rate (GFR) and hence increase serum creatinine; however, this change in serum creatinine will occur within days of drug initiation and then stabilize. In this case, the serum creatinine increased without a change in dose, suggesting an unrelated cause.

A 24-hour creatinine clearance may be helpful in estimating kidney function but will not change the evaluation at this time. Most studies show that the Chronic Kidney Disease Epidemiology (CKD-EPI) Collaboration equation or the Modification of Diet in Renal Disease (MDRD) study equation provides a more accurate estimated GFR (eGFR) compared with creatinine clearance.

Although this patient's CKD-EPI eGFR is reported as >60 mL/min/1.73 m², his increasing serum creatinine is consistent with a significantly declining eGFR. Although cystatin C will potentially add to the accuracy of the

CKD-EPI formula, it will not change the evaluation, as GFR is declining as documented by the serum creatinine elevation (and no baseline cystatin C is available to show otherwise).

- Indications for kidney biopsy include glomerular hematuria, severely increased albuminuria, acute or chronic kidney disease of unclear cause, and kidney transplant dysfunction or monitoring.

Bibliography

Hogan JJ, Mocanu M, Berns JS. The native kidney biopsy: update and evidence for best practice. Clin J Am Soc Nephrol. 2016;11:354-62. [PMID: 26339068]

Item 99   Answer: B

Educational Objective: Manage end-stage kidney disease in an elderly patient with multiple comorbidities and poor prognosis.

Discussion of conservative management and non-dialytic options is appropriate for this 82-year-old patient with end-stage kidney disease (ESKD) who has multiple comorbidities and poor prognosis. The life expectancy of some patients with ESKD with advanced age and severe comorbidities can be extremely short and may not be improved by dialysis. In elderly persons with progressing or advanced chronic kidney disease, decisions need to be made about the desires and plans to initiate renal replacement therapy and/or referral for evaluation for kidney transplantation. Several factors, including comorbid medical conditions, functional status, expected outcomes, and patient preferences regarding goals of care, should be considered. There is growing recognition that clinicians need to ensure maximal involvement of patients and their families in treatment decisions. This shared decision-making is a process whereby patients and providers can discuss the benefits and burdens of potential treatment strategies in the context of each patient's priorities and needs.

Patients with low comorbidity levels and a predicted survival of >3 years should be considered for all kidney disease treatment modalities, including kidney transplantation. In contrast, patients with a high 3- and 6-month expected mortality may choose to delay initiation and may be candidates for non-dialytic conservative management. Patients who choose conservative therapy have relatively preserved functional status until the last months of life. Conservative management may be a reasonable choice for patients whose primary goal is to maintain their independence and to avoid the time, pain, and discomfort related to dialysis, as well as for patients with poor functional status and a predicted post–dialysis initiation projected survival of <3 months.

- Non-dialytic therapy is a reasonable treatment option for elderly patients with end-stage kidney disease and multiple comorbidities; treatment focuses on symptom management.

Bibliography

Verberne WR, Geers AB, Jellema WT, Vincent HH, van Delden JJ, Bos WJ. Comparative survival among older adults with advanced kidney disease managed conservatively versus with dialysis. Clin J Am Soc Nephrol. 2016;11:633-40. [PMID: 26988748]

Item 100   Answer: B

Educational Objective: Manage difficult-to-control hypertension with the addition of a loop diuretic.

The addition of a loop diuretic such as furosemide is the most appropriate treatment. This patient has difficult-to-control hypertension in the setting of stage G4 chronic kidney disease (CKD), and his blood pressure is not at target. The American College of Cardiology/American Heart Association blood pressure guideline recommends a target blood pressure of <130/80 mm Hg for all patients, including those with CKD. The most appropriate treatment is the addition of a loop diuretic. Suboptimal blood pressure therapy in patients with difficult-to-control hypertension is frequently the result of not including a diuretic, which prevents or corrects extracellular volume expansion. Persistent volume expansion, even if not sufficient to produce clinically evident edema, contributes significantly to hypertension. This is particularly important in sodium-retentive, edematous conditions such as heart failure, liver cirrhosis, or CKD.

Although thiazide diuretics are frequently used as initial diuretic therapy, they are generally less effective in patients with lower glomerular filtration rates. At estimated glomerular filtration rates <30 mL/min/1.73 m^2, loop diuretics tend to be more effective at controlling extracellular volume expansion and should be used instead of (or added to) thiazide diuretics. The dosage of loop diuretics depends on the sodium intake and the severity of CKD. Generally, furosemide doses of 40 to 80 mg twice daily is initiated with a salt-restricted diet and adjusted according to the response. When it is appropriate to add a thiazide diuretic to a blood pressure regimen, chlorthalidone is often preferred because of its longer duration of action.

The patient is already on a maximum dose of the ACE inhibitor lisinopril, which is appropriate for the treatment of hypertension in patients with CKD. Although he still has albuminuria, addition of the angiotensin receptor blocker (ARB) losartan is inappropriate because several trials have shown that combination therapy with an ACE inhibitor and ARB may result in adverse events, such as acute kidney injury and hyperkalemia, and does not improve cardiovascular outcomes compared with treatment with an ACE inhibitor or ARB alone.

- Patients with difficult-to-control hypertension typically require the addition of a diuretic, which prevents or corrects extracellular volume expansion in sodium-retentive, edematous conditions (heart failure, liver cirrhosis, chronic kidney disease).

Bibliography

Braam B, Taler SJ, Rahman M, Fillaus JA, Greco BA, Forman JP, et al. Recognition and management of resistant hypertension. Clin J Am Soc Nephrol. 2017;12:524-535. [PMID: 27895136]

Item 101   Answer: B

Educational Objective: Diagnose cisplatin-induced acute kidney injury.

The patient has cisplatin-induced acute kidney injury (AKI). AKI due to renal tubular dysfunction can occur following administration of cisplatin and ifosfamide. High-dose methotrexate can also cause renal tubular injury, which can be avoided with aggressive intravenous hydration, forced diuresis, urine alkalization, and administration of leucovorin. Cisplatin induces direct cellular toxicity as a result of their transport through tubular cells, induction of mitochondrial injury, oxidative stress, and activation of apoptotic signaling pathways. Cisplatin-induced AKI develops 7 to 10 days after administration and is characterized by polyuria, tubular injury, hypomagnesemia, and proximal renal tubular acidosis (RTA) with Fanconi syndrome. Cisplatin nephrotoxicity results in volume depletion from urinary excretion of sodium and hypomagnesemia from urinary magnesium loss with ensuing hypokalemia and hypocalcemia. Fanconi syndrome in this patient is supported by the normal anion gap metabolic acidosis, hypophosphatemia, and urinary findings of glycosuria (in the setting of normal blood glucose) and proteinuria. In patients receiving cisplatin, serum electrolyte levels and kidney function must be carefully monitored because early recognition and prompt discontinuation of the drug are essential for renal recovery.

Bevacizumab and gemcitabine can cause hypertension and AKI due to thrombotic microangiopathy, which manifests as thrombocytopenia with hemolytic anemia, elevated lactate dehydrogenase, decreased haptoglobin, and schistocytes on peripheral smear. Urinary findings usually demonstrate significant proteinuria and hematuria. No laboratory findings in this patient support this diagnosis, and these drugs do not cause renal tubular injury.

Paclitaxel has been associated with subacute diffuse interstitial lung disease and peripheral neuropathy. Paclitaxel does not cause AKI or the electrolyte abnormalities as seen in this patient.

> **KEY POINT**
> - Cisplatin-induced acute kidney injury is characterized by polyuria, tubular injury, hypomagnesemia, and proximal renal tubular acidosis with Fanconi syndrome.

Bibliography

Rosner MH, Perazella MA. Acute kidney injury in patients with cancer. N Engl J Med. 2017;376:1770-1781. [PMID: 28467867]

Item 102   Answer: B

Educational Objective: Treat hypertension to a blood pressure target of <130/80 mm Hg in a patient with chronic kidney disease and hypervolemia.

The most appropriate management is to increase the furosemide dose. The patient has chronic kidney disease and proteinuria of 1000 mg/g, and he is taking prednisone for his primary focal segmental glomerulosclerosis. The pathophysiology of hypertension in kidney disease is complex, but sodium retention is the predominant mechanism and is related to a reduction in glomerular filtration rate (GFR), resistance to natriuretic peptides, and increased activity of the renin-angiotensin-aldosterone system. Control of sodium balance is an essential component of blood pressure management in patients with kidney disease. Dietary sodium restriction to <2000 mg/d combined with appropriate use of diuretics is advised. As the GFR declines, thiazide diuretics become less effective. Loop diuretics should be employed in such patients, with doses titrated to clinical response. Because this patient is hypervolemic (elevated jugular venous pressure, S_3, lower extremity edema), the dose of the loop diuretic needs to be increased.

Increasing the amlodipine dose is not the best option because it will not treat the underlying hypervolemia, and increasing the dose of amlodipine may worsen the lower extremity edema.

Adding an ACE inhibitor (such as lisinopril) is inappropriate because the patient is already on an angiotensin receptor blocker (losartan), and combination therapy with these agents and other renin-angiotensin system agents may result in adverse events such as hyperkalemia and acute kidney injury.

The 2017 American College of Cardiology/American Heart Association high blood pressure guideline recommends a target blood pressure of <130/80 mm Hg in patients with hypertension and chronic kidney disease. Therefore, maintaining this patient's current medication regimen would be inappropriate.

> **KEY POINT**
> - Control of sodium balance is an essential component of blood pressure management in patients with kidney disease; dietary sodium restriction to <2000 mg/d combined with appropriate use of diuretics is recommended.

Bibliography

Gargiulo R, Suhail F, Lerma EV. Hypertension and chronic kidney disease. Dis Mon. 2015;61:387-95. [PMID: 26328515]

Item 103   Answer: D

Educational Objective: Predict chronic kidney disease progression using the four-variable kidney failure risk equation.

A urine albumin-creatinine ratio is needed to complete the four-variable kidney failure risk equation (KFRE) for this patient with newly diagnosed chronic kidney disease (CKD). Not all patients with CKD will progress to end-stage kidney disease. In 2011, Tangri and colleagues developed and validated a set of risk prediction models for progression to kidney failure among Canadian patients with moderate to severe CKD. They demonstrated that using laboratory data that are routinely obtained in patients with CKD provided excellent discrimination for prediction of progression of CKD to kidney failure over a 2- to 5-year period. Several models and variables were tested. Ultimately, the highest-performing models were the four-variable KFRE (age, sex, estimated glomerular filtration rate, and urine albumin-creatinine ratio) and the eight-variable KFRE (previous four variables, plus serum calcium, phosphate, bicarbonate, and albumin). The addition of diabetes mellitus, hypertension, blood pressure, and body weight did not improve the ability to discriminate risk for kidney failure.

In 2016, the KFRE was validated in 31 international cohorts comprised of 721,357 patients with stage G3 to G5 CKD. Calculation of the area under the receiver operating characteristic (ROC) curve quantifies the performance of a diagnostic test and allows comparison of different tests. A perfect test has an area under the curve (AUC) equal to 1; the closer the AUC is to 1, the better the test. The pooled AUC for the four-variable KFRE was 0.90 (95% CI, 0.89-0.92) to predict kidney failure at 2 years and 0.88 (95% CI, 0.86-0.90) at 5 years. Use of the eight-variable KFRE did not add to the predictive accuracy (AUC for 2 years, 0.89 [95% CI, 0.88-0.91]; AUC for 5 years, 0.86 [95% CI, 0.84-0.87]). Thus, the four-variable original risk equation appears generalizable and highly accurate in most cohorts and can be easily implemented across multiple health care systems. The KFRE performs well across age, sex, race, and the presence or absence of diabetes. The use of this equation is consistent with the Kidney Disease: Improving Global Outcomes (KDIGO) guidelines, which recommend integration of risk prediction in the evaluation and management of CKD.

KEY POINT

- The kidney failure risk equation uses four variables (age, sex, estimated glomerular filtration rate, and albuminuria) to predict 2-year and 5-year risk of end-stage kidney disease in patients with stages G3 to G5 chronic kidney disease.

Bibliography

Tangri N, Grams ME, Levey AS, Coresh J, Appel LJ, Astor BC, et al; CKD Prognosis Consortium. Multinational Assessment of Accuracy of Equations for Predicting Risk of Kidney Failure: A Meta-analysis. JAMA. 2016;315:164-74. [PMID: 26757465]

Item 104   Answer: A

Educational Objective: Diagnose AA amyloidosis in a patient with rheumatoid arthritis.

AA amyloidosis is the most likely cause of this patient's proteinuria. Chronic inflammatory states, particularly rheumatoid arthritis, are associated with production of amyloid protein A. This acute phase reactant deposits in numerous tissues, most commonly the kidney (80%-90%) and heart, forming β-pleated sheets. In the kidney, amyloidosis presents with a bland urinary sediment and nephrotic-range proteinuria. Progression to end-stage kidney disease is frequent. Cardiac manifestations may include systolic or diastolic dysfunction

and heart failure; low voltage on electrocardiogram can be seen. Although serum amyloid P component scintigraphy can diagnose amyloid, it is not available in the United States. Confirmation would therefore require a kidney biopsy in this case. Current treatment strategies are aimed at the underlying disease. Tocilizumab, an anti–interleukin-6 antibody, has been used successfully in patients with AA amyloidosis from rheumatoid arthritis.

Both focal segmental glomerulosclerosis (FSGS) and minimal change glomerulopathy (MCG) are associated with the nephrotic syndrome. However, FSGS more frequently affects black persons, and MCG is the most common cause of the nephrotic syndrome in children. Finally, this patient's history of a chronic inflammatory disease and findings of heart failure and an abnormal electrocardiogram more strongly suggest the possibility of amyloidosis.

NSAIDs are associated with interstitial nephritis and the nephrotic syndrome due to MCG or membranous glomerulopathy; typical findings include hematuria, pyuria, leukocyte casts, proteinuria, and an acute rise in the plasma creatinine concentration. However, this patient has not been using NSAIDs for the past 6 months and her urinalysis is bland, making this diagnosis unlikely.

Proton pump inhibitors can cause acute interstitial nephritis but are not associated with nephrotic-range proteinuria.

KEY POINT

- AA amyloid is formed by serum amyloid A protein, an acute phase reactant produced in various inflammatory diseases such as rheumatoid arthritis; confirmation of AA renal amyloidosis requires a kidney biopsy.

Bibliography

Obici L, Raimondi S, Lavatelli F, Bellotti V, Merlini G. Susceptibility to AA amyloidosis in rheumatic diseases: a critical overview. Arthritis Rheum. 2009;61:1435-40. [PMID: 19790131]

Item 105   Answer: C

Educational Objective: Treat elevated blood pressure with lifestyle modification.

The most appropriate next step in management is lifestyle modification. According to the American College of Cardiology/American Heart Association (ACC/AHA) blood pressure guideline, this patient has elevated blood pressure (BP), defined as systolic BP between 120-129 mm Hg and diastolic BP <80 mm Hg. Meta-analysis of observational studies has demonstrated that elevated BP and hypertension (systolic BP >130 mm Hg or diastolic BP >80 mm Hg) are associated with an increased risk of cardiovascular disease, end-stage kidney disease, subclinical atherosclerosis, and all-cause death. Nonpharmacologic therapy alone is especially useful for prevention of hypertension, including in adults with elevated BP, and for management of high BP in adults with milder forms of hypertension. Recommended lifestyle modifications include weight loss in adults who are overweight or obese; a heart-healthy diet that facilitates achieving a desirable weight; reduced sodium intake; high potassium intake (unless contraindicated by the presence of chronic kidney disease or use of drugs that reduce potassium excretion); increase in physical activity; and limiting alcohol consumption of standard drinks to no more than two (men) or one (women) per day.

According to the ACC/AHA BP guideline, the use of antihypertensive medications is recommended for secondary prevention of recurrent coronary events in patients with clinical coronary vascular disease and an average systolic BP of ≥130 mm Hg or an average diastolic BP of ≥80 mm Hg. Drug therapy is also recommended for primary prevention in adults with an estimated 10-year atherosclerotic cardiovascular disease risk ≥10% and an average systolic BP ≥130 mm Hg or average diastolic BP ≥80 mm Hg. For initiation of antihypertensive drug therapy, first-line agents include thiazide diuretics, calcium channel blockers, and ACE inhibitors or angiotensin receptor blockers. Because this patient has elevated BP (not hypertension), initiation of drug therapy is not indicated at this time.

The ACC/AHA recommends that adults with an elevated BP, such as this patient, should be managed with nonpharmacologic therapy and have a repeat BP evaluation within 3 to 6 months. Patients with normal BP (systolic BP <120 mm Hg and diastolic BP <80 mm Hg) can be reevaluated in 1 year.

KEY POINT

- Nonpharmacologic therapy alone is especially useful for prevention of hypertension, including in adults with elevated blood pressure, and for management of high blood pressure in adults with milder forms of hypertension.

Bibliography

Whelton PK, Carey RM, Aronow WS, Casey DE Jr, Collins KJ, Dennison Himmelfarb C, et al. 2017 ACC/AHA/AAPA/ABC/ACPM/AGS/APhA/ASH/ASPC/NMA/PCNA guideline for the prevention, detection, evaluation, and management of high blood pressure in adults: a report of the American College of Cardiology/American Heart Association Task Force on Clinical Practice Guidelines. Hypertension. 2017. [PMID: 29133356]

Item 106   Answer: B

Educational Objective: Manage acquired cystic kidney disease with suspected renal cell carcinoma in a patient with end-stage kidney disease.

Bilateral radical nephrectomy is the most appropriate management for this patient with end-stage chronic kidney disease (ESKD) and bilateral kidney solid masses. Acquired kidney cysts often develop in patients with severe chronic kidney disease (CKD) and are frequently detected during routine kidney ultrasound or incidentally noted on abdominal CT or MRI scan. Acquired cystic kidney disease becomes more common and progresses during the course of ESKD, and some studies suggest that it may affect >50% of patients who have had ESKD for >3 years. The epithelial cells lining these cysts may undergo malignant transformation by poorly understood mechanisms. Patients with ESKD have a markedly increased

risk for renal cell carcinoma. Although current guidelines do not support routine screening for renal cell carcinoma in all patients with CKD, a high level of suspicion is warranted in patients with symptoms such as new-onset gross hematuria or unexplained flank pain.

Partial nephrectomy and nephron-sparing approaches would be indicated for less severe stages of CKD. However, this patient has ESKD, and maintaining residual kidney function is no longer a concern; therefore, radical nephrectomy would be the most appropriate option.

Kidney biopsy should be considered in patients with glomerular hematuria, severely increased albuminuria, acute or chronic kidney disease of unclear etiology, and kidney transplant dysfunction or monitoring. The role of kidney biopsy for a suspicious mass is more limited. It may be useful in the evaluation of a small mass if there is suspicion of a renal metastasis or lymphoma and is likely useful to confirm the diagnosis of renal cell carcinoma in patients who cannot tolerate surgery prior to initiating medical therapy. The best approach for this patient with a high likelihood of renal cell carcinoma is bilateral nephrectomy. The excised tissue will provide histological confirmation of the diagnosis and thus guide further therapy.

Surveillance ultrasonography would not be the best management of this patient with bilateral solid kidney masses. The new-onset hematuria and kidney masses in the context of advanced CKD are highly suspicious for renal cell carcinoma.

KEY POINT

- Patients with end-stage kidney disease have a markedly increased risk for renal cell carcinoma, and a high level of suspicion is warranted in patients with symptoms such as new-onset gross hematuria or unexplained flank pain.

Bibliography

Hu SL, Chang A, Perazella MA, Okusa MD, Jaimes EA, Weiss RH; American Society of Nephrology Onco-Nephrology Forum. The nephrologist's tumor: basic biology and management of renal cell carcinoma. J Am Soc Nephrol. 2016;27:2227-37. [PMID: 26961346]

Item 107   Answer: B

Educational Objective: Provide appropriate blood pressure screening for a patient at increased risk for cardiovascular disease.

Annual blood pressure screening is the most appropriate management. This patient is healthy, physically active, not overweight, and does not meet criteria for hypertension based on these office blood pressure (BP) readings measured during one visit. However, he is at risk for future hypertension given his age (>40 years), black race, and a positive family history of hypertension. In addition, according to the American College of Cardiology/American Heart Association (ACC/AHA) guideline, the patient has elevated BP, defined as systolic BP between 120-129 mm Hg and diastolic BP <80 mm Hg. Although no interventions are needed during this visit, the patient does need to be screened for high BP at least annually or more frequently. The U.S. Preventive Services Task Force (USPSTF) recommendations have not been updated since the release of the ACC/AHA guideline, with borderline and normal BP defined by older guidelines; however, the USPSTF recommends screening for hypertension in adults ≥18 years of age to identify those at increased risk for cardiovascular disease from hypertension and to begin early interventions to decrease this risk. Adults aged 18 to 39 years with normal BP and without cardiovascular risk factors should be rescreened every 3 to 5 years. Those who are ≥40 years of age and persons at increased risk for hypertension should be screened annually.

Beginning antihypertensive therapy with medications such as amlodipine or hydrochlorothiazide is inappropriate for this patient who does not meet the criteria for hypertension (defined by the ACC/AHA as a systolic BP ≥130 mm Hg and/or a diastolic BP ≥80 mm Hg). According to this guideline, patients with clinical cardiovascular disease and an average systolic BP ≥130 mm Hg or an average diastolic BP ≥80 mm Hg should be treated with lifestyle changes and medications for secondary prevention of cardiovascular events. Adults without clinical cardiovascular disease but an estimated 10-year atherosclerotic cardiovascular disease risk ≥10% and an average systolic BP ≥130 mm Hg or an average diastolic BP ≥80 mm Hg should also be treated with lifestyle interventions and pharmacologic therapy for primary prevention of cardiovascular disease.

> **KEY POINT**
>
> - Annual blood pressure screening is appropriate for patients who are ≥40 years of age and persons at increased risk for hypertension.

Bibliography

Siu AL; U.S. Preventive Services Task Force. Screening for high blood pressure in adults: U.S. Preventive Services Task Force recommendation statement. Ann Intern Med. 2015;163:778-86. [PMID: 26458123]

Item 108   Answer: A

Educational Objective: Manage stage G5 chronic kidney disease in a patient who will imminently require renal replacement therapy.

The most appropriate management for this patient with stage G5 chronic kidney disease (CKD) is to delay dialysis until she has uremic symptoms. She is not a candidate for transplant and has opted for hemodialysis for her renal replacement therapy (RRT). The decision of when to start RRT for CKD is complicated and requires frank discussion between providers and the patient and their families. For many years, consensus guidelines suggested that dialysis be initiated on the basis of estimated glomerular filtration rate (eGFR) cutoffs, ranging between 10 and 15 mL/min/1.73 m². In 2010, results were published from the IDEAL (Initiating Dialysis Early and Late) trial, which demonstrated no significant difference between the early dialysis group (eGFR, 10-15 mL/min/1.73 m²) and late dialysis group (eGFR, 5-7 mL/min/1.73 m²) in the frequency of adverse events (cardiovascular events, infections, or complications of dialysis). Although 76% of the late-start group ultimately initiated dialysis with eGFR >7.0 mL/min/1.73 m², the median delay in onset of dialysis was 5.6 months compared with the early start group. Thus, this study demonstrated that with careful clinical management, dialysis may be delayed until either the GFR drops below 7.0 mL/min/1.73 m² or more traditional clinical indicators (such as uremic symptoms or metabolic abnormalities) for the initiation of dialysis are present.

Discontinuation of diuretics is inappropriate because the patient does have some evidence of total body sodium and water overload (2+ edema) and thus needs continued diuretic therapy to avoid frank volume overload.

Referral for palliative care is not indicated because the patient is functioning well and is without signs of terminal illness or symptoms that require palliation; moreover, she has already chosen hemodialysis for future RRT. However, if her condition worsens over time, it is strongly encouraged to practice "kidney supportive care" or "patient-centered dialysis," in which treatment goals are closely aligned with patient preferences in a shared decision-making process.

> **KEY POINT**
>
> - There is no benefit in starting renal replacement therapy (RRT) in asymptomatic patients or at an arbitrary estimated glomerular filtration rate cutoff compared with careful clinical management and initiating RRT for symptoms or metabolic abnormalities that are refractory to medical treatment.

Bibliography

Cooper BA, Branley P, Bulfone L, Collins JF, Craig JC, Fraenkel MB, et al; IDEAL Study. A randomized, controlled trial of early versus late initiation of dialysis. N Engl J Med. 2010;363:609-19. [PMID: 20581422]

Index